IARC MONOGRAPHS
ON THE
EVALUATION OF THE CARCINOGENIC RISK
OF CHEMICALS TO MAN:

Some naturally occurring substances

Volume 10

This publication represents the views of an
IARC Working Group on the
Evaluation of the Carcinogenic Risk of Chemicals to Man
which met in Lyon,
7-13 October 1975

IARC WORKING GROUP ON THE EVALUATION OF THE CARCINOGENIC RISK OF CHEMICALS TO MAN: SOME NATURALLY OCCURRING SUBSTANCES

Lyon, 7-13 October 1975

Members[1]

Dr B.K. Armstrong, University Department of Medicine, Perth Medical Centre, Shenton Park 6008, Western Australia

Dr E.A. Bababunmi, Senior Lecturer in Biochemistry, University of Ibadan, Ibadan, Nigeria

Professor A.M. Clark, Professor of Biology & Pro-Vice-Chancellor, The Flinders University of South Australia, School of Biological Sciences, Bedford Park, South Australia 5042, Australia

Dr C.C.J. Culvenor, Commonwealth Scientific and Industrial Research Organization, Division of Animal Health, Animal Health Research Laboratory, Private Bag No. 1, Parkville, Victoria 3052, Australia

Professor F. Dickens, 15 Hazelhurst Crescent, Findon Valley, Worthing, Sussex BN14 0HW, UK

Dr H.L. Falk, Associate Director for Program, National Institute of Environmental Health Sciences, PO Box 12233, Research Triangle Park, North Carolina 27709, USA

Dr R.C. Garner, Cancer Research Unit, University of York, Heslington, York YO1 5DD, UK

Dr P. Krogh, National Food Institute, Division of Pesticides and Contaminants, 19 Mørkhøj Bygade, DK-2860 Søborg, Denmark

Dr M. Saito, Chairman and Professor, Department of Carcinogenesis and Cancer Susceptibility, The Institute of Medical Science, The University of Tokyo, PO Takanawa, Tokyo, Japan

Dr R. Saracci, Chief, Biostatistics and Clinical Epidemiology Section, CNR Laboratory for Clinical Physiology, University of Pisa, Via Savi 8, 56100 Pisa, Italy (*Vice-Chairman*)

Dr P. Shubik, Director, The Eppley Institute for Research in Cancer, University of Nebraska Medical Center, 42nd and Dewey Avenue, Omaha, Nebraska 68105, USA

---

[1]Unable to attend: Professor A. Lafontaine, Ministère de la Santé Publique, Institut d'Hygiène et d'Epidémiologie, 14 Rue Juliette Wytsman, B-1050 Brussels, Belgium; Dr F.M. Strong, 625 Anthony Lane, Madison, Wisconsin 53711, USA

Dr L. Teppo, Finnish Cancer Registry, The Institute for Statistical and Epidemiological Cancer Research, Liisankatu 21 B, SF-00170 Helsinki 17, Finland

Dr G.N. Wogan, Professor of Toxicology, Massachusetts Institute of Technology, Department of Nutrition and Food Science, Cambridge, Massachusetts 02139, USA (*Chairman*)

Dr F.K. Zimmermann, Technische Hochschule Darmstadt, Fachbereich Biologie, Schnittspahnstrasse 9 (Am Botanischen Garten), D-61 Darmstadt, FRG

Invited Guests[2]

Dr P.S. Elias, Principal Medical Officer, Department of Health and Social Security, Alexander Fleming House, Elephant and Castle, London SE1 6BY, UK

Dr O.H. Johnson, Senior Industrial Economist, Chemical-Environmental Program, Chemical Industries Center, Stanford Research Institute, Menlo Park, California 94025, USA (*Rapporteur sections 2.1 and 2.2*)

Dr F. Peers, Tropical Products Institute, 56-62 Grays Inn Road, London WC1, UK

Representative from the National Cancer Institute

Dr S. Siegel, Research Biologist, Carcinogen Bioassay and Program Resources Branch, National Cancer Institute, Bethesda, Maryland 20014, USA

Secretariat

    Dr C. Agthe, Unit of Chemical Carcinogenesis (*Secretary*)

    Dr H. Bartsch, Unit of Chemical Carcinogenesis (*Rapporteur section 3.2*)

    Dr L. Griciute, Chief, Unit of Environmental Carcinogens

    Dr C.A. Linsell, Chief, Interdisciplinary Programme and International Liaison

    Dr R. Montesano, Unit of Chemical Carcinogenesis (*Rapporteur section 3.1*)

    Mrs C. Partensky, Unit of Chemical Carcinogenesis (*Technical editor*)

    Mrs I. Peterschmitt, Unit of Chemical Carcinogenesis, Geneva (*Bibliographic researcher*)

---

[2]Unable to attend: Dr R. Kroes, Head of the Department of Oncology, Laboratory for Pathology, Rijks Instituut voor de Volksgezondheid, Postbus 1, Bilthoven, The Netherlands

Dr V. Ponomarkov, Unit of Chemical Carcinogenesis

Dr L. Tomatis, Chief, Unit of Chemical Carcinogenesis (*Head of the Programme*)

Mr E.A. Walker, Unit of Environmental Carcinogens (*Rapporteur sections 1 and 2.3*)

Mrs E. Ward, Montignac, France (*Editor*)

Mr J.D. Wilbourn, Unit of Chemical Carcinogenesis (*Co-secretary*)

Note to the reader

Every effort is made to present the monographs as accurately as possible without unduly delaying their publication. Nevertheless, mistakes have occurred and are still likely to occur. In the interest of all users of these monographs, readers are requested to communicate any errors observed to the Unit of Chemical Carcinogenesis of the International Agency for Research on Cancer, Lyon, France, in order that these can be included in corrigenda which will appear in subsequent volumes.

As stated in the preamble, great efforts are made to cover the whole literature, but some studies may have been inadvertently overlooked. Since the monographs are not intended to be a review of the literature and contain only data considered relevant by the Working Group, it is not possible for the reader to determine whether a certain study was considered or not. However, research workers who are aware of important published data which may change the evaluation are requested to make them available to the above-mentioned address, in order that they can be considered for a possible re-evaluation by a future Working Group.

CONTENTS

BACKGROUND AND PURPOSE OF THE IARC PROGRAMME ON THE EVALUATION
OF THE CARCINOGENIC RISK OF CHEMICALS TO MAN 11

SCOPE OF THE MONOGRAPHS 11

MECHANISM FOR PRODUCING THE MONOGRAPHS 12

    Priority for the preparation of monographs 12
    Data on which the evaluation is based 12
    The Working Group 13

GENERAL PRINCIPLES FOR THE EVALUATION 13

    Terminology 13
    Response to carcinogens 14
    Purity of the compounds tested 14
    Qualitative aspects 14
    Quantitative aspects 15
    Animal data in relation to the evaluation of risk to man 15
    Evidence of human carcinogenicity 15

EXPLANATORY NOTES ON THE MONOGRAPHS 16

GENERAL REMARKS ON THE SUBSTANCES CONSIDERED 25

THE MONOGRAPHS

    Actinomycins 29
    Adriamycin 43
    Aflatoxins 51
    Azaserine 73
    Cantharidin 79
    Chloramphenicol 85
    Cholesterol 99
    Coumarin 113
    Cycasin 121
    Cyclochlorotine 139
    Daunomycin 145

Griseofulvin	153
Luteoskyrin	163
Mitomycin C	171
Native carrageenans	181
Ochratoxin A	191
Parasorbic acid	199
Patulin	205
Penicillic acid	211
Reserpine	217
Safrole, isosafrole and dihydrosafrole	231
Sterigmatocystin	245
Tannic acid and tannins	253
Pyrrolizidine alkaloids:	
Hydroxysenkirkine	265
Isatidine	269
Jacobine	275
Lasiocarpine	281
Monocrotaline	291
Retrorsine	303
Riddelliine	313
Seneciphylline	319
Senkirkine	327
GENERAL INFORMATION AND CONCLUSIONS ON PYRROLIZIDINE ALKALOIDS	333
SUPPLEMENTARY CORRIGENDA TO VOLUMES 1-9	343
CUMULATIVE INDEX TO MONOGRAPHS	345

BACKGROUND AND PURPOSE OF THE IARC PROGRAMME ON THE EVALUATION OF THE CARCINOGENIC RISK OF CHEMICALS TO MAN

The International Agency for Research on Cancer (IARC) initiated in 1971 a programme on the evaluation of the carcinogenic risk of chemicals to man. This programme was supported by a Resolution of the Governing Council at its Ninth Session concerning the role of IARC in providing government authorities with expert, independent scientific opinion on environmental carcinogenesis. As one means to this end, the Governing Council recommended that IARC should continue to prepare monographs on the carcinogenic risk of individual chemicals to man.

In view of the importance of this programme and in order to expedite the production of monographs, the National Cancer Institute of the United States has provided IARC with additional funds for this purpose.

The objective of this programme is to elaborate and publish in the form of monographs a critical review of carcinogenicity and related data in the light of the present state of knowledge, with the final aim of evaluating the data in terms of possible human risk, and at the same time to indicate where additional research efforts are needed.

SCOPE OF THE MONOGRAPHS

The monographs summarize the evidence for the carcinogenicity of individual chemicals and other relevant information. The data are compiled, reviewed and evaluated by a Working Group of experts. No recommendations are given concerning preventive measures or legislation, since these matters depend on risk-benefit evaluation, which seems best made by individual governments and/or international agencies such as WHO and ILO.

Since 1971, when the programme was started, nine volumes have been published[1-9].

As new data on chemicals for which monographs have already been written and new principles for evaluation become available, re-evaluations will be made at future meetings, and revised monographs will be published as necessary. The monographs are being distributed to international and governmental agencies and will be available to industries and scientists dealing with these chemicals. They also form the basis of advice from IARC on carcinogenesis from these substances.

MECHANISM FOR PRODUCING THE MONOGRAPHS

As a first step, a list of chemicals for possible consideration by the Working Group is established. IARC then collects pertinent references regarding physico-chemical characteristics, production and use*, occurrence and analysis, and biological data** on these compounds. The material is summarized by an expert consultant or an IARC staff member, who prepares the first draft, which in some cases is sent to another expert for comments. The drafts are circulated to all members of the Working Group about one month before the meeting. During the meeting further additions to and deletions from the data are agreed upon, and a final version of comments and evaluation on each compound is adopted.

Priority for the Preparation of Monographs

Priority is given mainly to chemicals belonging to groups for which at least some suggestion of carcinogenicity exists from observations in animals and/or man and for which there is evidence of human exposure. However, neither human exposure nor potential carcinogenicity can be judged until all the relevant data have been collected and examined in detail, and *the inclusion of a particular compound in a volume does not necessarily mean that the substance is considered to be carcinogenic. Equally, the fact that a substance has not yet been considered does not imply that it is without carcinogenic hazard.*

Data on which the Evaluation is Based

With regard to the biological data, only published articles and papers already accepted for publication are reviewed. Every effort is made to

---

*Data provided by Chemical Information Services, Stanford Research Institute, Menlo Park, California, USA

**In the collection of original data reference was made to the publications "Survey of compounds which have been tested for carcinogenic activity"[10-15].

cover the whole literature, but some studies may have been inadvertently overlooked. The monographs are not intended to be a full review of the literature, and they contain only data considered relevant by the Working Group. Research workers who are aware of important data (published or accepted for publication) which may influence the evaluation are invited to make them available to the Unit of Chemical Carcinogenesis of the International Agency for Research on Cancer, Lyon, France.

The Working Group

The tasks of the Working Group are five-fold: (1) to verify that as far as feasible all data have been collected; (2) to select the data relevant for the evaluation; (3) to determine whether the data, as summarized, will enable the reader to follow the reasoning of the committee; (4) to judge the significance of results of experimental and epidemiological studies; and (5) to make an evaluation.

The members of the Working Group who participated in the consideration of particular substances are listed at the beginning of each publication. The members of the Working Group serve in their individual capacities as scientists, and not as representatives of their governments or of any organization with which they are affiliated.

GENERAL PRINCIPLES FOR THE EVALUATION

The general principles for the evaluation which are listed below were elaborated by previous Working Groups and were also applied to the substances listed in this volume.

Terminology

The term 'chemical carcinogenesis' in its widely accepted sense is used to indicate the induction or enhancement of neoplasia by chemicals. It is recognized that, in the strict etymological sense, this term means the induction of cancer; however, common usage has led to its employment to denote the induction of various types of neoplasms. The terms 'tumourigen', 'oncogen' and 'blastomogen' have all been used synonymously with 'carcinogen', although occasionally 'tumourigen' has been used specifically to denote the induction of benign tumours.

Response to Carcinogens

For present purposes, in general, no distinction is made between the induction of tumours and the enhancement of tumour incidence, although it is noted that there may be fundamental differences in mechanisms that will eventually be elucidated.

The response in experimental animals to a carcinogen may take several forms:

(1) a significant increase in the incidence of one or more of the same types of neoplasms as found in control animals;

(2) the occurrence of types of neoplasms not observed in control animals;

(3) a decreased latent period as compared with control animals.

Purity of the Compounds Tested

In any evaluation of biological data with respect to a possible carcinogenic risk, particular attention must be paid to the purity of the chemicals tested and to their stability under conditions of storage or administration. Information on purity and stability is given, when available, in the monographs.

Qualitative Aspects

The qualitative nature of neoplasia has been much discussed. In many instances, both benign and malignant tumours are induced by chemical carcinogens. There are so far few recorded instances in which only benign tumours are induced by chemicals that have been studied extensively. Their occurrence in experimental systems has been taken to indicate the possibility of an increased risk of malignant tumours also.

In experimental carcinogenesis, the type of cancer seen can be the same as that recorded in human studies (e.g., bladder cancer in man, monkeys, dogs and hamsters after administration of 2-naphthylamine). In other instances, however, a chemical can induce other types of neoplasms at different sites in various species (e.g., benzidine induces hepatic carcinoma in the rat, but bladder carcinoma in man).

Quantitative Aspects

Dose-response studies are important in the evaluation of human and animal carcinogenesis. The confidence with which a carcinogenic effect can be established is strengthened by the observation of an increasing incidence of neoplasms with increasing exposure. Such studies are the only ones on which a minimal effective dose can be established. The determination of such a dose allows a comparison with reliable data on human exposure.

Comparison of potency between compounds can only be made if and when substances have been tested simultaneously.

Animal Data in Relation to the Evaluation of Risk to Man

At the present time no attempt can be made to interpret the animal data directly in terms of human risk since no objective criteria are available to do so. The critical assessment of the validity of the animal data given in these monographs is intended to assist national and/or international authorities to make decisions concerning preventive measures or legislation. In this connection attention is drawn to WHO recommendations in relation to food additives[16], drugs[17] and occupational carcinogens[18].

Evidence of Human Carcinogenicity

Evaluation of the carcinogenic risk to man of suspected environmental agents rests on purely observational studies. Such studies require sufficient variation in the levels of human exposure to allow a meaningful relationship between cancer incidence and exposure to a given chemical to be established. Difficulties in isolating the effects of individual agents arise, however, since populations are exposed to multiple carcinogens.

The initial suggestion of a relationship between an agent and disease often comes from case reports of patients who have had similar exposures. Variations and time trends in regional or national cancer incidence, or their correlation with regional or national 'exposure' levels, may also provide valuable insights. Such observations by themselves, however, cannot in most circumstances be regarded as conclusive evidence of carcinogenicity. The most satisfactory epidemiological method is to compare the cancer risk (adjusted for age, sex and other confounding variables) among groups or cohorts, or among individuals exposed to various levels of the agent in question, and among control groups not so exposed. Ideally this is accomplished directly, by following such groups forward in time (prospectively) to determine time relationships, dose-response relationships and other aspects of cancer induction. Large cohorts and long observation periods are required to provide sufficient cases for a statistically valid comparison.

An alternative to prospective investigation is to assemble cohorts from past records and to evaluate their subsequent morbidity or mortality by means of medical histories and death certificates. Such occupational carcinogens as nickel, β-naphthylamine, asbestos and benzidine have been confirmed by this method. Another method is to compare the past exposures of a defined group of cancer cases with those of control cases from the hospital or general population. This does not provide an absolute measure of carcinogenic risk but can indicate the relative risks associated with different levels of exposure. The indirect means (e.g., interviews or tissue residues) used to measure exposures which may have commenced many years before can constitute a major source of error. Nevertheless such 'case-control' studies can often isolate one factor from several suspected agents. The carcinogenic effect of this substance could then be confirmed by cohort studies.

EXPLANATORY NOTES ON THE MONOGRAPHS

In sections 1, 2 and 3 of each monograph, except for minor remarks, the data are recorded as given by the author, whereas the comments by the Working Group are given in section 4, headed "Comments on Data Reported and Evaluation".

Chemical and Physical Data (section 1)

The Chemical Abstracts Registry Serial Number and the latest Chemical Abstracts Name are recorded in this section, together with other synonyms and trade names.

Chemical and physical properties include, in particular, data that might be relevant to carcinogenicity (for example, lipid solubility) and those that concern identification. Where applicable, data on solubility, volatility and stability are indicated. Data for which no reference is given are usually taken from standard reference books such as the *Merck Index*[19] or the *Handbook of Chemistry and Physics*[20]. All chemical data in this section refer to the pure substance, unless otherwise specified.

Production, Use, Occurrence and Analysis (section 2)

The ultimate purpose of this section is to give an idea of the extent of possible human exposure, and therefore data on production, use and occurrence are given when available. With regard to these data, IARC has collaborated with the Stanford Research Institute, USA, with the support of the National Cancer Institute of the USA, in order to obtain production figures of chemicals and their patterns of use.

The United States, Europe and Japan are reasonably representative areas of the world, and if data are available from these countries they are reported. It should *not*, however, be inferred that these nations are the sole sources or even the major sources of any individual chemical.

Production data are obtained from both governmental and trade publications in the three geographic areas. Information on use and occurrence is obtained by a comprehensive review of published data, complemented by direct contact with manufacturers of the chemicals in question.

Since cancer is a delayed toxic effect, past use and production data are also of importance. With respect to past and present use and production, regulatory actions in some countries are mentioned as examples only. Statements concerning regulations may not reflect the most recent situation, since such legislation is in a constant state of change; nor should it be taken to imply that other countries do not have similar regulations. In the cases of drugs, mention of the therapeutic uses of such chemicals does not necessarily represent presently accepted therapeutic indications, nor does it imply judgement as to their clinical efficacy.

It is hoped that in future revisions of these monographs, more information on production and use can be made available to IARC from other countries.

Biological Data Relevant to the Evaluation of Carcinogenic Risk to Man (section 3)

As pointed out earlier in this introduction, the monographs are not intended to consider all reported studies. Although every effort was made to review the whole literature, some studies were purposely omitted (a) because of their inadequacy, as judged from previously described criteria[21-24] (e.g., too short a duration, too few animals, poor survival or too small a dose); (b) because they only confirmed findings which have already been fully described; or (c) because they were judged irrelevant for the purpose of the evaluation. However, in certain cases, reference is made to studies which did not meet established criteria of adequacy, particularly when this information was considered a useful supplement to other reports or when it may have been the only data available. This does not, however, imply acceptance of the adequacy of experimental designs in these cases.

In general, the data recorded in this section are summarized as given by the author; however, certain shortcomings of reporting or of experimental design are also mentioned, and minor comments by the Working Group are given in square brackets.

The essential comments by the Working Group are made in section 4, "Comments on Data Reported and Evaluation".

Carcinogenicity and related studies in animals: Mention is usually made of all routes of administration by which the compound has been tested and of all species in which relevant tests have been carried out. In most cases the animal strains are given; general characteristics of mouse strains have been reported in a recent review[25]. Quantitative data are given in so far as they will enable the reader to realize the order of magnitude of the effective doses. In general, the doses are indicated as they appear in the original paper; sometimes conversions have been made for better comparison.

Other relevant biological data: The reporting of metabolic data is restricted to studies showing the metabolic fate of the chemical in animals and man. Comparison of animal and human data is made when possible. Other metabolic information (e.g., absorption, storage and excretion) is given when the Working Group considered that it would enable the reader to have a better understanding of the fate of the compound in the body. When the carcinogenicity of known metabolites has been tested, this also is reported.

Some LD_{50}'s are given, and other data on toxicity are included, if considered relevant.

Mutagenicity data are also included, and the reasons for including such data and the principles adopted by the Working Group for selection of the data are outlined below.

Many, but not all, mutagens are carcinogens and *vice versa*; the exact level of correlation is still under investigation. Nevertheless, practical use may be made of the available mutagenicity test procedures that combine microbial, mammalian or other animal cell systems as genetic targets with an *in vitro* or *in vivo* metabolic activation system. The results of relatively rapid and inexpensive mutagenicity tests on non-human organisms may help to pre-screen chemicals and may also aid in the selection of the most relevant animal species in which to carry out long-term carcinogenicity tests on these chemicals.

In seeking to make predictive use of, and to provide an explanation for, the observed correlation between carcinogenicity and mutagenicity, the ultimate goal is to detect genetic changes in the complete range of cell types in humans; but this is not attainable at present.

The role of genetic alterations in chemical carcinogenesis is not known, and therefore consideration must be given to a variety of changes. Although nuclear DNA has been defined as the main cellular target for the induction of genetic changes, other relevant targets have been recognized, e.g., mitochondrial DNA, enzymes involved in DNA synthesis, repair and recombination, and the spindle apparatus. Tests to detect the genetic activity of chemicals, including gene mutation, structural and numerical chromosomal changes and mitotic recombination, are available for non-human models; but not all such tests can be applied at present to human cells.

There are many genetic indicators and metabolic activation systems available for detecting mutagenic activity; they all, however, have individual advantages and limitations. Ideally, an appropriate mutagenicity test system would include the full metabolic competency of the intact human. Since the development or application of such a system appears to be impossible, the conclusion has been reached that a battery of test systems is needed in order to establish the mutagenic potential of chemicals.

Since many chemicals require metabolism to an active form, test systems which do not take this into account may fail to reveal the full range of genetic damage. Furthermore, since some reactive metabolites with a limited lifespan may fail to reach or to react with the genetic indicator, either because they are further metabolized to inactive compounds or because they react with other cellular constituents, mutagenicity tests in intact animals may give false negative results.

It is difficult in the present state of knowledge to select specific mutagenicity tests as being the most appropriate for the pre-screening of substances for possible carcinogenic activity. However, greater reliance may be placed on data obtained from those test systems which (a) permit the identification of the nature of induced genetic changes, and (b) demonstrate that the changes are transmitted to subsequent generations. Mutagenicity tests using organisms that are well-understood genetically, e.g., *Escherichia coli*, *Salmonella typhimurium*, *Saccharomyces* and *Drosophila*, meet these requirements.

Although a correlation has often been observed between the ability of a chemical to cause chromosome breakage and its ability to induce gene mutation, data on chromosomal breakage alone do not provide adequate evidence for mutagenicity, and therefore lesser weight should be given to pre-screening that is based on the use of peripheral leucocyte cultures.

Because of the complexity of factors that can contribute to reproductive failure, as well as the insensitivity of the method, the dominant lethal test in the mammal does not provide reliable data on mutagenicity.

A large-scale systematic screening of compounds to assess a correlation between mutagenicity and carcinogenicity has so far been carried out only with the bacterial/mammalian liver microsome system. Notwithstanding the demonstration of the mutagenicity of many known carcinogens to *Salmonella typhimurium* in the presence of liver microsomal systems, the possibility

of false-negative and false-positive results must not be overlooked.
False-negatives might arise as a consequence of mutagen specificity or
from failure to achieve optimal conditions for activation *in vitro*.
Alternative test systems must be used if there appear to be substantial
reasons for suspecting that a chemical which is apparently non-mutagenic
in a bacterial test system may nevertheless be potentially carcinogenic.
Conversely, some chemicals found to be mutagenic in this test may not in
fact have mutagenic activity in other systems.

For more detailed information, see references 26-33.

Observations in man: Epidemiological studies are summarized. Clinical
and other observations in man have been reviewed, when relevant.

Comments on Data Reported and Evaluation (section 4)

This section gives the critical view of the Working Group on the data
reported. It should be read in conjunction with the "General Remarks on the
Substances Considered".

Animal data: The animal species mentioned are those in which the
carcinogenicity of the substances was clearly demonstrated, irrespective of
the route of administration. In the case of inadequate studies, when
mentioned, comments to that effect are included. The route of administration
used in experimental animals that is similar to the possible human exposure
(ingestion, inhalation and skin exposure) is given particular mention. In
most cases tumour sites are also indicated. Experiments involving a possible action of the vehicle or a physical effect of the agent, such as in
subcutaneous injection or bladder implantation studies, are also mentioned;
however, the results of such tests require careful consideration, particularly if they are the only ones raising a suspicion of carcinogenicity. If
the substance has produced tumours on pre-natal exposure or in single-dose
experiments, this is also indicated. This sub-section should be read in
the light of comments made in the section, "Animal Data in Relation to the
Evaluation of Risk to Man" of this introduction.

Human data: In some cases, a brief statement is made on the possible
exposure of man. The significance of epidemiological studies and case
reports is discussed, and the data are interpreted in terms of possible
human risk.

References

1. IARC (1972) *IARC Monographs on the Evaluation of Carcinogenic Risk of Chemicals to Man*, *1*, Lyon

2. IARC (1973) *IARC Monographs on the Evaluation of Carcinogenic Risk of Chemicals to Man*, *2*, *Some Inorganic and Organometallic Compounds*, Lyon

3. IARC (1973) *IARC Monographs on the Evaluation of Carcinogenic Risk of Chemicals to Man*, *3*, *Certain Polycyclic Aromatic Hydrocarbons and Heterocyclic Compounds*, Lyon

4. IARC (1974) *IARC Monographs on the Evaluation of Carcinogenic Risk of Chemicals to Man*, *4*, *Some Aromatic Amines, Hydrazine and Related Substances, N-Nitroso Compounds and Miscellaneous Alkylating Agents*, Lyon

5. IARC (1974) *IARC Monographs on the Evaluation of Carcinogenic Risk of Chemicals to Man*, *5*, *Some Organochlorine Pesticides*, Lyon

6. IARC (1974) *IARC Monographs on the Evaluation of Carcinogenic Risk of Chemicals to Man*, *6*, *Sex Hormones*, Lyon

7. IARC (1974) *IARC Monographs on the Evaluation of Carcinogenic Risk of Chemicals to Man*, *7*, *Some Anti-thyroid and Related Substances, Nitrofurans and Industrial Chemicals*, Lyon

8. IARC (1975) *IARC Monographs on the Evaluation of Carcinogenic Risk of Chemicals to Man*, *8*, *Some Aromatic Azo Compounds*, Lyon

9. IARC (1975) *IARC Monographs on the Evaluation of Carcinogenic Risk of Chemicals to Man*, *9*, *Some Aziridines, N-, S- and O-Mustards and Selenium*, Lyon

10. Hartwell, J.L. (1951) *Survey of compounds which have been tested for carcinogenic activity*, Washington DC, US Government Printing Office (Public Health Service Publication No. 149)

11. Shubik, P. & Hartwell, J.L. (1957) *Survey of compounds which have been tested for carcinogenic activity*, Washington DC, US Government Printing Office (Public Health Service Publication No. 149: Supplement 1)

12. Shubik, P. & Hartwell, J.L. (1969) *Survey of compounds which have been tested for carcinogenic activity*, Washington DC, US Government Printing Office (Public Health Service Publication No. 149: Supplement 2)

13. Carcinogenesis Program National Cancer Institute (1971) *Survey of compounds which have been tested for carcinogenic activity* Washington DC, US Government Printing Office (Public Health Service Publication No. 149: 1968-1969)

14. Carcinogenesis Program National Cancer Institute (1973) *Survey of compounds which have been tested for carcinogenic activity*, Washington DC, US Government Printing Office (Public Health Service Publication No. 149: 1961-1967)

15. Carcinogenesis Program National Cancer Institute (1974) *Survey of compounds which have been tested for carcinogenic activity*, Washington DC, US Government Printing Office (Public Health Service Publication No. 149: 1970-1971)

16. WHO (1961) Fifth Report of the Joint FAO/WHO Expert Committee on Food Additives. Evaluation of carcinogenic hazard of food additives. *Wld Hlth Org. techn. Rep. Ser.*, No. 220, pp. 5, 18, 19

17. WHO (1969) Report of a WHO Scientific Group. Principles for the testing and evaluation of drugs for carcinogenicity. *Wld Hlth Org. techn. Rep. Ser.*, No. 426, pp. 19, 21, 22

18. WHO (1964) Report of a WHO Expert Committee. Prevention of cancer. *Wld Hlth Org. techn. Rep. Ser.*, No. 276, pp. 29, 30

19. Stecher, P.G., ed. (1968) *The Merck Index*, 8th ed., Rahway, NJ, Merck & Co.

20. Weast, R.C., ed. (1975) *CRC Handbook of Chemistry and Physics*, 56th ed., Cleveland, Ohio, Chemical Rubber Co.

21. WHO (1958) Second Report of the Joint FAO/WHO Expert Committee on Food Additives. Procedures for the testing of intentional food additives to establish their safety for use. *Wld Hlth Org. techn. Rep. Ser.*, No. 144

22. WHO (1961) Fifth Report of the Joint FAO/WHO Expert Committee on Food Additives. Evaluation of carcinogenic hazard of food additives. *Wld Hlth Org. techn. Rep. Ser.*, No. 220

23. WHO (1967) Scientific Group. Procedures for investigating intentional and unintentional food additives. *Wld Hlth Org. techn. Rep. Ser.*, No. 348

24. UICC (1969) Carcinogenicity testing. *UICC techn. Rep. Ser.*, 2

25. Committee on Standardized Genetic Nomenclature for Mice (1972) Standardized nomenclature for inbred strains of mice. Fifth listing. *Cancer Res.*, 32, 1609-1646

26. Bartsch, H. & Grover, P.L. (1976) Chemical carcinogenesis and mutagenesis. In: Symington, T. & Carter, R.L., eds, Scientific Foundations of Oncology, Vol. IX, Chemical Carcinogenesis, London, Heinemann Medical Books Ltd, pp. 334-342

27. Holländer, A., ed. (1971) Chemical Mutagens: Principles and Methods for Their Detection, Vols 1-3, New York, Plenum Press

28. Montesano, R. & Tomatis, L., eds (1974) Chemical Carcinogenesis Essays, IARC Scientific Publications, No. 10, Lyon, IARC

29. Ramel, C., ed. (1973) Evaluation of genetic risks of environmental chemicals, Report of a symposium held at Skokloster, Sweden, 1972, Ambio Special Report No. 3, Royal Swedish Academy of Sciences/Universitetsforlaget

30. Stoltz, D.R., Poirier, L.A., Irving, C.C., Stich, H.F., Weisburger, J.H. & Grice, H.C. (1974) Evaluation of short-term tests for carcinogenicity. Toxicol. appl. Pharmacol., 29, 157-180

31. WHO (1974) Report of a WHO Scientific Group. Assessment of the carcinogenicity and mutagenicity of chemicals. Wld Hlth Org. techn. Rep. Ser., No. 546

32. Montesano, R., Bartsch, H. & Tomatis, L., eds (1975) Screening Tests in Chemical Carcinogenesis, IARC Scientific Publications, No. 12, Lyon, IARC

33. Committee 17 (1975) Environmental mutagenic hazards. Science, 187, 503-514

GENERAL REMARKS ON SUBSTANCES CONSIDERED

This series of monographs is devoted to some naturally occurring substances. Since certain substances in this class, namely aflatoxins, cycasin, safrole and related compounds and sterigmatocystin, were included in the first volume of monographs, the available data on these substances have been updated, and new monographs are included in the present volume.

Some fungal metabolites which have been used as drugs (and as feed additives) have also been included, although they may have been mainly produced industrially under conditions which maximize yields.

Not all those naturally occurring substances so far shown to be carcinogenic have been included. The term 'naturally occurring' has *not* been used to include substances which are formed from natural products under extreme conditions, as of pressure and/or heat (e.g., polycyclic aromatic hydrocarbons).

Where the identification of a carcinogen(s) in a natural product is incomplete, or where the carcinogenic activity has been only partially explained by the presence of a certain chemical(s), the writing of a monograph has been postponed. Thus, natural products which contain unidentified carcinogens (e.g., bracken fern, betel, tobacco, certain alcoholic beverages and some fungi) have not been included, even though there are considerable data available. With respect to pyrrolizidine alkaloids, data from tests in which only plant material has been tested are recorded in the section, "General Information and Conclusions on Pyrrolizidine Alkaloids", p. 333. Common features of the pyrrolizidine alkaloids with respect to metabolism and toxicity have been taken into consideration in evaluating their carcinogenicity, and such data, together with general methods for their analysis, are also summarized in that section.

THE MONOGRAPHS

ACTINOMYCINS

There are several actinomycins, but only one, actinomycin D (which is identical with C_1), is known to be used commercially at this time. Actinomycin C, which is a mixture of C_1, C_2 and C_3, is reported to have been used as a drug in Europe until 1960. Actinomycins S and L, which may contain C_2 and C_3, have been investigated but are not in commercial use; however, information on them has been included because their chemical structures and biological properties are similar to those of actinomycin D.

1. Chemical and Physical Data

Actinomycin D

1.1 Synonyms and trade names

Chem. Abstr. Reg. Serial No.: 50-76-0

Chem. Abstr. Name: Actinomycin D

Actinomycin A_{IV}; actinomycin C_1; actinomycin D deriv. of 3H-phenoxazine; actinomycin D deriv. of 1H-pyrrolo(2,1-1) (1,4,7,10,13)oxatetraazacyclohexadecine; actinomycin I; actinomycin IV; actinomycin-(*threo*-val-pro-sar-meval); actinomycin X_1; 2-amino-N,N'-bis{hexadecahydro-6,13-diisopropyl-2,5,9-trimethyl-1,4,7,11,14-pentaoxo-1H-pyrrolo(2,1-1) (1,4,10,13)oxatetraazacyclohexadecin-10-yl}-4,6-dimethyl-3-oxo-3H-phenoxazine-1,9-dicarboxamide; 2-amino-N,N'-bis-{hexadecahydro-2,5,9-trimethyl-6,13-bis(1-methylethyl)-1,4,7,11,14-pentaoxo-1H-pyrrolo(2,1-1) (1,4,7,10,13)oxatetraazacyclohexadecin-10-yl}-4,6-dimethyl-3-oxo-3H-phenoxazine-1,9-dicarboxamide; 10,10'-{(2-amino-4,6-dimethyl-3-oxo-3H-phenoxazine-1,9-diyl)bis(carbonylimino)}bis{dodecahydro-6,13-diisopropyl-2,5,9-trimethyl-1H-pyrrolo-(2,1-1) (1,4,7,10,13)oxatetraazacyclohexadecine}-1,4,7,11,14-pentone; bis(XI-lactone)N,N'-{(2-amino-4,6-dimethyl-3-oxo-3H-phenoxazine-1,9-diyl)bis{carbonylimino(3-hydroxy-1-oxobutylidene)imino(3-methyl-1-oxobutylidene) (tetrahydro-1H-pyrrole-1,2-diyl)carbonyl(methylimino) (1-oxo-1,2-ethanediyl)}bis(N-methyl)L-valine; dactinomycin; dactinomycin D; dilactone actinomycin D acid; dilactone actinomycindioic D acid; HBF 386 meractinomycin; 1H-pyrrolo(2,1-1)-

(1,4,7,10,13)oxatetraazacyclohexadecine; stereoisomer of N,N'-{(2-amino-4,6-dimethyl-3-oxo-3H-phenoxazine-1,9-diyl)bis(carbonyl-imino{3-hydroxy-1-oxo-butylidene(tetrahydro-1H-pyrrole-1,2-diyl)carbonyl(methylimino)(1-oxo-1,2-ethanediyl)})bis(N-methyl-L-valine)bis-(ζ-lactone)}

Cosmegen; Oncostatin K

1.2 Chemical formula and molecular weight

$C_{62}H_{86}N_{12}O_{16}$ Mol. wt: 1255.5

1.3 Chemical and physical properties of the pure substance (as trihydrate)

(a) Description: Bright red, rhomboid prisms from absolute ethanol

(b) Melting-point: 241.5-243°C (decomposition)

(c) Spectroscopy data: λ_{max} 240-242 nm (E^1_1 = 26.8) and 422 nm (E^1_1 = 19.6); nuclear magnetic resonance spectra are given by Hollstein (1974)

(d) Optical rotation: $[\alpha]^{28}_D$ -315°C (2.5% in methanol)

(e) Solubility: Very soluble in ethanol; slightly soluble in ether and water (10°C); soluble in propylene glycol and in water/glycol mixtures

(f) <u>Stability</u>: Stable in distilled water at 5°C for 150 days. Appreciably degraded on autoclaving except in solution buffered to pH 5

(g) <u>Reactivity</u>: Reacts readily *in vitro* with DNA at pH 7; the absorption maximum of the DNA/actinomycin D complex is 465 nm (Kirk, 1960).

1.4 Technical products and impurities

The USP grade of actinomycin D contains not less than 90% of the stated amount of active ingredient. In the United States, actinomycin D destined for clinical use contains mannitol (Blacow, 1972) and must meet specifications laid down in the <u>US Code of Federal Regulations</u> (1974).

2. Production, Use, Occurrence and Analysis

For important background information on this section, see preamble, p. 17.

Two reviews on actinomycins have been published (Hollstein, 1974; Waksman, 1967).

2.1 Production and use

Actinomycin D is one of the antibiotics produced by various species of *Streptomyces*; it is the principal component of the mixture of actinomycins produced by *Streptomyces parvullus*. Unlike other species of *Streptomyces*, this organism yields an essentially pure substance that contains only traces of similar compounds differing in the amino acid content of the peptide side chain.

Actinomycin D was first isolated from broth cultures of *Streptomyces parvullus* by Mannaker *et al.* in 1954 (Mannaker *et al.*, 1955). Its structure was determined by Bullock & Johnson in 1957 (Bullock & Johnson, 1957), and it was synthesized by Brockmann & Manegold in 1964 (Brockmann & Manegold, 1964).

Actinomycin D was introduced commercially in the US in 1964 (Waksman, 1967); it is currently produced by only one company, by a fermentation process (Perlman, 1974). There are two reported producers of actinomycin D in Europe (Chemical Information Services, Ltd, 1975) and one (by fermentation) in Japan. The chemical was introduced commercially in Japan in 1969 (Fukai, 1974); the quantity produced in 1972 was 4.6 g, and that in 1973, 1.5 g (Japan Antibiotics Research Association, 1974; 1975).

Actinomycin D was the first antibiotic found to have anti-tumour activity; this was demonstrated in the early 1950s in the Federal Republic of Germany. In the US, the chemical has been used in the treatment of Wilms' tumour, gestational choriocarcinoma, testicular tumours, embryonal rhabdomyosarcomas, lymphomas, Ewing's sarcomas and acute leukaemia (Perry, 1974).

Toxic reactions to actinomycin D are frequent and may be severe, thus limiting in many instances the amount that may be given. The usual dosages for i.v. injections are 0.5 mg daily for a maximum of 5 days in adults and 0.015 mg/kg bw daily for 5 days in children. In both adults and children, a second course may be given after at least two weeks have elapsed, provided that all signs of toxicity have disappeared. When the isolation-perfusion technique is used, dosages of 0.035-0.05 mg/kg bw are given.

Total US sales of actinomycin D are estimated to be less than 1 kg annually.

2.2 Occurrence

Actinomycins are produced by several *Streptomyces* fungi, including *Streptomyces chrysomallus*, *Streptomyces antibioticus* and *Streptomyces parvullus*; but the extent to which actinomycin D occurs in nature is not known.

2.3 Analysis

A paper chromatographic method has been described (Vining & Waksman, 1954). Thin-layer chromatography has been employed for the separation of actinomycins D, C_2, C_3, F_1 and F_2; the individual compounds were recovered from the plates and determined colorimetrically (Cassani *et al.*, 1964). A general thin-layer chromatographic method for classification of 84 antibiotics includes actinomycins C_2 and C_3 (Aszalos *et al.*, 1968). Column chromatography on Sephadex G25 has been used to separate actinomycins D_1, C_2 and C_3, which are subsequently determined spectrophotometrically (Schmidt-Kastner, 1964). Reversed-phase high-pressure liquid chromatography can also be used (Rzeszotarski & Mauger, 1973).

3. Biological Data Relevant to the Evaluation of Carcinogenic Risk to Man

3.1 Carcinogenicity and related studies in animals

(a) <u>Subcutaneous and/or intramuscular administration</u>

<u>Mouse</u>: A group of 10 male btk mice[1] was given 35 twice weekly s.c. injections of 0.2 µg/animal <u>actinomycin D</u>. Local sarcomas occurred in 2/10 mice between 36 and 41 weeks after the start of treatment. In a concurrent positive control group, 10/10 mice which received s.c. injections of 0.4 mg methylcholanthrene developed local tumours within 8-24 weeks. No tumours were observed in 20 controls injected with olive oil or saline and observed for 66 weeks (Ikegami et al., 1967).

Four groups of 5-8 male btk mice were given s.c. injections of 9, 22.5, 67.5 or 250 µg/kg bw <u>actinomycin L</u> in saline twice weekly for up to one year. Because of toxic effects, mice given 250 µg/kg bw received 18 injections only. The numbers of local sarcomas were 0/8, 0/5, 5/8 and 0/5 in the respective groups; the first tumour occurred after 35 weeks. No subcutaneous sarcomas occurred in 41 non-treated or saline-injected controls observed for 40 weeks (Kawamata et al., 1959).

A group of 10 male btK mice and a group of 8 female ctK mice[2] were given twice weekly s.c. injections of 7.5 µg/kg bw <u>actinomycin S</u> in saline for up to 40 weeks. All ten btK males developed local sarcomas, the first tumour appearing at 22 weeks. Three females died prior to the appearance of the first tumour (28 weeks), and 4/5 remaining animals developed local sarcomas between 28-40 weeks. No local tumours were reported to have occurred in an unstated number of saline-injected controls (Kawamata et al., 1958).

In groups of 10 female and/or 10 male btK mice given twice weekly s.c. injections of 0.94, 7.5, 15, 30 or 125 µg/kg bw <u>actinomycin S</u> for up to one year, 2/8 males and 0/7 females given the lowest dose developed local sarcomas after 39 weeks. In groups given 7.5-30 µg/kg bw, the incidence

---

[1] Hybrids of C57Bl/He males paired with ta albino females
[2] Hybrids of C3H/He males paired with ta albino females

of sarcomas in both males and females was 70-100%. In those receiving the highest level, toxic effects occurred, and only 19 injections were given; 2/6 male mice developed local sarcomas, the first tumour appearing after 19 weeks. No subcutaneous tumours were observed in 41 untreated or saline-injected controls. Twice weekly s.c. injections of 7.5 µg/kg bw actinomycin S were also given to groups of male and female ctK, Swiss, ddO, C3H and C57BL mice. A high incidence of local sarcomas was observed in ctK males (9/9) and females (7/8). The incidences in male and female ddO, C57BL and Swiss mice were 4/8 and 4/10, 3/9 and 2/9, 1/10 and 1/8, respectively. Of the C3H mice, all males died early, and no local tumours occurred in 4 surviving females. No subcutaneous tumours occurred in approximately equal numbers of untreated or saline-injected controls (Kawamata et al., 1959).

(b) Intraperitoneal administration

Rat: Two groups, consisting of 11 and 15 male Fischer 344 rats, were given repeated i.p. injections of 0.025-0.05 or 0.05 mg/kg bw actinomycin D 2-5 times per week for up to 18 weeks (total doses, 0.65 and 0.8 mg), followed by observation for up to 50 weeks. Six and 12 mesenchymal tumours were observed, respectively; the time of the appearance of the first tumour was 23 weeks. A tumour of the same type was seen after 42 weeks in 1/9 rats given single injections of 2 mg/kg bw but in none of 15 rats given single injections of 0.5 or 1 mg/kg bw. No tumours occurred among 10 controls given i.p. injections of 0.9% saline thrice weekly for 50 weeks (Svoboda et al., 1970).

Two groups of 25 male and 25 female Charles River CD rats were given i.p. injections of 0.022 or 0.045 mg/kg bw actinomycin D thrice weekly for 6 months, followed by observation for a further 12 months, at which time the animals were killed. Peritoneal sarcomas developed in 32/38 males and 25/36 females (Weisburger et al., 1976).

(c) Intravenous administration

Rat: A group of 48 male BR46 rats received weekly i.v. injections of 7 mg/kg bw actinomycin C (7% of the LD_{50}) for 52 weeks, followed by observation for life. Of 35 rats alive at the appearance of the first tumour,

22 were examined pathologically: 4 were found to have developed benign tumours (3 thymomas and 1 adenoma of the kidney), and 2, malignant tumours (1 myeloblastic leukaemia and 1 angioendothelioma in the abdominal cavity) within 21±5 months. Among 65 controls, 3 (5%) developed benign tumours and 4 (6%), malignant tumours within 23±5 months (Schmähl & Osswald, 1970).

3.2 Other relevant biological data

In mice, the LD_{50} by i.p. injection of actinomycin D was 2-2.4 mg/kg bw; that by i.v. injection was 0.7 mg/kg bw (Stecher, 1968). Repeated i.p. injections of 75 μg/kg bw for 7 days resulted in the death of 60% of animals. The oral LD_{50} was above 7 mg/kg bw. In a dog, i.v. injection of 15 μg/kg bw for 5 days produced anorexia, dehydration from vomiting and haemorrhages and/or ulcers in the intestine and colon (DiPaolo et al., 1957). In rats, the LD_{50}'s by the i.v., i.p., s.c. and oral routes were 0.46, 0.40, 0.80 and 7.2 mg/kg bw, respectively. Actinomycin D was toxic to the blood-forming tissues, lymphoid tissues and intestinal epithelium in dogs (Phillips et al., 1960). The LD_{50} in rats of i.v. injections of actinomycin C was 100 mg/kg bw (Schmähl & Oswald, 1970). The LD_{50}'s of various fractions of actinomycin S in mice were reported to be about 0.5-0.9 mg/kg bw, but the route of administration was not stated (Kawamata & Fujita, 1958).

Inhibition of RNA synthesis, necrosis, hyperplasia and an altered mitotic index were observed in mouse skin within 4 days after six applications of 15 μg actinomycin D. After a single application of 1 μg, only RNA synthesis was inhibited (Flamm et al., 1966).

In rabbits given 1 mg/kg bw actinomycin D by i.v. injection, less than one-tenth of the initial concentration in the blood could be detected after 2 hours; after 10 hours a slight increase in the blood level was observed. Thirty minutes after its injection highest levels were found in the kidney, heart, spleen and liver; it was also present in the bile and urine (Fujita, 1971).

Actinomycin D had an inhibitory effect on the induction of mammary tumours by DMBA in rats (Anderson & Kellen, 1971; Gardner et al., 1973; Tominaga et al., 1973). Its topical application to mice inhibited the formation of skin tumours initiated by DMBA or β-propiolactone (Bates et al., 1968; Gelboin & Klein, 1964; Hennings & Boutwell, 1967; Hennings et al., 1968). Actinomycin D was reported to inhibit DNA synthesis in mouse skin (Bates et al., 1968; Flamm et al., 1966; Hennings et al., 1968).

Actinomycin D intercalates between deoxyguanosine residues in double-helical DNA (Gellert et al., 1965; Goldberg et al., 1962; Sobell, 1974). In mammalian cells it inhibits RNA synthesis (Goldberg & Rabinowitz, 1962; Goldberg & Reich, 1964; Hamilton et al., 1963); the growth of most RNA viruses is unaffected by this antibiotic (Reich, 1963). Actinomycin S binds reversibly to bacterial DNA *in vitro* but not to bacterial RNA (Kawamata & Imanishi, 1961).

In rats, doses of 50-100 µg/kg bw actinomycin D induced malformations of the CNS, viscera and skeleton; in rabbits, even small doses of actinomycin D were more embryotoxic and less teratogenic. In hamsters given 100 µg/kg bw on days 7 and 8 of pregnancy, embryotoxicity and teratogenicity on ossification were observed. With lower dose levels no embryotoxic or teratogenic effects occurred (Tuchmann-Duplessis et al., 1973).

Actinomycin D of unspecified origin and purity applied at concentrations of 5-10 mg/l induced mitotic crossing over in the soyabean *Glycine max* L. (Vig, 1973), and at a concentration of 50 mg/l it induced meiotic crossing over in barley (Sinha & Helgason, 1969). Fisher et al. (1970) reported the induction of forward mutations in the ad-3A and ad-3B regions of *Neurospora crassa*. Actinomycin D of unspecified purity injected into Oregon R *Drosophila melanogaster* females increased the frequencies of crossing over in meiotic and premeiotic cells (Suzuki, 1965).

An aqueous solution of actinomycin D of unspecified purity was injected intraperitoneally into ICR/Ha Swiss mice at doses of 0.34-1.67 mg/kg bw. A significant reduction in the number of implantation sites and an increase in early embryonic deaths was observed (Epstein et al., 1972). Actinomycin D of unspecified origin and purity induced chromatid breaks and translocations in short-time human peripheral leucocyte cultures, human epidermal fibroblasts and HeLa cells. Breaks were preferentially located in the centromere regions, and frequencies were dose-dependent (Ostertag & Kersten, 1965).

A solution of actinomycin C (100 mg/l) of unspecified origin and purity did not induce λ-bacteriophage in *Escherichia coli* K12 (Heinemann & Howard, 1964).

In man, actinomycin D has been reported to produce dermal folliculitis (Epstein & Lutzner, 1969).

3.3 Observations in man

No data were available to the Working Group.

4. Comments on Data Reported and Evaluation[1]

4.1 Animal data

Actinomycin D is carcinogenic in rats following its intraperitoneal injection: it produced malignant mesenchymal tumours in the peritoneal cavity. Actinomycins L and S produced sarcomas at the site of their subcutaneous injection in mice. Actinomycin C produced no carcinogenic effect in rats following its intravenous injection.

4.2 Human data

No case reports or epidemiological studies were available to the Working Group.

---

[1]See also the section "Animal Data in Relation to the Evaluation of Risk to Man" in the introduction to this volume, p. 15.

5. References

Anderson, K.M. & Kellen, J.A. (1971) Reduced incidence of DMBA-induced rat mammary tumors due to actinomycin D and the development of DMBA-induced hypertension. Oncology, 25, 446-454

Aszalos, A., Davis, S. & Frost, D. (1968) Classification of crude antibiotics by instant thin-layer chromatography (ITLC). J. Chromat., 37, 487-498

Bates, R.R., Wortham, J.S., Counts, W.B., Dingman, C.W. & Gelboin, H.V. (1968) Inhibition by actinomycin D of DNA synthesis and skin tumorigenesis induced by 7,12-dimethylbenz(a)anthracene. Cancer Res., 28, 27-34

Blacow, N.W., ed. (1972) Martindale, The Extra Pharmacopoeia, 26th ed., London, The Pharmaceutical Press, pp. 1181-1183

Brockmann, H. & Manegold, J.H. (1964) Partialsynthese von Actinomycin C_1 (D). Naturwissenschaften, 51, 383-384

Bullock, E. & Johnson, A.W. (1957) Actinomycin: the structure of actinomycin D. J. chem. Soc., 3280-3285

Cassani, G., Albertini, A. & Ciferri, O. (1964) Separation of actinomycins by thin-layer chromatography. J. Chromat., 13, 238-239

Chemical Information Services, Ltd (1975) Directory of Western European Chemical Producers, 1975/1976, Oceanside, NY

DiPaolo, J.A., Moore, G.E. & Niedbala, T.F. (1957) Experimental studies with actinomycin D. Cancer Res., 17, 1127-1134

Epstein, E.H., Jr & Lutzner, M.A. (1969) Folliculitis induced by actinomycin D. New Engl. J. Med., 281, 1094-1096

Epstein, S.S., Arnold, E., Andrea, J., Bass, W. & Bishop, Y. (1972) Detection of chemical mutagens by the dominant lethal assay in the mouse. Toxicol. appl. Pharmacol., 23, 288-325

Fisher, C.R., Malling, H.V. & de Serres, F.J. (1970) Mutagenicity of actinomycin D in *Neurospora crassa*. Genetics, 64, 20

Flamm, W.G., Banerjee, M.R. & Counts, W.B. (1966) Topical application of actinomycin D on mouse skin: effect on the synthesis of ribonucleic acid and protein. Cancer Res., 26, 1349-1360

Fujita, H. (1971) Comparative studies on the blood level, tissue distribution, excretion and inactivation of anticancer drugs. Jap. J. clin. Oncol., 12, 151-162

Fukai, S. (1974) Today's new medicinals, Tokyo, Yakuji Daily News, January 20, p. 654

Gardner, H.A., Kellen, J.A. & Anderson, K.M. (1973) Alterations in DMBA-induced rat mammary tumors by actinomycin D. J. nat. Cancer Inst., 50, 915-919

Gelboin, H.V. & Klein, M. (1964) Skin tumorigenesis by 7,12-dimethylbenz-(a)anthracene: inhibition by actinomycin D. Science, 145, 1321-1322

Gellert, M., Smith, C.E., Neville, D. & Felsenfeld, G. (1965) Actinomycin binding to DNA: mechanism and specificity. J. molec. Biol., 11, 445-457

Goldberg, I.H. & Rabinowitz, M. (1962) Actinomycin D inhibition of deoxyribonucleic acid-dependent synthesis of ribonucleic acid. Science, 136, 315-316

Goldberg, I.H. & Reich, E. (1964) Actinomycin inhibition of RNA synthesis directed by DNA. Fed. Proc., 23, 958-964

Goldberg, I.H., Rabinowitz, M. & Reich, E. (1962) Basis of actinomycin action. I. DNA binding and inhibition of RNA-polymerase synthetic reactions by actinomycin. Proc. nat. Acad. Sci. (Wash.), 48, 2094-2101

Hamilton, L.D., Fuller, W. & Reich, E. (1963) X-Ray diffraction and molecular model building studies of the interaction of actinomycin with nucleic acids. Nature (Lond.), 198, 538-540

Heinemann, B. & Howard, A.J. (1964) Induction of lambda-bacteriophage in *Escherichia coli* as a screening test for potential antitumor agents. Appl. Microbiol., 12, 234-239

Hennings, H. & Boutwell, R.K. (1967) On the mechanism of inhibition of benign and malignant skin tumor formation by actinomycin D. Life Sci., 6, 173-181

Hennings, H., Smith, H.C., Colburn, N.H. & Boutwell, R.K. (1968) Inhibition by actinomycin D of DNA and RNA synthesis and of skin carcinogenesis initiated by 7,12-dimethylbenz(a)anthracene or β-propiolactone. Cancer Res., 28, 543-552

Hollstein, U. (1974) Actinomycin. Chemistry and mechanism of action. Chem. Rev., 74, 625-652

Ikegami, R., Akamatsu, Y. & Haruta, M. (1967) Subcutaneous sarcomas induced by mitomycin C in mice: comparison of occurrence, transplantability and histology between sarcomas induced by actinomycin S and 3-methylcholanthrene. Acta path. jap., 17, 495-501

Japan Antibiotics Research Association (1974) The Japanese Journal of Antibiotics, Vol. 27, p. 252

Japan Antibiotics Research Association (1975) *The Japanese Journal of Antibiotics*, Vol. 28, p. 100

Kawamata, J. & Fujita, H. (1958) Separation and characterisation of actinomycin by the method of counter-current distribution. *Med. J. Osaka Univ.*, 8, 737-742

Kawamata, J. & Imanishi, M. (1961) Mechanism of action of actinomycin, with special reference to its interaction with deoxyribonucleic acid. *Biken's J.*, 4, 13-24

Kawamata, J., Nakabayashi, N., Kawai, A. & Ushida, T. (1958) Experimental production of sarcoma in mice with actinomycin. *Med. J. Osaka Univ.*, 8, 753-762

Kawamata, J., Nakabayashi, N., Kawai, A., Fujita, H., Imanishi, M. & Ikegami, R. (1959) Studies on the carcinogenic effect of actinomycin. *Biken's J.*, 2, 105-112

Kirk, J.M. (1960) The mode of action of actinomycin D. *Biochim. biophys. acta*, 42, 167-169

Mannaker, R.A., Gregory, F.J., Vining, L.C. & Waksman, S.A. (1955) Actinomycin. III. The production and properties of a new actinomycin. In: Welch, H. & Martilbanez, F., eds, *Antibiotics Annual 1954-1955*, New York, Medical Encyclopedia, Inc., pp. 853-857

Ostertag, W. & Kersten, W. (1965) The action of proflavine and actinomycin D in causing chromatid breakage in human cells. *Exp. Cell Res.*, 39, 296-301

Perlman, D. (1974) Prospects for the fermentation industries, 1974-1983, *Chemtech*, April, pp. 211, 216

Perry, S. (1974) Summation and general discussion. *Cancer Chemother. Rep.*, 58, 117-120

Phillips, F.S., Schwartz, H.S., Sternberg, S.S. & Tan, C.T.C. (1960) The toxicity of actinomycin D. *Ann. N.Y. Acad. Sci.*, 89, 348-360

Reich, E. (1963) Biochemistry of actinomycins. *Cancer Res.*, 23, 1428-1441

Rzeszotarski, W.J. & Mauger, A.B. (1973) Reversed-phase high-pressure liquid chromatography of actinomycins. *J. Chromat.*, 86, 246-249

Schmähl, D. & Osswald, H. (1970) Experimentelle Untersuchungen über carcinogene Wirkungen von Krebs-Chemotherapeutica und Immunosuppressiva. *Arzneimittel-Forsch.*, 20, 1461-1467

Schmidt-Kastner, G. (1964) Separation of actinomycin mixtures by chromatography on Sephadex. *Naturwissenschaften*, 51, 38-39

Sinha, R.P. & Helgason, S.B. (1969) The action of actinomycin D and diepoxybutane on recombination of two closely linked loci in *Hordeum*. Canad. J. Genet. Cytol., 11, 745-751

Sobell, H.M. (1974) The stereochemistry of actinomycin binding to DNA. Cancer Chemother. Rep., 58, 101-116

Stecher, P.G., ed. (1968) The Merck Index, 8th ed., Rahway, NJ, Merck & Co., pp. 319-320

Suzuki, D.T. (1965) Effects of actinomycin D on crossing over in *Drosophila melanogaster*. Genetics, 51, 11-21

Svoboda, D., Reddy, J. & Harris, C. (1970) Invasive tumors induced in rats with actinomycin D. Cancer Res., 30, 2271-2279

Tominaga, T., Taguchi, T. & Shiba, S. (1973) Effect of actinomycin-D and mitomycin-C on induction of rat mammary cancer with 7,12-dimethylbenz-(*a*)anthracene. Gann, 64, 301-303

Tuchmann-Duplessis, H., Hiss, D., Mottot, G. & Rosner, I. (1973) Embryotoxic and teratogenic effect of actinomycin D in the Syrian hamster. Toxicology, 1, 131-133

US Code of Federal Regulations (1974) Food and Drugs, Title 21, part 450.20a, Washington DC, US Government Printing Office, p. 679

Vig, B.K. (1973) Somatic crossing over in *Glycine max* (L.) Merrill: effect of some inhibitors of DNA synthesis on the induction of somatic crossing over and point mutations. Genetics, 73, 583-596

Vining, L.C. & Waksman, S.A. (1954) Paper chromatographic identification of the actinomycins. Science, 120, 389-390

Waksman, S., ed. (1967) Actinomycin, Nature, Formation and Activities, New York, Interscience Publishers

Weisburger, J.H., Griswold, D.P., Jr, Prejean, J.D., Casey, A.E., Wood, H.B., Jr & Weisburger, E.K. (1976) The carcinogenic properties of some of the principal drugs used in cancer chemotherapy. Recent Results Cancer Res. (in press)

ADRIAMYCIN

See also monograph on daunomycin, a closely related compound.

1. Chemical and Physical Data

1.1 Synonyms and trade names

Chem. Abstr. Reg. Serial No.: 23214-92-8

Chem. Abstr. Name: (8S-cis)-10-[(3-Amino-2,3,6-trideoxy-α-L-lyxo-hexapyranosyl)oxy]-7,8,9,10-tetrahydro-6,8,11-trihydroxy-8-(hydroxyacetyl)-1-methoxy-5,12-naphthacenedione

10-[(3-Amino-2,3,6-trideoxy-D-lyxohexopyranosyl)oxy]-8-glycolcyl-7,8,9,10-tetrahydro-6,8,11-trihydroxy-1-methoxy-5,12-naphthacenedione; doxorubicin; F.I. 106; 1,2,3,4,6,11-hexahydro-4β,5,12-trihydroxy-4-(hydroxyacetyl)-10-methoxy-6,11-dioxonaphthacen-1β-yl-3-amino-2,3,6-trideoxy-α-L-lyxohexopyranoside; 14-hydroxydaunomycin; 14'-hydroxydaunomycin; NSC 123127*

1.2 Chemical formula and molecular weight

$C_{27}H_{29}NO_{11}$ Mol. wt: 543.5

1.3 Chemical and physical properties of the pure substance (as hydrochloride)

(a) Description: Red, crystalline solid

(b) Melting point: 205°C (decomposition)

---

*Cancer Chemotherapy National Service Centre Number, NCI, NIH, USA

(c) Spectroscopy data: λ_{max} in methanol at 56°C of the dried substance:

λ_{max}	E^1_1
233 nm;	= 658
253	440
290	145
477	225
495	223
530	124

Arcamone *et al.* (1969)

Infra-red spectra of the hydrochloride are also reported by Arcamone *et al.* (1969).

(d) Identity and purity test: Adriamycin gives a purple colour with Marquis reagent. Solutions of adriamycin are orange-yellow at acid pH, orange-red at neutral pH and blue-violet at pH >9 (Clarke, 1975).

(e) Solubility: 1 g is soluble in 50 ml water (2%); soluble in aqueous alcohols; moderately soluble in anhydrous methanol; insoluble in non-polar organic solvents (Arcamone *et al.*, 1969)

(f) Stability: Neutral aqueous solutions are stable at room temperature.

(g) Optical rotation: $[\alpha]_D^{20}$ +248°C (0.1% in methanol) (Arcamone *et al.*, 1969)

1.4 Technical products and impurities

Technical adriamycin contains 90-110% of the quantity of the active drug, adriamycin hydrochloride, stated on the label, as determined by microbiological assay. It may contain up to 4% moisture. It is free of penicillin and contains no histamine or histamine-like impurities. Ampoules of adriamycin containing 10 mg of lyophilized adriamycin hydrochloride are available.

2. Production, Use, Occurrence and Analysis

For important background information on this section, see preamble, p. 17.

2.1 Production and use

Adriamycin is a cytotoxic antibiotic isolated from cultures of *Streptomyces peucetius* var. *caesius*, a mutant obtained by treating *Streptomyces peucetius* with N-nitroso-N-methylurethane. The antibiotic was first isolated in Italy in 1967 (Bonadonna et al., 1969) and is produced in submerged and aerated culture (Arcamone et al., 1969).

The only known producers of adriamycin are one company in Italy and one in Japan. Production in Japan in 1974 amounted to 140 g; the quantity produced in Italy is not known.

Adriamycin has been used in the treatment of the following neoplastic diseases: acute lymphoblastic leukaemia (Tan et al., 1973), Wilms' tumour (Mathé et al., 1970), soft tissue and osteogenic sarcomas (Cortes et al., 1974a), Ewing's sarcoma (Cortes et al., 1972) and bronchogenic carcinoma (Cortes et al., 1974b).

The recommended dosage schedule for adults is 60-75 mg/m^2 body surface as a single i.v. infusion administered at 21-day intervals, until a total dose of 550 mg/m^2 has been given.

2.2 Occurrence

No natural contamination by this compound was known to the Working Group.

2.3 Analysis

Spectrofluorometric methods have been used for identification and estimation of the drug in biological fluids and tissues (Dusonchet et al., 1971; Schwartz, 1973). A radioimmunoassay has been described for its determination in blood and tissue of experimental animals (Van Vunakis et al., 1974); the limit of detection was 2 pmol/ml. Adriamycin has also been isolated from cultures by paper and thin-layer chromatography; it was determined by extraction of the relevant zone and estimated spectrophotometrically (Arcamone et al., 1969).

3. Biological Data Relevant to the Evaluation of Carcinogenic Risk to Man

3.1 Carcinogenicity and related studies in animals

Intravenous administration

Rat: A group of 25 female Sprague-Dawley rats was given i.v. injections of a single dose of 8 mg/kg bw adriamycin. Eighteen animals died within one year, and one developed a mammary cancer. Of the 7 survivors killed after one year, 6 had mammary tumours (1 mammary adenocarcinoma and 6 fibroadenomas). The mean induction time was 223 days. No tumours developed in 25 controls (Bertazzoli et al., 1971).

3.2 Other relevant biological data

The i.v. LD_{50}'s for adriamycin were 9.4, 12.6 and 6 mg/kg bw for mice, rats and rabbits, respectively (Kiyohara et al., 1972). New Zealand rabbits given 200-400 mg/m² adriamycin developed chronic cardiomyopathy (Olson et al., 1974).

In mice, ³H-adriamycin was rapidly bound to tissues after i.v. injection of 5 mg/kg bw; after 30 minutes tissue concentrations were ten times greater than those in blood; 50% was excreted within 32 hours. Most of the radioactivity was excreted in the bile, but no metabolites were found (Di Fronzo et al., 1971). In rabbits, 17% of an i.v. dose of 5 mg/kg bw was excreted in the bile and 2% in the urine within 8 hours. The principal metabolite identified was adriamycinol; there were also several conjugates. Some glycosidic cleavage also takes place, particularly in the liver. Liver and kidney cytoplasmic enzymes reduce adriamycin to adriamycinol in a NADPH-dependent reaction (Bachur et al., 1974).

Adriamycin inhibits RNA and DNA metabolism by DNA intercalation (Meriwether & Bachur, 1972).

Transformation was observed in Fischer rat embryo cells grown for 4 weeks in a culture medium containing 0.15 ng/ml adriamycin. Local fibrosarcomas were produced in 3/10 and 4/10 newborn Fischer rats given s.c. injections of the transformed cells (Price et al., 1975). Adriamycin hydrochloride of unspecified purity induced reverse mutations in *Salmonella typhimurium* (McCann *et al.*, 1975).

In man, adriamycin causes baldness, stomatitis and bone-marrow aplasia. In addition, fatal disturbances in cardiac function have been reported (Lefrak *et al.*, 1970). The major metabolite identified in human urine is adriamycinol (Takanashi & Bachur, 1974).

A concentration of 0.02 µg/ml adriamycin induced a high frequency of chromatid and chromosome breaks and exchanges in cultures of human peripheral leucocytes (Vig, 1971).

3.3 Observations in man

No data were available to the Working Group.

4. Comments on Data Reported and Evaluation

4.1 Animal data

Adriamycin was tested only in rats by single intravenous injection. No evaluation of the carcinogenicity of this compound is possible on the basis of this limited study.

4.2 Human data

No case reports or epidemiological studies were available to the Working Group.

5. References

Arcamone, F., Cassinelli, G., Fantini, G., Grein, A., Orezzi, P., Pol, C. & Spalla, C. (1969) Adriamycin, 14-hydroxydaunomycin, a new antitumour antibiotic from *S. peucetius* var. *caesius*. Biotech. Bioeng., 11, 1101-1110

Bachur, N.R., Hildebrand, R.C. & Jaenke, R.S. (1974) Adriamycin and daunorubicin disposition in the rabbit. J. Pharmacol. exp. Ther., 191, 331-340

Bertazzoli, C., Chieli, T. & Solcia, E. (1971) Different incidence of breast carcinomas or fibroadenomas in daunomycin or adriamycin treated rats. Experientia, 27, 1209-1210

Bonadonna, G., Monfardini, S., de Lena, M. & Fossati-Bellani, F. (1969) Clinical evaluation of adriamycin, a new antitumour antibiotic. Brit. med. J., iii, 503-506

Clarke, E.G.C., ed. (1975) Isolation and Identification of Drugs, Vol. II, London, The Pharmaceutical Press

Cortes, E.P., Holland, J.F., Wang, J.J. & Sinks, L.F. (1972) Doxorubicin in disseminated osteosarcoma. J. Amer. med. Ass., 221, 1132-1138

Cortes, E.P., Holland, J.F., Wang, J.J., Sinks, L.F., Blom, J., Senn, H., Bank, A. & Glidewell, O. (1974a) Amputation and adriamycin in primary osteosarcoma. New Engl. J. Med., 291, 998-1000

Cortes, E.P., Takita, J. & Holland, J.F. (1974b) Adriamycin in advanced bronchogenic carcinoma. Cancer, 34, 518-525

Di Fronzo, G., Gambetta, R.A. & Lenaz, L. (1971) Distribution and metabolism of adriamycin in mice. Comparison with daunomycin. Rev. Europ. Et. clin. biol., 16, 572-576

Dusonchet, L., Gebbia, N. & Gerbasi, F. (1971) Spectrofluorometric characterization of adriamycin, a new anti-tumour drug. Pharmacol. Res. Commun., 3, 55-65

Kiyohara, A., Kubo, K., Okabe, M., Miyazaki, H., Baba, H., Iwata, H. & Takahira, H. (1972) General pharmacological effects of adriamycin. Oyo Yakuri, 6, 1075-1088

Lefrak, E.A., Pitha, J., Rosenheim, S. & Gottlieb, J.A. (1970) A clinicopathologic analysis of adriamycin cardiotoxicity. Cancer, 32, 302-314

Mathé, G., Amiel, S., Hayat, M., de Vassal, F., Schwarzenberg, L., Schneider, M., Jasmin, C. & Rosenfeld, C. (1970) Essai de l'adriamycine dans le traitement des leucémies aiguës. Nouv. Presse Méd., 78, 1997-1999

McCann, J., Choi, E., Yamasaki, E. & Ames, B.N. (1975) Detection of carcinogens as mutagens in the *Salmonella*/microsome test: assay of 300 chemicals. Proc. nat. Acad. Sci. (Wash.), 72, 5135-5139

Meriwether, W.D. & Bachur, N.R. (1972) Inhibition of DNA and RNA metabolism by daunorubicin and adriamycin in L1210 mouse leukaemia. Cancer Res., 32, 1137-1142

Olson, H.M., Young, D.M., Prieur, D.J., LeRoy, A.F. & Reagan, R.L. (1974) Electrolyte and morphologic alterations of myocardium in adriamycin-treated rabbits. Amer. J. Path., 77, 439-454

Price, P.J., Suk, W.A., Skeen, P.C., Chirigos, M.A. & Huebner, R.J. (1975) Transforming potential of the anticancer drug adriamycin. Science, 187, 1200-1201

Schwartz, H.S. (1973) A fluorometric assay for daunomycin and adriamycin in animal tissues. Biochem. Med., 7, 396-404

Takanashi, S. & Bachur, N.R. (1974) New adriamycin and daunorubicin metabolites in human urine. Proc. Amer. Ass. Cancer Res., 15, 76

Tan, C., Etcubanas, E., Wollner, N., Rosen, G., Gilladoga, A., Showell, J., Murphy, M.L. & Krakoff, I.H. (1973) Adriamycin - an antitumour antibiotic in the treatment of neoplastic diseases. Cancer, 32, 9-17

Van Vunakis, H., Langone, J.J., Riceberg, L.J. & Levine, L. (1974) Radio-immunoassays for adriamycin and daunomycin. Cancer Res., 34, 2546-2552

Vig, B.K. (1971) Chromosome aberrations induced in human leukocytes by the antileukemic antibiotic adriamycin. Cancer Res., 31, 32-38

AFLATOXINS

These substances were previously considered by an IARC Working Group in December 1971 (IARC, 1972). Since that time new data have become available, and these have been incorporated into the monograph and taken into account in the present evaluation.

1. Chemical and Physical Data

1.1 Synonyms and trade names

Aflatoxin B_1: Chem. Abstr. Reg. Serial No.: 1162-65-8

Chem. Abstr. Name: (6aR-*cis*)(2,3,6a,9a)Tetrahydro-4-methoxy-cyclopenta[*c*]furo[3',2':4,5]furo[2,3-*h*][*l*]benzopyran-1,11-dione

Aflatoxin B_2: Chem. Abstr. Reg. Serial No.: 7220-81-7

Chem. Abstr. Name: (6aR-*cis*)(2,3,6a,8,9,9a)Hexahydro-4-methoxy-cyclopenta[*c*]furo[3',2':4,5]furo[2,3-*h*][*l*]benzopyran-1,11-dione

Aflatoxin G_1: Chem. Abstr. Reg. Serial No.: 1165-39-5

Chem. Abstr. Name: (3,4,7a,10a)Tetrahydro-5-methoxy-1*H*,12*H*-furo-[3',2':4,5]furo[2,3-*h*]pyrano[3,4-*c*][*l*]benzopyran-1,12-dione

Aflatoxin G_2: Chem. Abstr. Reg. Serial No.: 7241-98-7

Chem. Abstr. Name: (7aR-*cis*)(3,4,7a,9,10,10a)Hexahydro-5-methoxy-1*H*,12*H*-furo[3',2':4,5]furo[2,3-*h*]pyrano[3,4-*c*][*l*]benzopyran-1,12-dione

1.2 Chemical formulae and molecular weights

B_1: $C_{17}H_{12}O_6$ Mol. wt: 312.3 B_2: $C_{17}H_{14}O_6$ Mol. wt: 314.3

G$_1$: C$_{17}$H$_{12}$O$_7$ Mol. wt: 328.3   G$_2$: C$_{17}$H$_{14}$O$_7$ Mol. wt: 330.3

1.3 Chemical and physical properties of the pure substances

(a) Description: Colourless to pale yellow crystals. Intensely fluorescent in ultra-violet light, emitting blue or yellow-green fluorescence, from which the designations B and G were derived.

(b) Melting-point and absorption spectroscopy: Data relating to these are given in the table below:

Aflatoxin	Melting-point (°C)	Ultraviolet absorption	
		λ_{max} (nm)	E^1_1
B$_1$	268-9	223 265 363	820 430 698
B$_2$	286-9	222 265 363	541 350 662
G$_1$	244-6	243 264 363	350 305 495
G$_2$	237-9	214 265 363	851 351 633

(c) <u>Identity and purity test</u>: Purity can conveniently be determined by visual examination under ultra-violet light of fluorescence on chromatograms.

(d) <u>Solubility</u>: Very slightly soluble in water (10-20 µg/ml); insoluble in non-polar solvents; freely soluble in moderately polar organic solvents (e.g., chloroform and methanol) and especially in dimethylsulphoxide

(e) <u>Stability</u>: Relatively unstable to light and air, particularly in solution in highly polar solvents. Fluorescent and non-fluorescent degradation products appear upon brief exposure of chromatograms to light. Chloroform solutions are stable for years if kept in the dark and cold.

(f) <u>Reactivity</u>: The lactone ring is susceptible to alkaline hydrolysis. Little or no destruction of aflatoxins occurs under ordinary cooking conditions, but they can be totally destroyed by drastic treatment such as autoclaving in the presence of ammonia or by treatment with hypochlorite.

1.4 Technical products and impurities

No data were available to the Working Group.

2. Production, Use, Occurrence and Analysis

For important background information on this section, see preamble, p. 17.

2.1 Production and use

Aflatoxins are produced in small quantities for experimental purposes only. Production is by large-scale fermentations on solid substrates or liquid media, from which aflatoxins are extracted and purified by chromatography. Total annual production probably does not exceed 100 g.

2.2 Occurrence

Aflatoxin-producing fungal strains appear to be distributed ubiquitously, except in colder climatic areas such as Northern Europe and Canada. Thus, virtually every foodstuff or food product is potentially susceptible to contamination, which may occur at any stage of food production or subsequent processing. Samples of nearly every major dietary staple have been found to contain some aflatoxin at one time or another. Adequate control measures involving especially rapid post-harvest drying of crops and storage at moisture contents of less than 10% can virtually eliminate contamination.

Under suitable conditions, contamination can occur in a given locality with great variability with regard to types of food affected, frequency of contamination and levels of aflatoxin present. However, the following generalizations can be made: (i) aflatoxin B_1 is most frequently present in contaminated samples; B_2 and G_1 are present much less frequently and almost never in the absence of B_1; (ii) dietary surveys in Uganda, Thailand and Swaziland revealed that peanuts, beans and corn were the principal vectors of aflatoxins, with many samples (up to 50% of market samples of peanuts) containing 0.1-1 mg/kg aflatoxins; other grains, such as rice, were rarely contaminated (Alpert et al., 1971; Keen & Martin, 1971; Shank et al., 1972c).

In different regions of Murang'a (Kenya) mean aflatoxin levels of 0.121-0.351 µg/kg of food and of 0.05-0.167 µg/l of beer have been detected (Peers & Linsell, 1973).

In some countries there are regulations limiting aflatoxin residues in foods, generally to levels of 20 µg/kg or less.

2.3 Analysis

Chemical assay methods are available for the detection and quantification of aflatoxins in various foods at concentrations of 1-5 µg/kg or more (Stoloff, 1972; 1975). Fluorimetric measurement of aflatoxin absorbed on florisil in minicolumns has been described (Velasco, 1975). Bioassays, mainly for confirmation of chemical assay results, have also been devised (Legator, 1969).

Methods originally developed for peanuts and peanut products have been adapted to many other commodities, such as cottonseed (Pons, 1975), roasted corn (Shannon & Shotwell, 1975) and nutmeg (Beljaars et al., 1975). Other procedures have been developed for determining aflatoxin M_1 in milk (Purchase et al., 1974; Stubblefield & Shannon, 1974).

3. Biological Data Relevant to the Evaluation of Carcinogenic Risk to Man

3.1 Carcinogenicity and related studies in animals

Aflatoxin carcinogenesis has been reviewed (Wogan, 1973).

(a) Oral administration

Mouse: Feeding of aflatoxin B_1 at a level of 1000 µg/kg of diet to random-bred and inbred mouse strains for 70 weeks failed to induce tumours (Wogan, 1969a).

Rat: Since the first report of hepatoma induction in rats by peanut meal involved in the original aflatoxicosis episodes (Lancaster et al., 1961), many studies in rats have demonstrated the carcinogenic potency of aflatoxins for the liver of rats.

A linear dose-response relationship was observed in rats fed diets containing various amounts of aflatoxins for 294 to 384 days; 5 µg/kg of diet failed to induce hepatomas (Newberne, 1965). When a diet containing 5000 µg aflatoxin B_1 per kg of diet was fed to Porton rats for 1 to 9 weeks early in their lifetime, the liver tumour frequency rose from 0 to 100% in groups of 6-14 animals. In male rats fed 500 or 100 µg per kg of diet for their lifetime, the frequencies of liver tumours were 100% and 50%, respectively, for groups of 15-34 animals; the frequency was lower in females (Butler & Barnes, 1968).

In studies involving the feeding of purified aflatoxins to Fischer rats, aflatoxin B_1 added to a semi-synthetic diet at levels of 15, 300 and 1000 µg/kg of diet induced liver-cell carcinomas. At the 15 µg/kg level tumours were induced in 12/12 animals surviving 68-80 weeks of feeding; higher dietary levels induced tumours after shorter feeding periods. No liver tumours were found in 25 controls (Wogan & Newberne, 1967).

A dose-response experiment of similar design subsequently revealed that a dietary level of 1 µg aflatoxin B_1 per kg of diet was carcinogenic to the livers of male Fischer rats (Wogan et al., 1974). Results of that experiment are summarized in the following table:

Dietary aflatoxin B_1 (µg/kg of diet)	Time of earliest tumour (wks)	Number of mice with	
		Hyperplastic nodules	Liver-cell carcinomas
0	-	1/18	0/18
1	104	7/22	2/22
5	93	5/22	1/22
15	96	13/21	4/21
50	82	15/25	20/25
100	54	12/28	28/28

In other, similar experiments, aflatoxin B_1 was fed at levels of 250, 500 and 1000 µg/kg of diet to male Wistar rats for 147 days; the animals were then kept without further treatment for their lifespan. Yields of liver tumours were 62%, 72% and 86% in the three treated groups, respectively (Epstein et al., 1969). When aflatoxin B_1 was administered in the drinking-water at concentrations of 3 and 1 µg/ml, it produced liver tumours in 19/30 MRC rats which had received a total of 2 mg/animal and in 3/10 animals receiving a total dose of 1 mg/animal (Butler et al., 1969).

Aflatoxin B_1 caused mainly hepatocellular carcinomas in these experiments. However, there are suggestions that it may also induce (in very low incidence) carcinomas of the glandular stomach (Butler & Barnes, 1966) and mucinous adenocarcinomas of the colon (Wogan & Newberne, 1967). It has recently been shown that the induction of colon carcinomas by aflatoxin B_1 is enhanced by lack of vitamin A (Newberne & Rogers, 1973). One rat strain (Wistar) also displayed a high incidence of renal epithelial neoplasias in response to highly purified aflatoxin B_1 (Epstein et al., 1969).

In a recent experiment, aflatoxin B_1 was fed at a level of 2000 µg/kg of diet to pregnant Fischer 344 rats and then to their offspring until death. In a parallel study, aflatoxin feeding was initiated when the rats were 6-7 weeks old. More than 75% of the animals which died from neoplasms had developed liver-cell carcinomas; 12/53 rats at risk also developed colon tumours. No liver or colon tumours were found in 18 control animals (Ward et al., 1975).

A mixture of crystalline aflatoxins containing 37.7% aflatoxin B_1, 56.4% aflatoxin G_1 and traces of aflatoxins B_2 and G_2, administered to rats in the drinking-water for 64 weeks, produced liver tumours in 6/6 rats receiving a dose of 300 μg/week and in 1/5 rats receiving 35 μg/week (Dickens et al., 1966).

Aflatoxin G_1 is a less potent hepatocarcinogen than aflatoxin B_1 for rats dosed orally, but it induces a significant incidence of kidney tumours (Butler et al., 1969; Wogan et al., 1971).

Aflatoxin B_2 is weakly active in inducing liver tumours in rats: doses more than 100 times higher than an effective dose of aflatoxin B_1 are required (Wogan et al., 1971).

Hepatocarcinogenesis in rats due to aflatoxin feeding is enhanced by dietary deficiency of lipotropic agents (Rogers & Newberne, 1969; 1971) and by cirrhosis (Newberne et al., 1966). However, rats are partially or totally protected from aflatoxin carcinogenesis by simultaneous administration of diethylstilboestrol (Newberne & Williams, 1969) or phenobarbitone (McLean & Marshall, 1971) or by dietary protein deficiency (Madhavan & Gopalan, 1968), hypophysectomy (Goodall & Butler, 1969) or castration (Cardeilhac & Nair, 1973).

Trout: Aflatoxin B_1 is hepatocarcinogenic to rainbow trout at very low dietary levels (Sinnhuber et al., 1968a). A linear dose-response relationship exists over the range of dietary levels of 0 to 1.5 μg aflatoxin B_1 per kg of diet fed continuously for 20 months. The minimal effective dose was calculated to be about 0.1 μg/kg of diet for a 10% tumour yield; no tumours occurred in control animals (Halver, 1969).

The response of rainbow trout to aflatoxin B_1 is enhanced by the simultaneous feeding of cyclopropenoid fatty acids (Sinnhuber et al., 1968b). These acids have little, if any, modifying effect on the aflatoxin response in rats (Friedman & Mohr, 1968; Lee et al., 1969; Nixon et al., 1974).

Aflatoxins G_1 and B_2 are carcinogenic to rainbow trout but are less potent than B_1 (Ayres et al., 1971).

Salmon: Hepatomas were induced in 45% of an unspecified number of sockeye salmon by a diet containing 12 μg aflatoxin B_1 per kg of diet and 50 mg cyclopropenoid fatty acids per kg of diet (Wales & Sinnhuber, 1972).

Guppy: Aflatoxin B_1 fed to guppies (*Lebistes reticulatus*) at a level of 6000 μg/kg of diet induced liver tumours in 9/16 animals within 11 months. No liver tumours were observed in 18 control animals (Sato *et al.*, 1973).

Duck: Continuous feeding of a diet containing aflatoxins derived from contaminated peanut meal, at a level of 30 μg/kg of diet, induced liver tumours in 8/11 ducks after 14 months (Carnaghan, 1965).

Monkey: A female rhesus monkey developed a primary liver carcinoma after ingesting a total of about 500 mg aflatoxin B_1 over a six-year period (Adamson *et al.*, 1973).

Other primates: Liver-cell carcinomas have been induced in 1/9 marmosets fed aflatoxin B_1 alone at a level of 2000 μg/kg in the diet (200 μg/kg bw) and surviving 9-55 weeks of treatment; such tumours were also produced in 2/7 animals injected with hepatitis virus during aflatoxin exposure and surviving 3-94 weeks of treatment (Lin *et al.*, 1974).

Intermittent feeding of a diet containing 2000 μg aflatoxin B_1 per kg of diet also produced hepatocellular carcinomas in 6/10 female and 3/8 male tree shrews (*Tupaia glis*) after 74-172 weeks of treatment (total dose, 24-66 mg) (Reddy & Svoboda, 1975).

(b) Intratracheal administration

Rat: A mixture of aflatoxins (37.7% B_1, 56.4% G_1 and traces of B_2 and G_2) was administered intratracheally to 6 male rats in doses of 300 μg suspended in 30 μl peanut oil twice weekly for 30 weeks. The rats were then held without further treatment up to 100 weeks. Three of the 6 animals developed squamous-cell carcinomas of the trachea within 37-62 weeks; 4/6 animals also developed hepatomas within 49-62 weeks (Dickens *et al.*, 1966).

(c) Subcutaneous administration

Mouse: Of mice injected twice weekly with 10 μg of a mixture of aflatoxins (37.7% B_1, 56.4% G_1 and traces of B_2 and G_2) suspended in oil, 15/17 animals developed sarcomas between 23 and 76 weeks (Dickens & Jones, 1965).

Rat: Injection of a mixture of aflatoxins (37.7% B_1, 56.4% G_1 and traces of B_2 and G_2) in oil twice weekly at a dose of 50 µg/injection for 60 weeks induced local sarcomas in 6/6 rats within 21-60 weeks. A dose of 500 µg given twice weekly for a period of only 8 weeks induced sarcomas in 5/5 rats within 20-30 weeks (Dickens & Jones, 1963).

Injection of the same mixture of aflatoxin B_1 and G_1 twice weekly at a dose of 2 µg/injection induced sarcomas in 5/6 rats within 44-69 weeks. Pure B_1 injected according to the same schedule at 20 µg/dose induced sarcomas in 6/6 rats within 18-37 weeks; G_1 was less potent (4/6 sarcomas within 30-50 weeks) (Dickens & Jones, 1965).

(d) Intraperitoneal administration

Mouse: Administration of aflatoxin B_1 in dimethylsulphoxide (DMSO) to female A/He mice in 12 thrice weekly doses for 4 weeks, up to a total average dose of 5.6 mg/animal, produced an average of 5.6 primary pulmonary adenomas in 14/14 animals 24 weeks after the start of treatment; no tumours occurred in untreated control animals. Of DMSO controls 25% had lung tumours, with an average of 0.3 tumours/mouse (Wieder et al., 1968).

Infant mouse: Hepatomas were induced in 82/105 inbred (C57BlxC3H)F_1 mice injected i.p. during the first 7 days after birth with doses as low as 1.25 µg/g bw aflatoxin B_1 and killed 82 weeks later. The incidence of hepatomas in the control group was 3/100 (Vesselinovitch et al., 1972).

Rat: A single, half-LD_{50} dose of aflatoxin B_1 (7.65 mg/kg bw) induced liver-cell carcinomas in 7/13 female Wistar rats surviving for 60-128 weeks after treatment (Carnaghan, 1967). Aflatoxin B_1 dissolved in DMSO was as potent in inducing hepatocellular carcinomas in rats when injected intraperitoneally as when administered by stomach tube (Wogan et al., 1971).

(e) Other experimental systems

Combined exposures: A male rhesus monkey was injected i.m. on 5 days/week with 50 then 100 µg mixed aflatoxins (44% B_1, 44% G_1, 2% B_2 and G_2) for one year. It was then given orally by gavage 200 µg/day mixed aflatoxins for 4.5 years. A hepatocellular carcinoma was found 2.5 years after the end of treatment (Gopalan et al., 1972). A female rhesus monkey treated identically, except that the oral dose was 100 µg/day, developed a metastasizing intrahepatic bile-duct carcinoma 5.25 years after the end of treatment (Tilak, 1975).

Pre and post-natal exposure: Six groups each of 10 female Wistar rats were fed a diet containing 25% or 50% toxic groundnut meal containing 10 mg/kg aflatoxin B_1 and 0.2 mg/kg aflatoxin B_2 from day 10 of pregnancy to parturition, or from 1 day post-partum to 10 days post-partum, or from day 10 of pregnancy to 10 days post-partum. Among 113 male and 95 female offspring observed for up to 36 months, 1 male exposed *in utero* from day 10 of pregnancy and 1 female exposed *via* the milk for 10 days post-partum, developed cholangiocarcinomas, and 2 females exposed *in utero* from day 10 of pregnancy and *via* the milk for 10 days post-partum developed liver-cell carcinomas. No liver tumours were reported in 50 male and 50 female controls obtained from mothers fed 25-50% soyabean meal in the diet during pregnancy (Grice *et al.*, 1973).

When rainbow trout embryos (15 days post-fertilization) were exposed for 1 hour to a solution containing aflatoxin B_1 at a concentration of 0.5 μg/ml, 40% of fish killed 321 days after hatching had hepatocellular carcinomas (Sinnhuber & Wales, 1974).

3.2 Other relevant biological data

(a) Experimental systems

The oral LD_{50} of aflatoxin B_1 in female rats is 16 mg/kg bw (Carnaghan, 1967). Studies of the effects of the various aflatoxins on human embryo and adult liver cells *in vitro* have demonstrated that the order of toxicity is $B_1 > G_1 > G_2 > B_2$.

Several features of the metabolism of aflatoxins in animals have been described (Wogan, 1969b). Two types of metabolic transformation are known to occur *in vivo*, and their products have been identified chemically. Aflatoxins M_1 and M_2, resulting from ring hydroxylation, were isolated from sheep urine and chemically identified (Holzapfel *et al.*, 1966). M_1 was also isolated from cows' milk (Masri *et al.*, 1967); it appears in the urine of all species after dosing with B_1, in general accounting for about 1-4% of the administered dose in 24 hours (Wogan, 1969b). Aflatoxin P_1, the *O*-demethylated derivative of B_1, was identified as the major urinary metabolite of B_1 in rhesus monkeys, in which it accounts for about 20% of an injected dose in 24 hours. It is present mainly as glucuronide or sulphate conjugates (Dalezios et al., 1971).

Investigations of the *in vitro* metabolism of aflatoxin B_1 by liver homogenates from humans and several animal species have identified aflatoxin B_{2a} (the hemiacetal of B_1), aflatoxicol (aflatoxin F_1) and aflatoxin Q_1 among the metabolic products present in the incubation medium (Buchi et al., 1974; Patterson, 1973); no evidence is available on their production *in vivo*. Similar investigations indicate that aflatoxin B_1-2,3 epoxide is produced by liver preparations from humans and from several animal species (Garner, 1973; Swenson et al., 1973; 1974).

Aflatoxin B_1 in the presence or absence of a rat-liver microsomal system induced unscheduled DNA repair synthesis in cultured human fibroblasts. In the same system, aflatoxin G_2 was inactive, and aflatoxin G_1 was positive only in the presence of rat liver microsomal preparations (San & Stich, 1975).

Aflatoxin B_1, G_1 and aflatoxicol showed lethal activity in *Salmonella typhimurium* only in the presence of a rat-liver microsomal system, while aflatoxin B_2, G_2, P_1, M_1 and B_{2a} were inactive (Garner & Wright, 1973).

Only a few studies on the induction of gene mutations by aflatoxins have been reported. Aflatoxin B_1 has been shown to induce mutations in transforming DNA of *Bacillus subtilis* (Maher & Summers, 1970), and B_1 as well as G_1 were mutagenic to vegetative cells (but not conidia) of *Neurospora crassa* (Ong, 1971) and to *Chlamydomonas reinhardii* (Schimmer & Werner, 1974). Aflatoxin B_1 has been shown to induce recessive lethal mutations in *Drosophila melanogaster* (Lamb & Lilly, 1971).

Incubation of aflatoxin B_1 with a rat- or human-liver microsomal system in the presence of tester strains of *Salmonella typhimurium* produced reverse mutations in the bacteria (Ames et al., 1973; Garner & Wright, 1973; Garner et al., 1972; McCann et al., 1975).

Aflatoxin B_1 did not induce chromosome aberrations in germ cells of male BALB/c mice (Leonard et al., 1975). Skin fibroblasts from xeroderma pigmentosum patients showed a greater sensitivity to chromosomal damage by aflatoxin B_1 than did fibroblasts from normal subjects (Stich & Laishes, 1975).

(b) *Man*

A number of episodes have provided circumstantial evidence of aflatoxin involvement in acute toxicoses in humans. Several of the earlier reports have been summarized by Kraybill & Shimkin (1964). More recently, it was reported that a child who died of acute hepatic disease had histological changes in the liver identical to those seen in aflatoxin poisoning in monkeys; circumstantial evidence suggested aflatoxin involvement (Serck-Hanssen, 1970).

It has been found that the tissues and body fluids of Thai children who died from an acute syndrome of unknown aetiology contained substantial quantities of un-metabolized aflatoxin B_1. Although a causal relationship was not established, pathological findings in the liver and other tissues resembled those induced in monkeys by aflatoxin B_1 (Shank *et al.*, 1971).

Two reports suggest that aflatoxins may play a role in this acute toxicity syndrome in Thailand (Bourgeois *et al.*, 1971) and may contribute to the development of cirrhosis in Indian children with kwashiorkor (Amla *et al.*, 1971). [In both instances agents other than aflatoxin may have been responsible for the observed effects.]

In parts of Western India there have recently been outbreaks of hepatitis with a high fatality rate, which are associated with the consumption of maize heavily contaminated with *Aspergillus flavus*. Analysis for aflatoxins suggested that some individuals could have consumed 2-6 mg aflatoxins daily over a period of one month (Krishnamachari *et al.*, 1975).

Aflatoxin M_1 is present in the urine of humans who ingest aflatoxin-contaminated foods (Campbell *et al.*, 1970).

(c) *Carcinogenicity of metabolites*

Aflatoxin M_1 induces liver-cell carcinomas in rainbow trout (Canton *et al.*, 1975; Sinnhuber *et al.*, 1974) and in rats (Wogan & Paglialunga, 1974) but is considerably less potent that B_1 in both species.

3.3 Observations in man

Published epidemiological studies have consisted of estimates of aflatoxin intake by populations in which the incidence or prevalence of primary liver cancer was determined simultaneously. In one such study in Uganda, the frequency of aflatoxin contamination of market food samples was positively associated with liver cancer incidence in localized population groups (Alpert et al., 1971).

A study in Thailand showed substantial variations in aflatoxin intake over three areas of the country and a threefold difference in liver cancer incidence between two of them; the aflatoxin levels and liver cancer incidence rates were positively correlated (Shank et al., 1972a,b). A study of similar design carried out in the Murang'a district of Kenya also showed a positive correlation between aflatoxin intake and liver cancer incidence (Peers & Linsell, 1973). High levels of aflatoxin in food have recently been found to be associated with the very high incidence of liver cancer in Mozambique (Van Rensburg et al., 1974). The results of these last three studies are summarized in the accompanying table.

Van Nieuwenhuize et al. (1973) reported results of an 11-year follow-up study of 67 men who had inhaled particles contaminated with aflatoxin while working in a mill crushing peanuts and other oil seeds. Two of 55 men aged more than 39 years on first exposure to aflatoxins developed fatal liver disease and 11 developed cancers of various organs. In one case it was thought that the cancer might have originated in the liver (possibly a cholangiocellular carcinoma). These 13 men had inhaled doses of aflatoxin estimated to be between 160 and 395 $\mu g/m^3$/man/week. In 55 matched control men, four cancers developed, and none died from liver disease. The excess of cancers observed in this study was not statistically significant, but the number of subjects was insufficient to exclude a significant positive correlation.

4. Comments on Data Reported and Evaluation

4.1 Animal data

Aflatoxins B_1 and G_1 have been shown to be carcinogenic in several animal species, including non-human primates. B_1 fed continuously is active at levels below 5 mg/kg of diet, and tumours have been induced in rats with 1 μg/kg of diet. Hepatocellular carcinoma is the main tumour type induced by aflatoxins, but tumours of the kidney and colon also result from exposure in some rat strains.

Aflatoxins M_1 and B_2 produced liver tumours in trout and rats.

4.2 Human data

The studies of liver cancer incidence in relation to aflatoxin intake provide circumstantial evidence of a causal relationship.

Population	Dietary aflatoxin intake (ng/kg bw/day)	Cases (per 10^5) of primary liver cancer/year[1]					
		In adults (> 15 years)				In total population Both sexes	
		Men		Women			
		No.	Incidence	No.	Incidence	No.	Incidence
Kenya (high altitude)	3-5	1	3.1	0	–		
Kenya (medium altitude)	6-8	13	10.8	6	3.3		
Thailand (Songkhla)	5-8					2	2.0
Kenya (low altitude)	10-15	16	12.9	9	5.4		
Thailand (Ratburi)	45-77					6	6.0
Mozambique	222						25.4[2]

[1] The periods covered were 4 years in Kenya, 1 year in Thailand and 3 years in Mozambique.

[2] Men – 35.0; women – 15.7; number of cases not available

5. References

Adamson, R.H., Correa, P. & Dalgard, D.W. (1973) Occurrence of a primary liver carcinoma in a rhesus monkey fed aflatoxin B_1. J. nat. Cancer Inst., 50, 549-553

Alpert, M.E., Hutt, M.S.R., Wogan, G.N. & Davidson, C.S. (1971) Association between aflatoxin content of food and hepatoma frequency in Uganda. Cancer, 28, 253-260

Ames, B.N., Durston, W.E., Yamasaki, E. & Lee, F.D. (1973) Carcinogens are mutagens: a simple test system combining liver homogenates for activation and bacteria for detection. Proc. nat. Acad. Sci. (Wash.), 70, 2281-2285

Amla, I., Kamala, C.S., Gopalakrishna, G.S., Jayaraj, A.P., Sreenivasamurthy, V. & Parpia, H.A.B. (1971) Cirrhosis in children from peanut meal contaminated by aflatoxin. Amer. J. clin. Nutr., 24, 609-614

Ayres, J.L., Lee, D.J., Wales, J.H. & Sinnhuber, R.O. (1971) Aflatoxin structure and hepatocarcinogenicity in rainbow trout (*Salmo gairdneri*). J. nat. Cancer Inst., 46, 561-564

Beljaars, P.R., Schumans, J.C.H.M. & Koken, P.J. (1975) Quantitative fluorodensitometric determination and survey of aflatoxins in nutmeg. J. Ass. off. analyt. Chem., 58, 263-271

Bourgeois, C.H., Shank, R.C., Grossman, R.A., Johnsen, D.O., Wooding, W.L. & Chandavimol, P. (1971) Acute aflatoxin B_1 toxicity in the macaque and its similarities to Reye's syndrome. Lab. Invest., 24, 206-216

Büchi, G.H., Müller, P.M., Roebuck, B.D. & Wogan, G.N. (1974) Aflatoxin Q_1: a major metabolite of aflatoxin B_1 produced by human liver. Res. Comm. Chem. Path. Pharmacol., 8, 585-592

Butler, W.H. & Barnes, J.M. (1966) Carcinoma of the glandular stomach in rats given diets containing aflatoxin. Nature (Lond.), 209, 90

Butler, W.H. & Barnes, J.M. (1968) Carcinogenic action of groundnut meal containing aflatoxin in rats. Fd Cosmet. Toxicol., 6, 135-141

Butler, W.H., Greenblatt, B. & Lijinsky, W. (1969) Carcinogenesis in rats by aflatoxins B_1, G_1 and B_2. Cancer Res., 29, 2206-2211

Campbell, T.C., Caedo, J.P., Jr, Bulatao-Jayme, J., Salamat, L. & Engel, R.W. (1970) Aflatoxin M_1 in human urine. Nature (Lond.), 227, 403-404

Canton, J.H., Kroes, R., Van Logten, M.J., Van Schothorst, M., Stavenuiter, J.F. & Verhülsdonk, C.A.H. (1975) The carcinogenicity of aflatoxin M_1 in rainbow trout. Fd Cosmet. Toxicol., 13, 441-443

Cardeilhac, P.T. & Nair, K.P.C. (1973) Inhibition by castration of aflatoxin-induced hepatoma in carbon tetrachloride-treated rats. Toxicol. appl. Pharmacol., 26, 393-397

Carnaghan, R.B.A. (1965) Hepatic tumours in ducks fed a low level of toxic ground-nut meal. Nature (Lond.), 208, 308

Carnaghan, R.B.A. (1967) Hepatic tumours and other chronic liver changes in rats following a single oral administration of aflatoxin. Brit. J. Cancer, 21, 811-814

Dalezios, J., Wogan, G.N. & Weinreb, S.M. (1971) Aflatoxin P_1: a new aflatoxin metabolite in monkeys. Science, 171, 584

Dickens, F. & Jones, H.E.H. (1963) The carcinogenic action of aflatoxin after its subcutaneous injection in the rat. Brit. J. Cancer, 17, 691-698

Dickens, F. & Jones, H.E.H. (1965) Further studies on the carcinogenic action of certain lactones and related substances in the rat and mouse. Brit. J. Cancer, 19, 392-403

Dickens, F., Jones, H.E.H. & Waynforth, H.B. (1966) Oral, subcutaneous and intratracheal administration of carcinogenic lactones and related substances: the intratracheal administration of cigarette tar in the rat. Brit. J. Cancer, 20, 134-144

Epstein, S.M., Bartus, B. & Farber, E. (1969) Renal epithelial neoplasms induced in male Wistar rats by oral aflatoxin B_1. Cancer Res., 29, 1045-1050

Friedman, L. & Mohr, H. (1968) Absence of interaction between cyclopropenoid fatty acids and aflatoxin in rats. Fed. Proc., 27, 551

Garner, R.C. (1973) Chemical evidence for the formation of a reactive aflatoxin B_1 metabolite, by hamster liver microsomes. Fed. Europ. Biochem. Soc. Lett., 36, 261-264

Garner, R.C. & Wright, C.M. (1973) Induction of mutations in DNA-repair deficient bacteria by a liver microsomal metabolite of aflatoxin B_1. Brit. J. Cancer, 28, 544-551

Garner, R.C., Miller, E.C. & Miller, J.A. (1972) Liver microsomal metabolism of aflatoxin B_1 to a reactive derivative toxic to *Salmonella typhimurium* TA 1530. Cancer Res., 32, 2058-2066

Goodall, C.M. & Butler, W.H. (1969) Aflatoxin carcinogenesis: inhibition of liver cancer induction in hypophysectomized rats. Int. J. Cancer, 4, 422-429

Gopalan, C., Tulpule, P.G. & Krishnamurthi, D. (1972) Induction of hepatic carcinoma with aflatoxin in the rhesus monkey. Fd Cosmet. Toxicol., 10, 519-521

Grice, H.C., Moodie, C.A. & Smith, D.C. (1973) The carcinogenic potential of aflatoxin or its metabolites in rats from dams fed aflatoxin pre- and post-partum. Cancer Res., 33, 262-268

Halver, J.E. (1969) Aflatoxicosis and trout hepatoma. In: Goldblatt, L.A., ed., Aflatoxin: Scientific Background, Control and Implications, New York, Academic Press, pp. 265-306

Holzapfel, C.W., Steyn, P.S. & Purchase, I.F.H. (1966) Isolation and structure of aflatoxins M_1 and M_2. Tetrahedron Lett., 25, 2799-2803

IARC (1972) IARC Monographs on the Evaluation of Carcinogenic Risk of Chemicals to Man, 1, Lyon, pp. 145-156

Keen, P. & Martin, P. (1971) Is aflatoxin carcinogenic in man? The evidence in Swaziland. Trop. geogr. Med., 23, 44-53

Kraybill, H.F. & Shimkin, M.B. (1964) Carcinogenesis related to foods contaminated by processing and fungal metabolites. Advanc. Cancer Res., 8, 191-248

Krishnamachari, K.A.V.R., Bhat, R.V., Nagarajan, V. & Tilak, T.B.G. (1975) Hepatitis due to aflatoxicosis: an outbreak in Western India. Lancet, i, 1061-1063

Lamb, M.J. & Lilly, L.J. (1971) Induction of recessive lethals in *Drosophila melanogaster* by aflatoxin B_1. Mutation Res., 11, 430-433

Lancaster, M.C., Jenkins, F.P. & Philp, J. McL. (1961) Toxicity associated with certain samples of groundnuts. Nature (Lond.), 192, 1095-1096

Lee, D.J., Wales, J.H. & Sinnhuber, R.O. (1969) Hepatoma and renal tubule adenoma in rats fed aflatoxin and cyclopropenoid fatty acids. J. nat. Cancer Inst., 43, 1037-1044

Legator, M.S. (1969) Biological assay for aflatoxins. In: Goldblatt, L.A., ed., Aflatoxin: Scientific Background, Control and Implications, New York, Academic Press, pp. 107-149

Leonard, A., DeKnudt, G. & Linden, G. (1975) Mutagenicity tests with aflatoxins in the mouse. Mutation Res., 28, 137-139

Lin, J.J., Liu, C. & Svoboda, D.J. (1974) Long-term effects of aflatoxin B_1 and viral hepatitis on marmoset liver. Lab. Invest., 30, 267-278

Madhavan, T.V. & Gopalan, C. (1968) The effect of dietary protein on carcinogenesis of aflatoxin. Arch. Path., 85, 133-137

Maher, V.M. & Summers, W.C. (1970) Mutagenic action of aflatoxin B_1 on transforming DNA and inhibition of DNA template activity *in vitro*. Nature (Lond.), 225, 68-70

Masri, M.S., Lundin, R.E., Page, J.R. & Garcia, V.C. (1967) Crystalline aflatoxin M_1 from urine and milk. Nature (Lond.), 215, 753-755

McCann, J., Spingarn, N.E., Kobori, J. & Ames, B.N. (1975) Detection of carcinogens as mutagens: bacterial tester strains with R factor plasmids. Proc. nat. Acad. Sci. (Wash.), 72, 979-983

McLean, A.E.M. & Marshall, A. (1971) Reduced carcinogenic effects of aflatoxin in rats given phenobarbitone. Brit. J. exp. Path., 52, 322-329

Newberne, P.M. (1965) Carcinogenicity of aflatoxin-contaminated peanut meals. In: Wogan, G.N., ed., Mycotoxins in Foodstuffs, Cambridge, Mass., Massachusetts Institute of Technology Press, pp. 187-208

Newberne, P.M. & Rogers, A.E. (1973) Rat colon carcinomas associated with aflatoxin and marginal vitamin A. J. nat. Cancer Inst., 50, 439-448

Newberne, P.M. & Williams, G. (1969) Inhibition of aflatoxin carcinogenesis by diethylstilboestrol in male rats. Arch. environm. Hlth, 19, 489-498

Newberne, P.M., Harrington, D.H. & Wogan, G.N. (1966) Effects of cirrhosis and other liver insults on induction of liver tumours by aflatoxin in rats. Lab. Invest., 15, 962-969

Nixon, J.E., Sinnhuber, R.O., Lee, D.J., Landers, M.K. & Harr, J.R. (1974) Effect of cyclopropenoid compounds on the carcinogenic activity of diethylnitrosamine and aflatoxin B_1 in rats. J. nat. Cancer Inst., 53, 453-458

Ong, T. (1971) Mutagenic activities of aflatoxin B_1 and G_1 in *Neurospora crassa*. Mol. Gen. Genet., 111, 159-170

Patterson, D.S.P. (1973) Metabolism as a factor in determining the toxic action of the aflatoxins in different animal species. Fd Cosmet. Toxicol., 11, 287-294

Peers, F.G. & Linsell, C.A. (1973) Dietary aflatoxins and liver cancer: a population-based study in Kenya. Brit. J. Cancer, 27, 473-484

Pons, W.A., Jr (1975) Collaborative study of a rapid method for determining aflatoxins in cottonseed products. J. Ass. off. analyt. Chem., 58, 746-753

Purchase, I.F.H., Stubblefield, R.D. & Altenkirk, B.A. (1974) Collaboration study of the determination of aflatoxin M_1 in milk. IUPAC Information Bulletin, Technical Rep. No. 11

Reddy, J.K. & Svoboda, D.J. (1975) Aflatoxin B_1-induced liver tumors in *Tupaia glis* (tree shrews), a nonhuman primate. Fed. Proc., 34, 827

Rogers, A.E. & Newberne, P.M. (1969) Aflatoxin B_1 carcinogenesis in lipotrope-deficient rats. Cancer Res., 29, 1965-1972

Rogers, A.E. & Newberne, P.M. (1971) Nutrition and aflatoxin carcinogenesis. Nature (Lond.), 229, 62-63

San, R.H.C. & Stich, H.F. (1975) DNA repair synthesis of cultured human cells as a rapid bioassay for chemical carcinogens. Int. J. Cancer, 16, 284-291

Sato, S., Matsushima, T., Tanaka, N., Sugimura, T. & Takashima, F. (1973) Hepatic tumors in the guppy (Lebistes reticulatus) induced by aflatoxin B_1, dimethylnitrosamine, and 2-acetylaminofluorene. J. nat. Cancer Inst., 50, 765-778

Schimmer, O. & Werner, R. (1974) Mutagenic effect of aflatoxin B_1 on nuclear and extranuclear DNA in Chlamydomonas reinhardii. Mutation Res., 26, 423-425

Serck-Hanssen, A. (1970) Aflatoxin-induced fatal hepatitis? A report from Uganda. Arch. environm. Hlth, 20, 729-731

Shank, R.C., Bourgeois, C.H., Keschamras, N. & Chandavimol, P. (1971) Aflatoxins in autopsy specimens from Thai children with an acute disease of unknown etiology. Fd Cosmet. Toxicol., 9, 501-507

Shank, R.C., Bhamarapravati, N., Gordon, J.E. & Wogan, G.N. (1972a) Dietary aflatoxins and human liver cancer. IV. Incidence of primary liver cancer in two municipal populations in Thailand. Fd Cosmet. Toxicol. 10, 171-181

Shank, R.C., Gordon, J.E., Wogan, G.N., Nondasuta, A. & Subhamani, B. (1972b) Dietary aflatoxins and human liver cancer. III. Field survey of rural Thai families for ingested aflatoxins. Fd Cosmet. Toxicol., 10, 71-84

Shank, R.C., Wogan, G.N., Gibson, J.E. & Nondasuta, A. (1972c) Dietary aflatoxins and human liver cancer. II. Aflatoxins in market foods and foodstuffs in Thailand and Hong Kong. Fd Cosmet. Toxicol., 10, 61-69

Shannon, G.M. & Shotwell, D.L. (1975) A quantitative method for determination of aflatoxin B_1 in roasted corn. J. Ass. off. analyt. Chem., 58, 743-745

Sinnhuber, R.O. & Wales, J.H. (1974) Aflatoxin B_1 hepatocarcinogenicity in rainbow trout embryos. Fed. Proc., 33, 247

Sinnhuber, R.O., Wales, J.H., Ayres, J.L., Engebrecht, R.H. & Amend, D.L. (1968a) Dietary factors and hepatoma in rainbow trout (Salmo gairdneri). I. Aflatoxins in vegetable protein feedstuffs. J. nat. Cancer Inst., 41, 711-718

Sinnhuber, R.O., Lee, D.J., Wales, J.H. & Ayres, J.L. (1968b) Dietary factors and hepatoma in rainbow trout (*Salmo gairdneri*). II. Co-carcinogenesis by cyclopropenoid fatty acids and the effect of gossypol and altered lipids on aflatoxin-induced liver cancer. J. nat. Cancer Inst., 41, 1293-1301

Sinnhuber, R.O., Lee, D.J., Wales, J.H., Landers, M.K. & Keyl, A.C. (1974) Hepatic carcinogenesis by aflatoxin M_1 in rainbow trout (*Salmo gairdneri*) and its enhancement by cyclopropene fatty acids. J. nat. Cancer Inst., 53, 1285-1288

Stich, H.F. & Laishes, B.A. (1975) The response of xeroderma pigmentosum cells and controls to the activated mycotoxins, aflatoxins and sterigmatocystin. Int. J. Cancer, 16, 266-274

Stoloff, L. (1972) Analytical methods for mycotoxins. Clin. Toxicol., 5, 465-494

Stoloff, L. (1975) Report on mycotoxins. J. Ass. off. analyt. Chem., 58, 213-217

Stubblefield, R.D. & Shannon, G.M. (1974) Aflatoxin M_1 : analysis in dairy products and distribution in dairy foods made from artificially contamined milk. J. Ass. off. analyt. Chem., 57, 847-851

Swenson, D.H., Miller, J.A. & Miller, E.C. (1973) 2,3-Dihydro-2,3-dihydroxy-aflatoxin B_1 : an acid hydrolysis product of an RNA-aflatoxin B_1 adduct formed by hamster and rat liver microsomes *in vitro*. Biochem. biophys. Res. Commun., 53, 1260-1267

Swenson, D.H., Miller, E.C. & Miller, J.A. (1974) Aflatoxin B_1-2,3-oxide: evidence for its formation in rat liver *in vivo* and by human liver microsomes *in vitro*. Biochem. biophys. Res. Commun., 60, 1036-1043

Tilak, T.B.G. (1975) Induction of cholangiocarcinoma following treatment of a rhesus monkey with aflatoxin. Fd Cosmet. Toxicol., 13, 247-249

Van Nieuwenhuize, J.P., Herber, F.M., De Bruin, A., Meyer, P.B. & Duba, W.C. (1973) Aflatoxinen: Epidemiologish onderzoek naar carcinogeniteit bij langdurige 'low level' expositie van een fabriekspopulatie. II. Eigen onderzoek. T. soc. Geneesk., 51, 754-760

Van Rensburg, S.J., Van der Watt, J.J., Purchase, I.F.H., Pereira Coutinho, L. & Markham, R. (1974) Primary liver cancer rate and aflatoxin intake in a high cancer area. S. Afr. med. J., 48, 2508a-2508d

Velasco, J. (1975) Fluorometric measurement of aflatoxin adsorbed on florisil in minicolumns. J. Ass. off. analyt. Chem., 58, 757-763

Vesselinovitch, S.D., Mihailovich, N., Wogan, G.N., Lombard, L.S. & Rao, K.V.N. (1972) Aflatoxin B_1, a hepatocarcinogen in the infant mouse. Cancer Res., 32, 2289-2291

Wales, J.H. & Sinnhuber, R.O. (1972) Hepatomas induced by aflatoxin in the sockeye salmon (*Oncorhynchus nerka*). J. nat. Cancer Inst., 48, 1529-1530

Ward, J.M., Sontag, J.M., Weisburger, E.K. & Brown, C.A. (1975) Effect of lifetime exposure to aflatoxin B_1 in rats. J. nat. Cancer Inst., 55, 107-113

Wieder, R., Wogan, G.N. & Shimkin, M.B. (1968) Pulmonary tumors in strain A mice given injections of aflatoxin B_1. J. nat. Cancer Inst., 40, 1195-1197

Wogan, G.N. (1969a) Naturally occurring carcinogens in foods. Progr. exp. Tumor Res. (Basel), 11, 134-162

Wogan, G.N. (1969b) Metabolism and biochemical effects of aflatoxins. In: Goldblatt, L.A., ed., Aflatoxin: Scientific Background, Control and Implications, New York, Academic Press, pp. 151-186

Wogan, G.N. (1973) Aflatoxin carcinogenesis. Methods Cancer Res., 7, 309-344

Wogan, G.N. & Newberne, P.M. (1967) Dose-response characteristics of aflatoxin B_1 carcinogenesis in the rat. Cancer Res., 27, 2370-2376

Wogan, G.N. & Paglialunga, S. (1974) Carcinogenicity of synthetic aflatoxin M_1 in rats. Fd Cosmet. Toxicol., 12, 381-384

Wogan, G.N., Edwards, G.S. & Newberne, P.M. (1971) Structure-activity relationships in toxicity and carcinogenicity of aflatoxins and analogs. Cancer Res., 31, 1936-1942

Wogan, G.N., Paglialunga, S. & Newberne, P.M. (1974) Carcinogenic effects of low dietary levels of aflatoxin B_1 in rats. Fd Cosmet. Toxicol., 12, 681-685

AZASERINE

1. Chemical and Physical Data

1.1 Synonyms and trade names

Chem. Abstr. Reg. Serial No.: 115-02-6

Chem. Abstr. Name: Serine diazoacetate

L-Azaserine; diazoacetate (ester) L-serine; L-diazoacetate (ester) serine; diazoacetic acid ester with serine; O-diazoacetyl-L-serine

1.2 Chemical formula and molecular weight

$$N_2CH-COO-CH_2-CH(NH_2)-COOH$$

$C_5H_7N_3O_4$ Mol. wt: 173.1

1.3 Chemical and physical properties of the pure substance

(a) Description: Light yellow-green crystals

(b) Melting-point: 146-162°C (decomposition)

(c) Refractive index: $[\alpha]_D^{27.5}$ -0.5° (8.46% in water at pH 5.18)

(d) Spectroscopy data: λ_{max} 250.5 nm (E_1^1 = 1140) (pH 7); λ_{max} 252 nm (E_1^1 = 1230) (after 30 min in 0.1 N sodium hydroxide)

(e) Solubility: Very soluble in water; only slightly soluble in absolute methanol, absolute ethanol and acetone in the cold, but soluble in warm aqueous solutions of these solvents

(f) Stability: Relatively stable in neutral solutions

1.4 Technical products and impurities

No data were available to the Working Group.

2. Production, Use, Occurrence and Analysis

For important background information on this section, see preamble, p. 17.

A review on azaserine has been published (Pittillo & Hunt, 1967).

2.1 Production and use

Azaserine is an antibiotic produced by *Streptomyces fragilis*; its isolation and synthesis were first reported in 1954 (Bartz et al., 1954; Wittle et al., 1954). The synthesis was accomplished by selective diazotization of O-glycyl-L-serine which was prepared by the reaction of N-carboxyglycine anhydride with N-carbobenzoxy-L-serine.

One company in the US produced azaserine in 1955-1965; another started production in about 1970 and at present is believed to be producing less than 50 g per year for use in biochemical research.

Azaserine has been tested as an inhibitor of purine synthesis, and, in conjunction with mercaptopurine, in the treatment of acute childhood leukaemia (American Society of Hospital Pharmacists, 1962).

2.2 Occurrence

Azaserine is produced by *Streptomyces fragilis*, but the extent to which it may occur in nature is unknown.

2.3 Analysis

Microbiological assays have been developed (Pittillo & Hunt, 1967).

3. Biological Data Relevant to the Evaluation of Carcinogenic Risk to Man

3.1 Carcinogenicity and related studies in animals

Intraperitoneal administration

Rat: Two groups of 60 Charles River Wistar rats of both sexes were given weekly or twice weekly i.p. injections of 5 mg/kg bw azaserine in saline for 6 months. Of 23 rats given the i.p. injections twice weekly and autopsied 12 or more months after the initial treatment, 9 had adenocarcinomas of the pancreas and 3 had probable carcinomas. Among 18 rats given weekly i.p. injections and killed 12 or more months after the initial treatment, 5 adenocarcinomas of the pancreas and 1 probable carcinoma were observed. Metastases in the liver occurred in 5 rats. In addition, renal tumours (classified as papillary epithelial tumours, clear-cell tumours and tubular adenomas) occurred in similar numbers of rats from the two groups. No pancreatic or kidney tumours occurred in 17 control rats, injected with saline, which had been autopsied at the time of reporting (Longnecker & Curphey, 1975).

In a preliminary study, doses of 5-25 mg/kg bw were given once or twice weekly in saline for 6 weeks to 6 months. All of 18 Charles River Wistar rats autopsied 4, 6 or 8 months after start of treatment had developed hyperplastic nodules in the pancreas, and acinar-cell adenomas were observed in 3 animals. One of 6 control rats had a hyperplastic nodule in the pancreas (Longnecker & Crawford, 1974).

3.2 Other relevant biological data

Oral LD_{50}'s were reported to be 150 mg/kg bw in mice and 170 mg/kg in rats (Stecher, 1968). Single i.p. LD_{50}'s were 100 mg/kg bw in mice and 147 mg/kg bw in rats. When repeated doses were given by i.p. injection on five successive days the LD_{50} in rats was 25 mg/kg bw (Sternberg & Philips, 1957).

Pancreatic acinar-cell injury has been reported in rats treated with azaserine (Hruban et al., 1965); after treatment of rats with ^{3}H-azaserine the pancreas has been shown to attain high levels of radioactivity (Longnecker & Crawford, 1974). Toxic changes in the kidneys, salivary glands and prostate were observed in dogs given azaserine by i.v. perfusion (Fleischman et al., 1972).

Azaserine inhibits *de novo* purine synthesis (Pittillo & Hunt, 1967).

In Long-Evans rats given i.p. injections of 2.5-10 mg/kg bw azaserine, doses of 5 mg/kg bw on the 8th day of gestation and of 10 mg/kg bw on the 8th or 11th-12th day of gestation destroyed the entire litter. Of the foetuses which survived the lower dosage a high proportion had gross malformations (Thiersch, 1957).

Azaserine of unspecified origin and purity at a concentration range of 0.01-5 µg/ml increased the spontaneous reverse mutation frequency in *Escherichia coli* (strain Sd4-73) by 1000 times after treatment for 2 hours, with negligible cell killing (Iyer & Szybalski, 1958). It was mutagenic in *Escherichia coli* and several *Salmonella* strains (Longnecker & Curphey, 1975; Longnecker *et al.*, 1974) and has been shown to induce recessive lethal mutations in *Drosophila* (Altenburg & Browning, 1964).

3.3 Observations in man

No data were available to the Working Group.

4. Comments on Data Reported and Evaluation[1]

4.1 Animal data

Azaserine is carcinogenic in rats following its intraperitoneal injection, the only species and route tested: it produced adenocarcinomas of the pancreas and tumours of the kidney.

4.2 Human data

No case reports or epidemiological studies were available to the Working Group.

---

[1]See also the section "Animal Data in Relation to the Evaluation of Risk to Man" in the introduction to this volume, p. 15.

5. References

Altenburg, E. & Browning, L.S. (1964) The rate of gonadal mosaicism for lethals in late broods of *Drosophila* as compared with early when induced by X-rays, azaserine and quinacrine mustard. Genetics, 50, 232

American Society of Hospital Pharmacists (1962) Hospital Formulary, Section 10.00, Washington DC

Bartz, Q.R., Elder, C.C., Johannessen, D.W., Haskell, T.H., Ryder, A., Frohardt, R.P. & Fusari, S.A. (1954) Azaserine, a new tumor-inhibitory substance. Isolation and characterization. J. Amer. chem. Soc., 76, 2878-2881

Fleischman, R.W., Baker, J.R., Schaeppi, U., Thompson, G.R., Rosenkrantz, H., Cooney, D.A. & Davis, R.D. (1972) Azaserine-induced pathology in dogs. Toxicol. appl. Pharmacol., 22, 595-606

Hruban, Z., Swift, H. & Slesers, A. (1965) Effect of azaserine on the fine structure of the liver and pancreatic acinar-cells. Cancer Res., 25, 708-723

Iyer, V.N. & Szybalski, W. (1958) The mechanism of chemical mutagenesis. I. Kinetic studies on the action of triethylene melamine (TEM) and azaserine. Proc. nat. Acad. Sci. (Wash.), 44, 446-456

Longnecker, D.S. & Crawford, B.G. (1974) Hyperplastic nodules and adenomas of exocrine pancreas in azaserine-treated rats. J. nat. Cancer Inst., 53, 573-577

Longnecker, D.S. & Curphey, T.J. (1975) Adenocarcinoma of the pancreas in azaserine-treated rats. Cancer Res., 35, 2249-2258

Longnecker, D.S., Curphey, T.J., James, S.T., Daniel, D.S. & Jacobs, N.J. (1974) Trial of a bacterial screening system for rapid detection of mutagens and carcinogens. Cancer Res., 34, 1658-1663

Pittillo, R.F. & Hunt, D.E. (1967) Azaserine and 6-diazo-5-oxo-L-norleucine (DON). In: Gottlieb, D. & Shaw, P.D., eds, Antibiotics, 1, Mechanism of Action, Berlin, Heidelberg, New York, Springer-Verlag, pp. 481-493

Stecher, P.G., ed. (1968) The Merck Index, 8th ed., Rahway, NJ, Merck & Co., p. 114

Sternberg, S.S. & Philips, F.S. (1957) Azaserine: pathological and pharmacological studies. Cancer, 10, 889-901

Thiersch, J.B. (1957) Effects of *O*-diazo-acetyl-L-serine on rat litter. Proc. Soc. exp. Biol. (N.Y.), 94, 27-32

Wittle, E., Westland, R., Nicolaides, E., Dice, J. & Moore, J. (1954) Azaserine synthetic studies. I. J. Amer. chem. Soc., 76, 2884-2887

CANTHARIDIN

1. Chemical and Physical Data

1.1 Synonyms and trade names

Chem. Abstr. Reg. Serial No.: 56-25-7

Chem. Abstr. Name: (3aα,4β,7β,7aα)Hexahydro-3a,7a-dimethyl-4,7-epoxyisobenzofuran-1,3-dione

Cantharides camphor; cantharidine; 2,3-dimethyl-7-oxabicyclo-(2.2.1)heptane-2,3-dicarboxylic anhydride; exo-1,2-*cis*-dimethyl-3,6-epoxyhexahydrophthalic anhydride; hexahydro-3a,7a-dimethyl-4,7-epoxyisobenzofuran-1,3-dione; hexahydro-3α,7α-dimethyl-(3α,4β,7β,7aα)-4,7-epoxy-isobenzofuran-1,3-dione

Cantharone®

1.2 Chemical formula and molecular weight

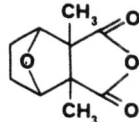

$C_{10}H_{12}O_4$ Mol. wt: 196.2

1.3 Chemical and physical properties of the pure substance

(a) Description: Orthorhombic plates

(b) Melting-point: 218°C

(c) Solubility: Practically insoluble in cold water, slightly soluble in hot water; soluble in oils. One g dissolves in 40 ml acetone, 65 ml chloroform, 560 ml ether or 150 ml ethyl acetate.

(d) Volatility: Sublimes at 12 mm at 100°C

(e) Reactivity: Hydrolysed to cantharinic acid

1.4 Technical products and impurities

Cantharidin is used commercially in the form of the crude product, cantharides, from which it is derived, or in a collodion formulation. It is present to the extent of 0.6-1.0% in each of these forms. In addition to cantharidin, cantharides contains 10-15% fat, the balance being resinous substances, acetic acid and uric acid (Medical Economics Co., 1975; Stecher, 1968).

2. Production, Use, Occurrence and Analysis

For important background information on this section, see preamble, p. 17.

2.1 Production and use

Cantharidin, the active irritant in the crude drug cantharides, is obtained from the dried insects *Cantharis vesicatoria* (Goodman & Gilman, 1970). Cantharidin was synthesized by Ziegler *et al.* (1942) through a long series of reactions, starting with butadiene and dimethyl maleic anhydride.

In human medicine cantharidin is used for the removal of benign epithelial warts (Kastrup, 1972). It is estimated that the total annual sales of cantharidin in the US for this use are less than 10 kg. Cantharidin in the form of cantharides was formerly used as a counter-irritant and vesicant, but undesirable side effects were encountered (Stecher, 1968).

Cantharidin in the form of cantharides was used in veterinary medicine as a vesicant for the treatment of small umbilical hernias and as a counter-irritant in certain diseases of bones, joints, ligaments and tendons (Stecher, 1968).

2.2 Occurrence

Cantharides occurs at a concentration of less than 1% in Spanish flies, the common blister beetle (*Cantharis vesicatoria*), and in telini flies (*Myleabris cichorii*).

2.3 Analysis

Cantharidin has been determined in plasters containing crude preparations of cantharides by gas chromatography (Rollet *et al.*, 1973).

3. Biological Data Relevant to the Evaluation of Carcinogenic Risk to Man

3.1 Carcinogenicity and related studies in animals

Skin application

Mouse: A group of Hr/hr hairless mice of both sexes, 8-10 weeks old, received twice weekly skin applications to the dorsal skin of a solution of 0.016% cantharidin in benzene for lifespan (mean survival, 18.8 months). Thirty-two mice survived the appearance of the first tumour, and 10 mice (31%) developed skin tumours, including two squamous-cell carcinomas. Internal tumours were present in 17 animals (51.6%), and 9 mice (28%) had reticulum-cell tumours or malignant lymphomas. In the control group, painted with benzene alone, only 7.3% of an unspecified number of mice had developed skin papillomas after 10-14 months (Laerum & Iversen, 1972).

In parallel experiments in which cantharidin was investigated as a promoter of skin carcinogenesis, 0.1 ml of a 0.1% solution of methyl cholanthrene (MCA) in benzene was applied to the skin 2 weeks before the start of cantharidin applications. A higher incidence of skin-tumour-bearing mice (59.5%) and an increased incidence of reticulum-cell tumours or malignant lymphomas (56.1%) were observed. The incidence of skin-tumour-bearing mice did not differ from that in tests in which benzene was applied following initiation by MCA (55.9%), but only half as many (25%) reticulum-cell tumours or malignant lymphomas were found in the benzene-treated compared to the cantharidin-treated animals following initiation by MCA. Skin carcinomas occurred in only 2.9% of animals treated with MCA and benzene, whereas cantharidin painting after initiation by MCA produced squamous carcinomas in 6.3% of animals. During the initiation-promotion experiments, cantharidin painting reduced the number of papilloma-bearing animals for the first 18 months but had increased it rapidly by 22 months (Laerum & Iversen, 1972).

A group of 20 male 'S' mice, 7-9 weeks old, received 9 weekly applications of 0.3 ml of a 0.01% solution of cantharidin in acetone, followed by 6 weekly applications of a 0.02% solution in acetone (total dose, 630 µg/animal). Croton-oil treatment was begun 17 days after the start of cantharidin applications and consisted of 18 weekly applications of 0.3 ml of a 0.5%

solution in acetone. At the end of the croton-oil treatment, 17 mice survived, and 4 had developed a total of 6 papillomas. In the croton-oil control group, 1/20 survivors had 3 skin tumours. The difference was not statistically significant (Roe & Salaman, 1955).

In an experiment on female 'skin-tumour-susceptible' mice, 6-8 weeks old, Hennings & Boutwell (1970) studied the tumour-promoting ability of cantharidin. Dimethylbenzanthracene (DMBA), cantharidin and croton oil were prepared in acetone. In one experiment the initiating dose of DMBA was 25 µg, and 50 µg cantharidin were applied 1-5 times weekly to different groups of 30 animals. The promotion treatment was started one week after initiation, and experiments were continued for 32 weeks. In the experiment in which the frequency of painting with cantharidin was greatest (5 times/week), no papillomas were observed, but only 1 mouse survived 32 weeks. When painting was carried out three times weekly, 4 mice survived and developed 5 skin papillomas; however, when 1-2 weekly paintings were given, 22 and 20 mice survived, and 8 and 11 mice developed a total of 10 and 20 skin papillomas. The promoting activity of cantharidin was compared to that of weekly paintings with 0.2 ml of a 0.5% solution of croton oil in acetone, following initiation by 18 µg DMBA; this procedure produced a total of 398 papillomas in all 30 animals after only 12 weeks of treatment. In a control study, in which no initiator was used, a dose of 50 µg cantharidin was applied once weekly for 1-12 weeks and thrice weekly from week 13 to the end of the experiment. Among 20 survivors, 1 mouse had a papilloma (Hennings & Boutwell, 1970).

3.2 Other relevant biological data

The rate of incorporation of tritiated thymidine into mouse skin DNA during a 30-minute period was studied in animals treated with 0.2 ml acetone containing 20, 50, 100, or 200 µg cantharidin. Mice were killed at intervals of 1, 3, 5 and 7 days. With lower levels of cantharidin treatment (20, 50 and 100 µg) the specific activity of DNA increased to 200 and 300% that of controls during the first day but returned to normal by the third day. With the highest dose (200 µg), a decline in thymidine incorporation occurred during the first day followed by a steady increase to a maximum of 400% on the third day and reaching normal levels only after 7 days.

Treatment with cantharidin also stimulated the synthesis of rapidly-labelled RNA measured 2 hours after treatment; this seemed to be correlated with a slight stimulation of transfer-RNA synthesis and a greater stimulation of ribosomal-RNA synthesis (Hennings & Boutwell, 1970).

A carcinogenic tar (unspecified) was applied by painting with a camel-hair brush on small area of skin in the intra-scapular region of 50 mice, and cantharidin was applied at a concentration of 0.25% in acetone; 42 animals survived after 15 weeks, compared to 45 in a control group painted with tar alone, and 3 of the animals had papillomas, compared with 18 controls (Berenblum, 1935).

Six mice were painted on days 0 and 2 on the right flank with 0.03 ml of a 0.075% solution of cantharidin in acetone. Both flanks of the mice were then painted with 0.02 ml of a 0.3% solution of benzo[a]pyrene in acetone on days 4, 6 and 8. Finally, both sides were painted twice a week for 20 weeks with croton oil in acetone. On the side that had not been treated with cantharidin, fifteen tumours developed, compared to none on the cantharidin side. The author suggested that cantharidin inhibits the induction of tumours produced by short exposures to benzo[a]pyrene (Mottram, 1944).

3.3 Observations in man

No data were available to the Working Group.

4. Comments on Data Reported and Evaluation

4.1 Animal data

Cantharidin was tested only by skin application in mice; it produced an increased incidence of skin papillomas and a low incidence of skin carcinomas.

4.2 Human data

No case reports or epidemiological studies were available to the Working Group.

5. References

Berenblum, I. (1935) Experimental inhibition of tumour induction by mustard gas and other compounds. J. Path. Bact., 40, 549-558

Goodman, L.S. & Gilman, A., eds (1970) The Pharmacological Basis of Therapeutics, 4th ed., London, Toronto, MacMillan, p. 994

Hennings, H. & Boutwell, R.K. (1970) Studies on the mechanism of skin tumor promotion. Cancer Res., 30, 312-320

Kastrup, E.K., ed. (1972) Facts and Comparisons, St. Louis, Missouri, p. 494b

Laerum, O.D. & Iversen, O.H. (1972) Reticuloses and epidermal tumors in hairless mice after topical skin applications of cantharidin and asiaticoside. Cancer Res., 32, 1463-1469

Medical Economics Co. (1975) Physicians Desk Reference, Oradell, NJ, p. 826

Mottram, J.C. (1944) A sensitising factor in experimental blastogenesis. J. Path. Bact., 56, 391-402

Roe, F.J.C. & Salaman, M.H. (1955) Further studies on incomplete carcinogenesis: triethylene melamine (TEM), 1,2-benzanthracene and β-propiolactone, as initiators of skin tumour formation in the mouse. Brit. J. Cancer, 9, 177-203

Rollet, M., Moisson, M. & Moiroux, G. (1973) Contribution au dosage de la cantharidine dans les milieux complexes, type emplâtre de cantharide mitagé. Utilisation de la chromatographie gazeuse. J. Pharm. Belg., 28, 359-372

Stecher, P.G., ed. (1968) The Merck Index, 8th ed., Rahway, NJ, Merck & Co., p. 201

Ziegler, K., Schenck, G., Krockow, E.W., Siebert, A., Wenz, A. & Weber, H. (1942) Synthesis of cantharidin. Justus liebigs Ann. Chem., 551, 1-79

CHLORAMPHENICOL

1. Chemical and Physical Data

1.1 Synonyms and trade names

Chem. Abstr. Reg. Serial No.: 56-75-7

Chem. Abstr. Name: [R-(R*,R*)]-2,2-Dichloro-*N*-[2-hydroxy-1-(hydroxymethyl)-2-(4-nitrophenyl)ethyl]acetamide

D-(−)-Threo-2-dichloroacetamido-1-*p*-nitrophenyl-1,3-propanediol; D-threo-*N*-dichloroacetyl-1-*p*-nitrophenyl-2-amino-1,3-propanediol; D-threo-(−)-2,2-dichloro-*N*-[β-hydroxy-α-(hydroxymethyl)-*p*-nitrophenethyl]acetamide; D-threo-*N*-(1,1'-dihydroxy-1-*p*-nitrophenylisopropyl)-dichloroacetamide; D-(−)-threo-*p*-nitrophenyl-1-dichloroacetamido-2-propanediol-(1,3)

Alficetyn; Ambofen; Amphicol; Amseclor; Aquamycetin; Austracol; Biocetin; Biophenicol; CAF; CAM; CAP; Catilan; Chemicetina; Chlomin; Chlomycol; Chloramex; Chloramsaar; Chlorasol; Chlora-Tabs; Chloricol; Chloroamphenicol; Chlorocaps; Chlorocid; Chlorocol; Chloromycetin; Chloronitrin; Chloroptic; Chloro-25 Vetag; Cidocetine; Ciplamycetin; Cloramficin; Cloramicol; Cloramidina; Clorocyn; Cloromisan; Clorosintex; Comycetin; Cylphenicol; Desphen; Detreomycine; Dextromycetin; Doctamicina; Embacetin; Emetren; Enicol; Enteromycetin; Erbaplast; Ertilen; Farmicetina; Fenicol; Globenicol; Glorous; Halomycetin; Hortfenicol; Intramycetin; Isicetin; Ismicetina; Isophénicol; Isopto Fenicol; Juvamycetin; Kamaver; Kemicetina; Kémicétine; Klorita; Leukomycin; Levomicetina; Levomycetin; Loromisan; Médiamycétine; Micloretin; Micochlorine; Micoclorina; Microcetina; Mycinol; Novochlorocap; Novomycetin; Novophenicol; Oftalent; Oleomycetin; Opelor; Ophtochlor; Otachron; Otophen; Pantovernil; Paraxin; Pentamycetin; Quemicetina; Rivomycin; Romphenil; Septicol; Sificetina; Sintomicetina; Sintomycétine; Stanomycetin; Synthomycetine; Synthomycine; Tevcocin; Tifomycin; Tifomycine; Treomicetina; Unimycetin; Veticol

1.2 Chemical formula and molecular weight

$$O_2N-\underset{}{\bigcirc}-\underset{NH-CO-CHCl_2}{\overset{OH}{CH}-CH-CH_2-OH}$$

$C_{11}H_{12}Cl_2N_2O_5$ Mol. wt: 323.1

1.3 Chemical and physical properties of the pure substance

(a) Description: White to greyish-white needles with bitter taste

(b) Melting-point: 150.5-151.5°C (sublimes in high vacuum)

(c) Spectroscopy data: λ_{max} 278 nm (E_1^1 = 298) (in water)

(d) Optical rotation: $[\alpha]_D^{27}$ +18.6° (4.86% in ethanol)

(e) Identity test: Methods of identification are given in the British Pharmacopoeia (British Pharmacopoeia Commission, 1973).

(f) Solubility: 1 g dissolves in 400 ml water or 6 ml propylene glycol at 25°C; very soluble in methanol, ethanol, butanol, ethyl acetate, acetone; fairly soluble in ether

(g) Stability: Aqueous solutions are stable if protected from light.

(h) Reactivity: The nitro group is readily converted to the amine by reduction.

1.4 Technical products and impurities

Chloramphenicol is listed in the British Pharmacopoeia (British Pharmacopoeia Commission, 1973) and is often formulated as the cinnamate, palmitate or sodium succinate salt. Data on physical properties of these salts are given by Cole (1969). Preparations are available as capsules (250 mg), ear-drops (5% solution in propylene glycol), eye-drops (0.5% solution) or eye-ointment (1% chloramphenicol). Chloramphenicol palmitate or cinnamate are water-insoluble powders formulated to overcome the bitter taste of chloramphenicol; on hydrolysis they release the free drug: 1.7 g of the palmitate are equivalent to 1.0 g chloramphenicol.

USP grade chloramphenicol is available in the United States; chloramphenicol capsules containing 90-120% of the labelled amount of active ingredient are available in doses of 50, 100 and 250 mg. Chloramphenicol ointment (1%) for ophthalmic use contains 90-130% of the labelled amount of active ingredient; an ophthalmic solution (0.5%) is available as a sterile, dry mixture of chloramphenicol and suitable buffers and contains 90-130% of the labelled amount of chloramphenicol (US Pharmacopeial Convention, Inc., 1975). USP grade chloramphenicol palmitate is sold as a suspension for oral administration, and chloramphenicol sodium succinate is prepared for injection (American Society of Hospital Pharmacists, 1971).

Chloramphenicol is available in Japan in the form of tablets, capsules, syrups and for injection. Chloramphenicol succinate is also made up for injection, and the stearoyl glycolate is sold as a syrup (Fukai, 1974).

In Europe, chloramphenicol is available in forms for ophthalmic and otic use, for injection, in capsules for oral use, in suppositories, as a syrup, and in combination with vitamins (Bundesverband der Pharmazeutischen Industrie, 1969; Council of Europe, 1971; Dictionnaire Vidal, 1975).

2. Production, Use, Occurrence and Analysis

For important background information on this section, see preamble, p. 17.

2.1 Production and use

Chloramphenicol is an antibiotic produced by *Streptomyces venezuelae*, an organism first isolated by Burkholder in 1947 from a soil sample collected in Venezuela (Ehrlich *et al.*, 1947). The crystalline antibiotic substance was isolated by Bartz in 1948 (Goodman & Gilman, 1970), and in 1949 its structural determination (Rebstock *et al.*, 1949) and chemical synthesis (Controulis *et al.*, 1949) were reported.

The method believed to be used for commercial production involves the following steps: condensation of *para*-nitrobenzoyl chloride with ethyl malonate to give *para*-nitroacetophenone; bromination in acetic acid to form *para*-nitro-α-bromoacetophenone; reaction of this with hexamethylene tetramine, followed by hydrolysis to give *para*-nitro-α-aminoacetophenone; acetylation of the amine group, followed by condensation with formaldehyde to give an hydroxymethyl group *alpha* to the amine group; treatment with aluminium isopropylate to reduce the keto group to a secondary alcohol; and, after deacetylation, condensation of the amine group with methyl dichloroacetate to give chloramphenicol (Anon., 1969).

Commercial production of chloramphenicol was first reported to the US Tariff Commission in 1948 (US Tariff Commission, 1949). In 1973 only two US companies reported production, and imports through the principle US customs districts in that year were reported to have been 1.6 thousand kg (US Tariff Commission, 1974). Total US sales of chloramphenicol in its various forms for use in human medicine are estimated to be in the order of 6000 kg annually, mostly in capsule form for oral ingestion.

In 1971 a plant using a fermentation process started production in Japan. The process resulted from the discovery and isolation of a new strain of microbe and is claimed to be superior to the synthetic process since separation of stereoisomers is not required (Anon., 1972). There are currently five producers of chloramphenicol in Japan (Anon., 1974). Production between 1969 and 1972 was in the range of 27-75 thousand kg per year and in 1973 amounted to 42 thousand kg (Ministry of Health and Welfare, 1973).

There are reported to be producers of chloramphenicol in the Federal Republic of Germany, France, Italy, Spain, Switzerland and the United Kingdom (Chemical Information Services Ltd, 1975).

The commercial production of chloramphenicol in 1948 made available for the first time a broad-spectrum antibiotic effective against both Gram-positive and Gram-negative bacteria. Rickettsiae and organisms of the psittacosis-lymphogranuloma group are also sensitive to chloramphenicol; most fungi and yeasts are resistant.

Chloramphenicol is still mainly used for the treatment of *Salmonella* infections, as well as for many other infectious diseases (Dunne *et al.*, 1973). The dose of chloramphenicol given to adults with typhoid fever is 2 g initially, followed by 1 g every six hours for 4 weeks, while the doses used for other infections are usually lower. For rickettsial diseases, the first dose of chloramphenicol is 50 mg/kg bw, followed by 1 g every 8 hours or 0.5 g orally every 4 hours.

Chloramphenicol has also been used in veterinary medicine, functioning as a broad-spectrum antibiotic treatment against many bacteria and certain viruses and rickettsiae (Stecher, 1968). It should not be used for any purpose that might result in the presence of residues in food for human consumption (FAO/WHO, 1969).

2.2 Occurrence

Although chloramphenicol is produced by *Streptomyces venezuelae* and has recently been isolated from a microbe in Japan, there are no data on its occurrence in nature.

In some countries food regulations require withdrawal periods in animals so as to avoid antibiotic residues in the final product. No figures on levels of chloramphenicol found in foods were available to the Working Group.

2.3 Analysis

Colorimetric methods for the determination of chloramphenicol have been described (Döll, 1955; Glazko *et al.*, 1949a; Masterson, 1968). A microbiological method is given in The US Pharmacopeia (US Pharmacopeial Convention, Inc., 1975); an almost similar one is outlined by Banerjee *et al.* (1973). An ultra-violet absorption method for analysis of chloramphenicol preparations was described by Summa (1965), who also compared microbiological, polarographic and spectrophotometric methods. Chloramphenicol may also be determined by gas chromatography of its trimethylsilyl derivative (Janssen & Vanderhaeghe, 1973; Margosis, 1970). The use of combined gas chromatography-mass spectrometry for determination of chloramphenicol, thiamphenicol and their metabolites in urine is described by Nakagawa *et al.* (1975) (limit of detection, 0.05 mg/l).

3. Biological Data Relevant to the Evaluation of Carcinogenic Risk to Man

3.1 Carcinogenicity and related studies in animals

No adequate data were available to the Working Group.

3.2 Other relevant biological data

The LD_{50}'s for single doses of chloramphenicol in albino mice were about 200 mg/kg bw by i.v. injection and 1320 mg/kg bw by i.p. injection. The i.v. LD_{50} in rats was 170 mg/kg bw. Maximum tolerated doses of chloramphenicol given daily to mice for 2-4 weeks were 385-425 mg/kg bw/day in the diet or by cannula, 100 mg/kg bw/day by s.c. injection and 250 mg/kg bw/day by i.p. injection; in guinea-pigs, 250 mg/kg bw/day in the diet; and in dogs, more than 200 mg/kg bw/day in the form of capsules given orally for 3-5 weeks. Lethal or near-lethal amounts of chloramphenicol given orally or parenterally produced respiratory depression or failure accompanied by a fall in blood pressure and anoxia (Gruhzit *et al.*, 1949).

Three groups of 10 three-month-old Swiss mice were given daily i.p. injections of 20, 40 or 100 mg/kg bw chloramphenicol for 3 months. During the second month, groups given 40 and 100 mg/kg bw developed splenomegaly, hepatomegaly, adenopathy and hypertrophy of the thymus. These pathological alterations were not found in animals receiving the lowest dose until after the third month (German & Loc, 1962).

Metabolites identified in the urine of rats and dogs are unchanged chloramphenicol, a glucuronide conjugate of the terminal OH group and a hydrolysis product (Glazko *et al.*, 1950). The major route of metabolism in the rat is *via* biliary excretion, mainly as the glucuronide; gut bacteria can hydrolyse this metabolite, so that free chloramphenicol can be absorbed from the caecum and large intestine (Glazko *et al.*, 1952). After chloramphenicol administration to rats (100 mg/kg bw by s.c. administration in propylene glycol) highest tissue concentrations of the nitro compounds were found in the kidney and liver between 1 and 2 hours after administration. In the guinea-pig, the liver and kidneys contained low amounts of nitro derivatives and high concentrations of aryl amines, due to the capacity of this species to reduce nitro groups in the liver (Glazko *et al.*, 1949b).

Chloramphenicol exerts its antibiotic effects by inhibiting bacterial protein biosynthesis by binding specifically to bacterial ribosomes to prevent peptide chain extension. At low concentrations it affects only prokaryotic synthesis and not that of eukaryotes, although mitochondrial protein synthesis in eukaryotic cells is inhibited (Hahn, 1967).

Inhibition of carcinogenicity by chloramphenicol has been shown for a number of liver carcinogens, including N-2-fluorenyl-diacetamide (Oster et al., 1971; Puron & Firminger, 1965), 4-dimethylaminoazobenzene (Lacassagne & Hurst, 1967), nitrosodiethylamine (Alonso & Herranz, 1970) and 3'-methyl-4-dimethylaminoazobenzene (Blunk, 1971).

Chloramphenicol failed to induce any embryotoxic or teratogenic effects in the offspring when given by stomach tube to rats on the third and sixth day of pregnancy. On the 9th-11th days of gestation the same dose caused malformations which included hydrocephaly and cleft palate (Dyban & Chebotar, 1971).

No preferential growth inhibition was found in the pol-A$^-$ system of *Escherichia coli* p3478 with 30 µg chloramphenicol per plate (Slater et al., 1971). A preparation of unspecified origin and purity (3 mg/ml) induced petite mutants (mitochondrially inherited respiratory deficiency) in several yeast strains (Williamson et al., 1971).

Chloramphenicol injected i.p. into male ICR/Ha Swiss mice at doses of 333 and 666 mg/kg bw caused no increase in early foetal deaths or pre-implantation losses (Epstein et al., 1972). A preparation of unspecified origin and purity injected i.p. into hybrid (101 x C3H)F$_1$ male mice at a concentration of 1.5 mg/kg bw produced no evidence of induction of dominant lethal mutations (Ehling, 1971). No significant increase in the number of chromosomal aberrations was induced by chloramphenicol in the rat *in vivo* in the bone-marrow cytogenetic test or in cultures of human peripheral lymphocytes (Jensen, 1972).

The primary toxic effect associated with chloramphenicol therapy is bone-marrow damage. Among 487 patients with aplastic or hypoplastic anaemia or generalized cytopaenia, a history of drug exposure was obtained for 209 people, 26 of whom had taken chloramphenicol alone and 66 of whom had taken it in conjunction with other drugs (Welch et al., 1954). The incidences of blood disorders after chloramphenicol therapy in 1958 were estimated to be one in 156,000 and in 1959 one in 227,000 (Leikin et al., 1961); the incidence was higher in females (1.6:1, females:males) (Yunis & Bloomberg, 1964). More recent data suggest that the risk is considerably greater: in the order of one in 40,800 to one in 24,500 (Wallerstein et al., 1969).

Chloramphenicol-induced leucopenia, thrombocytopenia and aplasia of the marrow with fatal generalized cytopenia do not appear to be related to dose. Nausea, vomiting, unpleasant taste and diarrhoea are also associated with chloramphenicol therapy. Fatal toxicity may occur in newborn infants after drug treatment, due to failure to glucuronidate the compound, with a consequent build-up of high blood levels and failure to excrete the unconjugated drug.

In man, about 90% of a single oral dose of 1.5 g chloramphenicol is recovered as inactive nitro derivatives in the urine within 24 hours, only about 10% of the drug being excreted as unchanged chloramphenicol (Glazko et al., 1949b). The bulk of the excreted drug is in the form of the glucuronide. In a study of absorption characteristics in man receiving an oral dose of 500 mg, maximum blood levels (9 µg/ml) were found between 0.5 and 4 hours (Glazko et al., 1968). The plasma half-life for man given a 3 g oral dose was found to be in the order of 6 hours (Glazko et al., 1949b).

A metabolite not found in adults, D(-)-threo-2-hydroxyacetamido-1-p-nitrophenyl-1,3-propanediol, was excreted in serum and urine (Weiss et al., 1960).

3.3 Observations in man

Case reports

A large number of cases of bone-marrow depression and aplastic anaemia have been reported in subjects given chloramphenicol (Leikin et al., 1961; Pisciotta, 1971; Wallerstein et al., 1969; Welch et al., 1954; Yunis & Bloomberg, 1964). In 1955, Lebon & Messerschmitt (1955) reported the case of a 5-year old boy who died of acute myeloblastic leukaemia following a one-year history of aplastic anaemia after administration of chloramphenicol. In 1957, Mukherji (1957) reported that a man aged 63 who received 12 g chloramphenicol developed marrow depression 4 months later, which was followed after 3 months by acute myeloblastic leukaemia. A similar case was reported by Cohen & Greger (1967) of a woman aged 34 who received 40 g chloramphenicol over a 3-month period; she developed generalized cytopenia a year later and acute myeloblastic leukaemia after 7 years. Three further cases were described by Brauer & Dameshek (1967) in 3 women (aged 38, 57 and 61) given doses of chloramphenicol ranging from 15 to 175 g over periods of 6 weeks to 8 years, who developed hypoplastic anaemia after an interval ranging from a few weeks to 8 years after the initial administration; acute myeloblastic leukaemia followed in two cases and acute granulocytic leukaemia in one, after a further interval ranging from 8 months to 8 years.

In a follow-up study of 126 patients with bone-marrow depression following (after an interval of 3 weeks to 8 months) chloramphenicol use, Fraumeni (1967) identified 3 cases of leukaemia (1 acute myeloid in a female of 67, 1 chronic myeloid in a male of 57 and 1 acute lymphatic in a 2-year old girl) occurring between 5 months and $3\frac{1}{2}$ years after first use of the drug. The estimated dose of the drug ranged between 5 and 14 g, given over a period of 3 days to 8 months. In the same paper 5 new cases of myeloid leukaemia (2 acute, 2 acute stem-cell and 1 chronic), not included in the follow-up study, were reported to have occurred after bone-marrow depression subsequent (at intervals ranging from 1 week to several years) to chloramphenicol use. Four were in women, aged 17-60 years, and occurred between 1 month to 15 years after initial treatment with chloramphenicol at total doses ranging from 7-200 g; 1 was in a 14-year old child and occurred 1 month after initial treatment with 10 g.

Three children aged $4\frac{1}{2}$ - $9\frac{1}{2}$ developed acute leukaemia (1 lymphatic, 2 stem-cell) 8 months to 4 years after treatment with chloramphenicol (alone or with other drugs) at total doses of 18-230 g over periods ranging from 20 days to 3 years (Gadner et al., 1973). A further case of acute myeloblastic leukaemia was observed in a 6-year old girl 6 months after receiving 5 g chloramphenicol (Awwaad et al. 1975).

4. Comments on Data Reported and Evaluation

4.1 Animal data

No adequate tests of the carcinogenicity of chloramphenicol were available to the Working Group.

4.2 Human data

The available case reports suggest that aplastic anaemia due to chloramphenicol use is associated with subsequent development of leukaemia.

5. References

Alonso, A. & Herranz, G. (1970) Der Einfluss von Chloramphenicol auf die Leber-Cancerisierung durch Diäthylnitrosamin. *Naturwissenschaften*, 57, 249

American Society of Hospital Pharmacists (1971) *Hospital Formulary*, Section 8:1208, Washington DC

Anon. (1969) Leading world manufacturers of chloramphenicol. *Informations Chimie*, March/April, pp. 47-52

Anon. (1972) New manufacturing process for chloramphenicol. *Chemical Economy and Engineering Review*, 4, 51

Anon. (1974) *Essentials for Pharmaceuticals, 1971*, Tokyo, Yakugyo News Co., p. 1085

Awwaad, S., Khalifa, A.S. & Kamel, K. (1975) Vacuolization of leukocytes and bone marrow aplasia due to chloramphenicol toxicity. *Clin. Ped.*, 14, 499-506

Banerjee, S., Chakrabarti, K. & Haldar, A.K. (1973) Determination of chloramphenicol palmitate in pharmaceutical suspensions. *J. pharm. Sci.*, 62, 1841-1844

Blunk, J.M. (1971) Inhibition by chloramphenicol of aminoazo dye carcinogenesis in rat liver: morphological studies. *Pathology*, 3, 99-106

Brauer, M.J. & Dameshek, W. (1967) Hypoblastic anaemia and myeloblastic leukaemia following chloramphenicol therapy. *New Engl. J. Med.*, 277, 1003-1005

British Pharmacopeia Commission (1973) *British Pharmacopoeia*, London, HMSO, pp. 94-95

Bundesverband der pharmazeutischen Industrie (1969) *Rote Liste*, Frankfurt, pp. 231-232

Chemical Information Services, Ltd (1975) *Directory of Western European Chemical Producers, 1975/1976*, Oceanside, NY

Cohen, T. & Greger, W.P. (1967) Acute myeloid leukaemia following seven years of aplastic anaemia induced by chloramphenicol. *Amer. J. Med.*, 43, 762-770

Cole, E.G.C., ed. (1969) *Isolation and Identification of Drugs*, Vol. 1, London, The Pharmaceutical Press, p. 246

Controulis, J., Rebstock, M.C. & Crooks, H.M., Jr (1949) Chloramphenicol (chloromycetin). V. Synthesis. *J. Amer. chem. Soc.*, 71, 2463-2468

Council of Europe (1971) European Pharmacopoeia, European Treaty Series No. 50, Vol. 2, Paris, Maisonneuve, p. 180

Dictionnaire Vidal (1975) 51st ed., Paris, Office de Vulgarisation Pharmaceutique, p. 511

Döll, W. (1955) Eine einfache kolorimetrische Bestimmungsmethode für chloromycetin (Chloramphenicol, Leukomycin) in wässriger Lösung. Arzneimittel-Forsch., 5, 97-99

Dunne, M., Herxheimer, A., Newman, M. & Ridley, H. (1971) Indications and warnings about chloramphenicol. Lancet, ii, 781-783

Dyban, A.P. & Chebotar, N.A. (1971) Can cleft palate be induced by chloramphenicol (levomycetin) at early stages of embryogenesis in the rat? Arkh. Anat. Gistol. Embriol., 60, 25-29

Ehling, U.H. (1971) Comparison of radiation- and chemically-induced dominant lethal mutations in male mice. Mutation Res., 11, 35-44

Ehrlich, J., Bartz, Q.R., Smith, R.M., Joslyn, D.A. & Burkholder, P.R. (1947) Chloromycetin, a new antibiotic from a soil actinomycete. Science, 106, 417

Epstein, S.S., Arnold, E., Andrea, J., Bass, W. & Bishop, Y. (1972) Detection of chemical mutagens by the dominant lethal assay in the mouse. Toxicol. appl. Pharmacol., 23, 288-325

FAO/WHO (1969) Specifications for the identity and purity of food additives and their toxicological evaluation : some antibiotics. Wld Hlth Org. techn. rep. Ser., No. 430

Fraumeni, J.F. (1967) Bone marrow depression induced by chloramphenicol or phenylbutazone. J. Amer. med. Ass., 201, 150-156

Fukai, S. (1974) Today's new medicinals, Tokyo, Yakuji Daily News, January 20, p. 654

Gadner, H., Gethmann, U., Jessenberger, K. & Riehm, H. (1973) Akute Leukämie nach Chloramphenicol Exposition? Ein kasuistischen Beitrag mit Literaturübersicht. Mschr. Kinderheilk., 121, 590-594

German, A. & Loc, T.B. (1962) Induction d'une tumeur transplantable chez des souris de lignée Swiss par injections répetées de chloramphenicol. Ann. pharm. franç., 20, 116-120

Glazko, A.J., Wolf, L.M. & Dill, W.A. (1949a) Biochemical studies on chloramphenicol (chloromycetin). I. Colorimetric methods for the determination of chloramphenicol and related nitro compounds. Arch. Biochem., 23, 411-418

Glazko, A.J., Wolf, L.M., Dill, W.A. & Bratton, A.C. (1949b) Biochemical studies on chloramphenicol (chloromycetin). II. Tissue distribution and excretion studies. J. Pharmacol. exp. Ther., 96, 445-449

Glazko, A.J., Dill, W.A. & Rebstock, M.C. (1950) Biochemical studies on chloramphenicol (chloromycetin). III. Isolation and identification of metabolic products in urine. J. biol. Chem., 183, 679-691

Glazko, A.J., Dill, W.A. & Wolf, L.M. (1952) Observations on the metabolic disposition of chloramphenicol (chloromycetin) in the rat. J. Pharmacol. exp. Ther., 104, 452-458

Glazko, A.J., Kinbel, A.W., Alegnani, W.C. & Holmes, E.L. (1968) An evaluation of the absorption characteristics of different chloramphenicol preparations in normal human subjects. Clin. Pharmacol. Ther., 9, 472-483

Goodman, L.S. & Gilman, A., eds (1970) The Pharmacological Basis of Therapeutics, 4th ed., London, Toronto, MacMillan, pp. 1269-1274

Gruhzit, O.M., Fisken, R.A., Reutner, T.F. & Martino, E. (1949) Chloramphenicol (chloromycetin), an antibiotic. Pharmacological and pathological studies in animals. J. clin. Invest., 28, 943-952

Hahn, F.E. (1967) Chloramphenicol. In: Gottlieb, D. & Shaw, P.W., eds, Antibiotics, Vol. 1, Mechanism of Action, Berlin, Springer-Verlag, pp. 308-330

Janssen, G. & Vanderhaeghe, H. (1973) Preparation of trimethylsilyl derivatives of chloramphenicol for gas-liquid chromatography. J. Chromat., 82, 297-306

Jensen, M.K. (1972) Phenylbutazone, chloramphenicol and mammalian chromosomes. Humangenetik, 12, 61-64

Lacassagne, A. & Hurst, L. (1967) Action retardatrice du chloramphénicol sur le processus de cancérisation du foie du rat par le p-diméthylaminoazobenzène (DAB). Bull. Cancer, 54, 405-408

Lebon, J. & Messerschmitt, J. (1955) Myélose, aplastique d'origine médicamenteuse, myéloblastose aigue terminal, reflexions pathogeniques. Le Sang, 26, 799-804

Leikin, S.L., Welch, H. & Guin, G.H. (1961) Aplastic anaemia due to chloramphenicol. Clin. Proc. Child. Hosp. (Wash.)., 17, 171-181

Margosis, M. (1970) Analysis of antibiotics by gas chromatography. II. Chloramphenicol. J. Chromat., 47, 341-347

Masterson, D.S., Jr (1968) Colorimetric assay for chloramphenicol using 1-naphthol. J. pharm. Sci., 57, 305-308

Ministry of Health and Welfare (1973) *Annual Statistical Report of Production in the Pharmaceutical Industry*, Tokyo, Medical Department, p. 46

Mukherji, P.S. (1957) Acute myeloblastic leukaemia following chloramphenicol treatment. *Brit. med. J.*, ii, 1286-1287

Nagakawa, T., Masada, M. & Uno, T. (1975) Gas chromatographic determination and gas chromatographic-mass spectrometric analysis of chloramphenicol, thiamphenicol and their metabolites. *J. Chromat.*, 111, 355-364

Oster, W.F., Firminger, H.I. & Morrison, D.M. (1971) Inhibition of N-fluorenyldiacetamide-induced hepatic carcinogenesis in rats by chloramphenicol: a dose-related phenomenon with reduced protein binding of carcinogens. *Yale J. Biol. Med.*, 43, 297-306

Pisciotta, A.V. (1971) Drug-induced leukopenia and aplastic anaemia. *Clin. Pharmacol. Ther.*, 12, 13-43

Puron, R. & Firminger, H.I. (1965) Protection against induced cirrhosis and hepatocellular carcinoma in rats by chloramphenicol. *J. nat. Cancer Inst.*, 35, 29-37

Rebstock, M.C., Crooks, H.M., Jr, Controulis, J. & Bartz, Q.R. (1949) Chloramphenicol (chloromycetin). IV. Chemical studies. *J. Amer. chem. Soc.*, 71, 2458-2462

Slater, E.E., Anderson, M.D. & Rosenkranz, H.S. (1971) Rapid detection of mutagens and carcinogens. *Cancer Res.*, 31, 970-973

Stecher, P.G., ed. (1968) *The Merck Index*, 8th ed., Rahway, NJ, Merck & Co., p. 233

Summa, A.F. (1965) Polarographic determination of chloramphenicol preparations. *J. pharm. Sci.*, 54, 442-444

US Pharmacopeial Convention, Inc. (1975) *The US Pharmacopeia*, 19th rev., Easton, Pa, Mack, pp. 77-79

US Tariff Commission (1949) *Synthetic Organic Chemicals, US Production and Sales 1948*, Second Series, Report No. 164, Washington DC, US Government Printing Office, p. 103

US Tariff Commission (1974) *Imports of Benzenoid Chemicals and Products, 1973*, TC Publication 688, Washington DC, US Government Printing Office, p. 78

Wallerstein, R.O., Condit, P.K., Kasper, C.K., Brown, J.W. & Morrison, F.R. (1969) Statewide study of chloramphenicol therapy and fatal aplastic anaemia. *J. Amer. med. Ass.*, 208, 2045-2050

Weiss, C.F., Glazko, A.J. & Weston, J.K. (1960) Chloramphenicol in the newborn infant. *New Engl. J. Med.*, 262, 787-794

Welch, H., Lewis, C.N. & Kerlan, I. (1954) Blood dyscrasias, a nationwide survey. Antibiot. Chemother., 4, 607-623

Williamson, D.H., Maroudas, N.G. & Wilkie, D. (1971) Induction of cytoplasmic petite mutation in *Saccharomyces cerevisiae* by the antibacterial antibiotics erythromycin and chloramphenicol. Molec. gen. Genet., 111, 209-223

Yunis, A.A. & Bloomberg, G.R. (1964) Chloramphenicol toxicity : clinical features and pathogenesis. Progr. Hematol., 4, 138-159

CHOLESTEROL

1. Chemical and Physical Data

1.1 Synonyms and trade names

Chem. Abstr. Reg. Serial No.: 57-88-5

Chem. Abstr. Name: Cholest-5-en-3-ol(3β)

Cholest-5-en-3β-ol; 5-cholesten-3β-ol; 5:6-cholesten-3β-ol; (3β)cholest-5-en-ol; cholesterin; cholesterol base H; dythol; hydrocerin; 3β-hydroxycholest-5-ene; provitamin D

Cordulan; Dusoline; Dusoran; Kathro; Lanol; Nimco Cholesterol Base H; Nimco Cholesterol Base No. 712; Super Hartolan; Tegolan

1.2 Chemical formula and molecular weight

$C_{27}H_{46}O$ Mol. wt: 386.6

1.3 Chemical and physical properties of the pure substance (as monohydrate)

(a) Description: White or faintly yellow, almost odourless, pearly leaflets or granules

(b) Melting-point: 148.5°C (anhydrous form)

(c) Boiling-point: 360°C (decomposition)

(d) Optical rotation: $[\alpha]_D^{20}$ -31.5° (in ether); -39.5° (in chloroform)

(e) Identity and purity test: Methods for identification have been published in The US Pharmacopeia (US Pharmacopeial Convention, Inc., 1970).

(f) _Solubility_: Practically insoluble in water (0.2 mg/100 ml); 28 g/100 ml in 96% ethanol; 1 g/2.8 ml in ether; 1 g/4.5 ml in chloroform; soluble in benzene, petroleum ether, oils, fats and aqueous solutions of bile salts

(g) _Stability_: Unstable in air; the autoxidation of cholesterol has been reviewed by Bergström & Samuelsson (1961).

(h) _Reactivity_: Yields hydroperoxides on photo-oxidation or heating beyond its melting-point in the dark in the presence of molecular oxygen

1.4 Technical products and impurities

Specifications for USP grade cholesterol have been published (US Pharmacopeial Convention, Inc., 1970). Cholesterol from animal sources always contains cholestanol (dihydrocholesterol) and other saturated sterols (Stecher, 1968). Cholesterol is listed in the European Pharmacopoeia (Council of Europe, 1969).

2. Production, Use, Occurrence and Analysis

A review on cholesterol has been published (Kritchevsky, 1958).

2.1 Production and use

Cholesterol is one of the most widely disseminated organic compounds in the animal kingdom and one of the oldest from the standpoint of isolation and recognition: it was isolated from gallstones by Poulletier de la Salle in about 1763. Progress towards elucidation of its structure was made in the 19th century by Berthelot, Wislecenus then Moldenhaur (Kritchevsky, 1958). The synthesis of cholesterol was reported by Robinson *et al*. (Cardwell *et al*., 1953). Woodward *et al*. (1952) achieved the total synthesis of compounds convertible to cholesterol by a series of known reactions based upon 4-methoxytoluquinone: this was converted by a twenty-step synthesis to DL-$\Delta^{9(11),16}$-bisdehydro-20-norprogesterone, convertible to cholesterol by established methods. A total synthesis was reported by Keana & Johnson (1964).

Cholesterol is prepared commercially by extraction of the non-saponifiable matter from the spinal cord of cattle with petroleum ether. It is also produced from wool grease (Stecher, 1968).

Cholesterol is a constituent of many cosmetic products, including lipstick, lubricating creams, bath oils, shampoos, hair dressings and tonics, suntan lotions, rouge and blush make-up, eye shadows, lotions and creams and eyebrow pencil.

2.2 Occurrence

Cholesterol occurs in all body tissues of higher animals, especially brain and spinal cord, and in animal fats and oils. It is the main constituent of gallstones. The total cholesterol content of a 64 kg man is 210 g.

Oxidation products of cholesterol have also been isolated from natural sources.

2.3 Analysis

A method for the determination of cholesterol and its esters was described by Boutwell (1961). For histochemical detection of cholesterol the method of Schultz (1924/25) has been found satisfactory and is still used. A gas-liquid chromatographic method has been developed for qualitative determination of cholesterol and its esters in dairy products (LaCroix *et al.*, 1972). A gas chromatographic method has also been proposed for the analysis of cholesterol and other sterols as free alcohols, acetates or trimethylsilyl ethers (Evans, 1972).

3. Biological Data Relevant to the Evaluation of Carcinogenic Risk to Man

3.1 Carcinogenicity and related studies in animals

(a) Oral administration

Mouse: A number of feeding studies were carried out using diets containing lard supplemented by cholesterol (Szepsenwol, 1963; 1969), and in another experiment, egg yolk was used as the source of dietary cholesterol (Szepsenwol, 1963). [These experiments were difficult to interpret with regard to tumour incidence because of the uncertain composition of the lard administered in the first two and the presence of unidentified contaminants which may have arisen from the animal feed in all three.]

Mice of the TM strain given cholesterol in the diet had a high incidence of lung adenocarcinomas (76%) compared to that in the control group (13%), and the incidence of mammary cancers was 9% compared to 7% in the controls. Three squamous-cell carcinomas of the skin were found only in mice of the treated group; none occurred in controls. Survival times of both treated and control groups were similar, being 665 and 676 days, respectively (Szepsenwol, 1966).

(b) Subcutaneous and/or intramuscular administration

Mouse: In a series of experiments in which mice were injected s.c. with either of the solvents olive oil and tricaprylin, only 2 local sarcomas were found in 464 mice injected with olive oil and 1 in 30 mice injected with tricaprylin. The incidence of sarcomas at the site of injection of cholesterol dissolved in olive oil, tricaprylin or other solvents varied over a period of 2 years from 0-24% (Hieger, 1957; 1958; 1959; 1962; Hieger & Orr, 1954). [It was not possible to evaluate these findings because of variations in other parameters unrelated to the administration of cholesterol.]

(c) Other experimental systems

Cholesterol has been used as a standard vehicle for local administration of carcinogens at many experimental sites, e.g., urinary and gall bladders, brain, kidney and embryonic tissues. None of these studies were directly concerned with the effect of cholesterol itself, and in most studies little attention was paid to the actual amount of cholesterol introduced.

In experiments in which cholesterol pellets were implanted into mouse bladders for 30 weeks, 5 malignant and 4 benign bladder tumours were observed among 77 mice (Boyland et al., 1964). Similarly, of 55 mice surviving 40 weeks after bladder implantation, 5 malignant and 1 benign bladder tumours were observed (Clayson et al., 1958). In experiments in large groups of mice, extending for up to 1½ years, the reported ratios of malignant to benign tumours varied from 4:2 to 1:9 (Bryan et al., 1964). Clayson & Cooper (1970) have reviewed such experiments. In guinea-pigs, the implantation of cholesterol pellets weighing 20-40 mg into the gall bladder produced no changes by 41 weeks (Desforges et al., 1950).

(d) Co-carcinogenesis experiments

Mouse: Female mice of the DDD strain were fed a diet containing 1% cholesterol and 0.5% cholic acid (a gallstone-inducing diet) for 18 weeks. The bile ducts and gall bladders of these mice showed marked proliferative and inflammatory changes. One mouse died of an adenocarcinoma originating from the ampulla orifice of the common bile duct after 553 days. The experiment served as control to evaluate the effect of the cholesterol/cholic acid diet on the carcinogenicity of 2-acetylaminofluorene (AAF) or its metabolite N-hydroxy-AAF. No effects were observed with AAF (total dose, 130-300 mg fed over 15-18 weeks) when the mice were sacrificed at 34 weeks. Feeding of N-hydroxy-AAF produced many tumours of the urinary bladder, oesophagus, forestomach and liver. The presence of cholesterol and cholic acid in the N-hydroxy-AAF diet enhanced the incidence and reduced the latent period of development of liver-cell tumours (adenomas and carcinomas) as well as that of hyperplastic nodules; it enhanced the proliferation of the bile duct and gall bladder (Enomoto et al., 1974).

Hamster: Male hamsters were given gall bladder implants of cholesterol pellets and nitrosodiethyl- and nitrosodimethylamine (NDEA and NDMA) in drinking-water; dose levels of 0.159 NDEA or 0.02 ml NDMA per 1000 ml water were administered. When the experiments were terminated, at 22 weeks, hepatocellular carcinomas were seen in 50% and cholangiocarcinomas in 100% of NDEA-exposed animals, whether the animals had a cholesterol pellet implant or not. In the NDMA groups, 40% had hepatocellular carcinomas and 60% had cholangiocarcinomas, independent of pellet implants. However, in NDMA-exposed animals the incidence of carcinoma in the gall bladder depended on the presence of a cholesterol pellet, the incidence being 68% with pellet and 6% without. No carcinomas of the gall bladder were seen in NDEA groups (Kowalewski & Todd, 1971).

3.2 Other relevant biological data

Cholesterol, lathosterol and methostenol were found in the small intestine, caecum and faeces of germ-free rats, together with plant sterols from the diet: campesterol, stigmasterol and β-sitosterol. In normal rats, coprostanol was the major sterol found in caecum and faeces; but cholesterol, lathosterol, methostenol, 24α-ethyl-coprostanol and β-sitosterol were also found in the faeces (Gustafsson *et al.*, 1966).

Cholesterol introduced into the caecum of rats is changed to lithocholic and isolithocholic acids, 6% of which are excreted in the faeces. In the guinea-pig, the gut bacteria can metabolize 1.7% of a dose of cholesterol to oestradiol and oestrone, which are excreted in the urine; the reaction also takes place *in vitro* (Goddard & Hill, 1974).

Studies with ^{14}C-cholesterol in the rat showed that both placental transfer and foetal synthesis of cholesterol can occur (Chevallier, 1964). It has been shown to induce foetal malformations in albino rats (Buresh & Urban, 1964; 1967).

Coprostanol, 5α-cholestan-3-β-ol and cholesta-5,7-dien-3β-ol were injected s.c. as 0.133% solutions in tricaprylin into female NMRI mice, 0.5 ml 3 times at intervals of 2 weeks. Of the 47 animals injected with coprostanol, 4 had sarcomas and 5, tumours of liver, spleen and kidney. No sarcomas were produced by the stereoisomer of coprostanol or with the solvent alone. Cholesta-5,7-dien-3β-ol induced 1 sarcoma among 25 mice (Pfeiffer, 1973).

Male C_{57} black and albino mice were given 10 weekly s.c. injections of 2 mg 5α-cholest-6-ene or 5α-cholesta-1,3,6-triene in 0.2 ml olive oil; controls were injected with olive oil only. 5α-Cholesta-1,3,6-triene produced a fibrosarcoma in 1 C_{57} black mouse at the end of 50 weeks. Both compounds were co-carcinogenic when used in conjunction with dibenz[*a,h*]-anthracene (de Kock & Barnardt, 1970).

Bryson & Bischoff (1963) showed that cholesterol-(α)-oxide was carcinogenic in Evans rats and Marsh mice following its s.c. injection in isotonic saline but inactive following its i.p. injection or injection into the thymus. After testicular injection of 10 mg cholesterol-(α)-oxide in saline suspension, 7/89 Marsh mice had fibro- or myosarcomas.

In lifetime feeding experiments in 248 Holtzmann white rats of both sexes and in 252 C57Bl/6 mice of both sexes fed cholesterol-(α)-oxide, no increase in tumour frequency was found over that in control groups (Seelkopf & Salfelder, 1962).

Black & Douglas (1972) reported the formation of cholesterol-(α)-oxide by ultra-violet irradiation on the skin of hairless mice; this effect had already been demonstrated on human skin (Black & Lo, 1971).

Bischoff *et al.* (1955) tested a number of pure oxidation products of cholesterol for their carcinogenicity in Marsh-Buffalo mice; 33 mice were used in each group; males received Δ^4-cholesten-3,6-dione, 6-hydroxy-Δ^4-cholesten-3-one or sesame oil, and castrated females received cholesterol-(α)-oxide or sesame oil. The doses were not reported, but s.c. injection produced a 19% incidence of sarcomas with 6-hydroxy-Δ^4-cholesten-3-one, 34% with Δ^4-cholesten-3,6-dione and 43% with cholesterol-(α)-oxide; no sarcomas were observed in the two sesame-oil control groups.

AB (Agnes Blum) mice of both sexes and C_{57} black females were given total doses of 20 mg Δ^4-cholesten-3,6-dione in 3 s.c. injections at intervals of two weeks; the 50% survival times were 20 and 16 months for female and male AB mice and 26 months for male C_{57} black mice. One local malignant tumour was observed in each experimental group, and 5 malignant mammary tumours were observed in the female AB mice (Bruns *et al.*, 1963).

Three s.c. injections of 5 mg 6β-hydroperoxy-Δ^4-cholesten-3-one in sesame oil were given to 32 Marsh-Buffalo mice (age unspecified). Fibrosarcomas appeared at the site of injection in 13 mice at 12 months of age; 17 mice were still tumour-free. No tumours were seen in groups of littermates given the compound in aqueous colloidal solution nor in sesame-oil controls (Fieser *et al.*, 1955).

Koch & Schenk (1961) gave i.p. injections of 30 mg Δ^6-cholesten-3β-ol-5α-hydroperoxide in olive oil and X-irradiation to male white rats. After 2 years, 1 fibroadenoma, 4 carcinomas and 5 sarcomas at various locations were observed, representing a 9.5% tumour incidence. In similar groups given i.p. injections of cholesterol plus X-irradiation, 3 carcinomas and 5 sarcomas were observed (17.5%). None of the results were considered proof of carcinogenic activity for the two substances. Δ^6-Cholesten-3β-ol-5α-hydroperoxide was also tested in a mouse strain which has a spontaneous tumour incidence of 0% in males and 10.2% in females. The substance was dissolved in olive oil, and doses of 25 mg/kg bw were injected intraperitoneally in females: after 2 years a tumour incidence of 35% (1 fibroma, 1 adenoma, 9 sarcomas and 12 carcinomas) was observed, as compared to 10% with cholesterol (Koch, 1963).

Because of carcinogenic effects reported after the feeding of a diet supplemented with boiled egg yolk, Hradec & Kruml (1960) set out to isolate, characterize and identify the responsible component. The substance was obtained from tissues, in particular the liver, of tumour-bearing rats. Doses of 3 mg of the substance in olive oil were injected s.c. into 50 8-month old male and female Wistar rats; 14 months after the start of the experiment no tumours were seen in the controls, while in the experimental group there were already 3 local sarcomas (latent periods, 5, 9 and 11 months), 2 carcinomas and 2 mammary adenomas. The substance was named 'carcinolipin' and was characterized as cholesteryl-(+)-14-methylhexadecanoate (Hradec & Dolejs, 1968).

Shabad *et al.* (1973) studied the transplacental carcinogenic effect of carcinolipin in A strain mice by giving 5-18 mg of the compound in 1-4 injections in olive oil during the last third of pregnancy. Lung adenomas were seen in 2/6 offspring dying before 1 year and in 7/13 killed at 14-18 months (47.3%). The incidence among control animals was 10.7%. Post-natal treatment of mice with carcinolipin produced only 5 lung tumours in 27 animals (18.5%). No multiple lung adenomas were observed.

In man on a liquid diet, the reduction of cholesterol to coprostanol was almost completely abolished due to changes in the intestinal flora. A study of the ability of bacteria to metabolize cholesterol showed that none of 20 strains of *Escherichia coli* or *Streptococcus faecalis* could reduce cholesterol, but 9/20 strains of *Clostridium*, 12/18 strains of *Bacteroides* and 9/12 strains of *Bifidobacterium* could (Crowther *et al.*, 1973).

Cholesterol-(α)-oxide, coprostanol, β-sitosterol, cholest-4-en-3-one and cholesta-4,6-dien-3-one have been isolated and identified in human serum. The levels of cholesterol-(α)-oxide were very low in normal serum; however, in the serum of patients with hypercholesterolaemia such levels were found to range from 250-3250 µg/100 ml serum and in pooled samples, up to 4450 µg/100 ml serum. The cholesterol level in the sera of the hypercholesterolaemics ranged from 316-454 mg/100 ml serum (Gray et al., 1971).

3.3 Observations in man

No case reports or epidemiological studies of the relationship of exogenous cholesterol to cancer risk in man were available to the Working Group. Data which bear indirectly on this subject are available, as from studies of possible relationships between cancer and dietary fat (Armstrong & Doll, 1975; Carroll et al., 1968; Ederer et al., 1971; Lea, 1966; Wynder, 1974; 1975), serum cholesterol levels (Rose et al., 1974) and bacterial metabolism of biliary steroids (Hill et al., 1975).

4. Comments on Data Reported and Evaluation

4.1 Animal data

There are no adequate feeding studies with pure cholesterol available to evaluate its carcinogenicity. Experiments involving subcutaneous injection of cholesterol in various vehicles cannot be evaluated because of variations in parameters unrelated to the dose of cholesterol administered. Implantation experiments using cholesterol are difficult to interpret, because the effects of the physical factors must be taken into consideration.

On the basis of the experimental evidence available no assessment of the carcinogenicity of cholesterol is possible.

4.2 Human data

No data are available to assess the carcinogenicity of exogenous cholesterol in man. Studies of cancer in relation to dietary fat, serum cholesterol levels and the degradation of biliary steroids are not directly relevant to this question.

5. References

Armstrong, B. & Doll, R. (1975) Environmental factors and cancer incidence and mortality in different countries with special reference to dietary practices. Int. J. Cancer, 15, 617-631

Bergström, S. & Samuelsson, B. (1961) The autoxidation of cholesterol. In: Lundberg, ed., Autoxidation and Antioxidants, Vol. 1, Chichester, UK, Interscience, pp. 233-248

Bischoff, F., Lopez, G., Rupp, J.J. & Gray, C.L. (1955) Carcinogenic activity of cholesterol degradation products. Fed. Proc., 14, 590

Black, H.S. & Douglas, D.R. (1972) A model system for the evaluation of the role of cholesterol-α-oxide in ultraviolet carcinogenesis. Cancer Res., 32, 2630-2632

Black, H.S. & Lo, W.-B. (1971) Formation of a carcinogen in human skin irradiated with ultraviolet light. Nature (Lond.), 234, 306-308

Boutwell, J.H., Jr (1961) Clinical Chemistry. Laboratory Manual and Methods, Philadelphia, Lea & Febiger, pp. 175-183

Boyland, E., Busby, E.R., Dukes, C.E., Grover, P.L. & Manson, D. (1964) Further experiments on implanation of materials into the urinary bladder of mice. Brit. J. Cancer, 18, 575-581

Bruns, V.G., Schubert, K., Zschiesche, W. & Rose, G. (1963) Die Kritik am Cancerogentest mit Δ-4-Cholesten-3,6-dion. Arch. Geschwulstforsch., 22, 52-71

Bryan, G.T., Brown, R.R. & Price, J.M. (1964) Mouse bladder carcinogenicity of certain tryptophan metabolites and other aromatic nitrogen compounds suspended in cholesterol. Cancer Res., 24, 596-602

Bryson, G. & Bischoff, F. (1963) Carcinogenesis in Marsh mice by testicular injection of cholesterol *alpha* oxide. Proc. Amer. Ass. Cancer Res., 4, 29

Buresh, J.J. & Urban, T.J. (1964) The teratogenic effect of the steroid nucleus in the rat. J. dent. Res., 43, 548-554

Buresh, J.J. & Urban, T.J. (1967) Cholesterol-induced palatal clefts in the rat. Arch. oral Biol., 12, 1221-1228

Cardwell, H.M.E., Cornforth, J.W., Duff, S.R., Holtermann, H. & Robinson, R. (1953) Experiments on the synthesis of substances related to the sterols. LI. Completion of the synthesis of androgenic hormones and of the cholesterol group of sterols. J. chem. Soc., 361-384

Carroll, K.K., Gammal, E.B. & Plunkett, E.R. (1968) Dietary fat and mammary cancer. Canad. med. Ass. J., 98, 590-593

Chevallier, F. (1964) Transferts et synthèse du cholestérol chez le rat au cours de sa croissance. Biochim. biophys. acta, 84, 316-339

Clayson, D.B. & Cooper, E.H. (1970) Cancer of the urinary tract. Advanc. Cancer Res., 13, 271-381

Clayson, D.B., Jull, J.W. & Bonser, G.M. (1958) The testing of *ortho* hydroxyamines and related compounds by bladder implantation and a discussion of their structural requirements for carcinogenic activity. Brit. J. Cancer, 12, 222-230

Council of Europe (1969) European Pharmacopoeia, European Treaty Series No. 50, Vol. 1, Paris, Maisonneuve, p. 147

Desforges, G., Desforges, J. & Robbins, S.L. (1950) Carcinoma of the gall bladder. An attempt at experimental production. Cancer, 3, 1088-1096

Ederer, F., Leren, P., Turpeinen, O. & Frantz, I.D. (1971) Cancer among men on cholesterol-lowering diets. Experience from five clinical trials. Lancet, ii, 203-206

Enomoto, M., Nase, S., Harada, M., Miyata, K., Saito, M. & Noguchi, Y. (1974) Carcinogenesis in extrahepatic bile duct and gall-bladder. Carcinogenic effect of *N*-hydroxy-2-acetamidofluorene in mice fed a gallstone-inducing diet. Japan. J. exp. Med., 44, 37-54

Evans, J.R. (1972) The gas chromatography of calciferol, dihydrotachysterol and cholesterol. Clin. chim. acta, 42, 167-174

Fieser, L.F., Greene, T.W., Bischoff, F., Lopez, G. & Rupp, J.J. (1955) A carcinogenic oxidation product of cholesterol. J. Amer. chem. Soc., 77, 3928-3929

Goddard, P. & Hill, M.J. (1974) The *in vivo* metabolism of cholesterol by gut bacteria in the rat and guinea-pig. J. Steroid Biochem., 5, 569-572

Gray, M.F., Lawrie, T.D.V. & Brooks, C.J.W. (1971) Isolation and identification of cholesterol α-oxide and other minor sterols in human serum. Lipids, 6, 836-843

Gustafsson, B.E., Gustafsson, J.A. & Sjovall, J. (1966) Intestinal and fecal sterols in germfree and conventional rats. Bile acids and steroids 172. Acta chem. scand., 20, 1827-1835

Hieger, I. (1957) Cholesterol as a carcinogen. Proc. roy. Soc. (Lond.), Ser. B, 147, 84-89

Hieger, I. (1958) Cholesterol carcinogenesis. Brit. med. Bull., 14, 159-160

Hieger, I. (1959) Carcinogenesis by cholesterol. Brit. J. Cancer, 13, 439-451

Hieger, I. (1962) Cholesterol as carcinogen. I. Sarcoma induction by cholesterol in a sensitive strain of mice. II. Croton oil a complete carcinogen. Brit. J. Cancer, 16, 716-721

Hieger, I. & Orr, S.F.D. (1954) On the carcinogenic activity of purified cholesterol. Brit. J. Cancer, 8, 274-290

Hill, M.J., Drasar, B.S., Williams, R.E.O., Meade, T.W., Cox, A.G., Simpson, J.E.P. & Morson, B.C. (1975) Faecal bile-acids and *Clostridia* in patients with cancer of the large bowel. Lancet, i, 535-538

Hradec, J. & Dolejs, L. (1968) The chemical constitution of carcinolipin. Biochim. J., 107, 129-134

Hradec, J. & Kruml, J. (1960) Carcinolipin: an endogenous carcinogenic substance. Nature (Lond.), 185, 55

Keana, J.F.W. & Johnson, W.S. (1964) Racemic cholesterol. Steroids, 4, 457-462

Koch, R. (1963) Zur Cancerogenität des Cholesterins und seins 5.-bzw. 7.-Hydroperoxydes. Arzneimittelforsch., 15, 1116-1117

Koch, R. & Schenk, G.O. (1961) Möglichkeiten des Eingreifens sensibilisierender und desensibilisiereunder Zusätze in der Strahlenchemie und Strahlenbiologie. III. Die Beeinflussung der Strahlensensibilität und des Tumorwachstumsdurch Cholesterin und Cholesterinhydroperoxyd. Strahlentherapie, 116, 364-373

de Kock, D.H. & Barnardt, J.H. (1970) Tumour-promoting properties and metabolism of 5α-cholest-6-ene and 5α-cholesta-1,3,6-triene. S. Afr. med. J., 44, 1274-1276

Kowalewski, K. & Todd, E.F. (1971) Carcinoma of the gallbladder induced in hamsters by insertion of cholesterol pellets and feeding dimethylnitrosamine. Proc. Soc. exp. Biol. (N.Y.), 136, 482-486

Kritchevsky, D. (1958) Cholesterol, New York, John Wiley and Sons

LaCroix, D.E., Feeley, R.M., Wong, N.P. & Alford, J.A. (1972) Comparison of two extraction procedures for the determination of cholesterol in dairy products. J. Ass. off. analyt. Chem., 55, 972-974

Lea, A.J. (1966) Dietary factors associated with death rates from certain neoplasms in man. Lancet, ii, 332-333

Pfeiffer, E.H. (1973) Zur Kanzerogenität des Koprosterins, eines intestinalen Reduktionsprodukts des Cholesterins. Naturwissenschaften, 11, 525-526

Rose, G., Blackburn, H., Keys, A., Taylor, H.L., Kannel, W.B., Paul, O., Reid, D.D. & Stamler, J. (1974) Colon cancer and blood-cholesterol. Lancet, i, 7850-7852

Schultz, A. (1924/5) Eine Methode des mikrochemischen Cholesterin-Nachweises am Gewebsschnitt. Zbl. allgemeine Path. Anat., 35, 314-317

Seelkopf, C. & Salfelder, K. (1962) Tierversuche zur Frage cancerogener Eigenschaften einiger Epoxyde in überhitzten Fetten. Z. Krebsforsch., 64, 459-464

Shabad, L.M., Kolesnichenko, T.S. & Savluchinskaya, L.A. (1973) Transplacental effect of carcinolipin in mice. Neoplasma, 20, 347-348

Stecher, P.G., ed. (1968) The Merck Index, 8th ed., Rahway, NJ, Merck & Co., p. 253

Szepsenwol, J. (1963) Carcinogenic effect of egg white, egg yolk and lipids in mice. Proc. Soc. exp. Biol. (N.Y.), 112, 1073-1076

Szepsenwol, J. (1966) Carcinogenic effect of cholesterol in mice. Proc. Soc. exp. Biol. (N.Y.), 121, 168-171

Szepsenwol, J. (1969) Brain nerve cell tumors in mice on diets supplemented with various lipids. Path. Microbiol., 34, 1-9

US Pharmacopeial Convention, Inc. (1970) The US Pharmacopeia, 18th rev., Easton, Pa, Mack, pp. 131-132

Woodward, R.B., Sondheimer, F., Taub, D., Heusler, K. & McLamore, W.M. (1952) The total synthesis of steroids. J. Amer. chem. Soc., 74, 4223-4251

Wynder, E.L. (1974) Diet and colon cancer. Ostomy Quarterly, 11, 61-62

Wynder, E.L. (1975) An epidemiological evaluation of the causes of cancer of the pancreas. Cancer Res., 35, 2228-2233

COUMARIN

1. Chemical and Physical Data

1.1 Synonyms and trade names

Chem. Abstr. Reg. Serial No.: 91-64-5

Chem. Abstr. Name: 2H-1-Benzopyran-2-one

1,2-Benzopyrone; *cis-o*-coumarinic acid lactone; coumarinic anhydride; cumarin; *o*-hydroxycinnamic acid-δ-lactone; 2-oxo-2H-1-benzopyran; Tonka bean camphor

1.2 Chemical formula and molecular weight

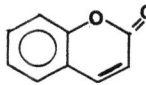

$C_9H_6O_2$ Mol. wt: 146.1

1.3 Chemical and physical properties of the pure substance

(a) *Description*: Orthorhombic rectangular plates; fragrant odour; burning taste

(b) *Boiling-point*: 303°C; 139°C at 5 mm Hg

(c) *Melting-point*: 70.6°C

(d) *Spectroscopy data*: λ_{max} 209 nm, 272 nm, 310 nm (in 95% ethanol) (Schepartz *et al.*, 1972)

(e) *Solubility*: 1 g is soluble in 400 ml water at 25°C and in 50 ml water at 100°C; freely soluble in ethanol, chloroform, ether and oils

(f) *Stability*: Converted to a dimer on long exposure to light

(g) *Reactivity*: Can be halogenated, nitrated and hydrogenated (in presence of catalysts)

1.4 Technical products and impurities

One commercial grade of coumarin has the form of white prismatic crystals of characteristic odour; melting-point, 68.8°C; 1 g dissolves in 10 ml ethanol; maximum moisture content 0.10%; practically colourless when molten or solidified (DeGarmo & Raizman, 1967).

The impurities are usually the starting materials in the manufacturing process, depending on the process used, e.g., phenols, salicylaldehyde and chlorinated products (DeGarmo & Raizman, 1967).

2. Production, Use, Occurrence and Analysis

For important background information on this section, see preamble, p. 17.

A review on coumarin has been published (DeGarmo & Raizman, 1967).

2.1 Production and use

Coumarin was first synthesized by Perkin in 1868 (DeGarmo & Raizman, 1967) by heating the sodium derivative of salicylaldehyde with acetic anhydride or by boiling salicylaldehyde, acetic anhydride and anhydrous sodium acetate. Most of the coumarin used commercially is produced synthetically (DeGarmo & Raizman, 1967); high-quality grades of coumarin are isolated from Tonka beans (Hawley, 1971).

The production of synthetic coumarin doubled in the US during the decade 1958-1967. In 1967, the last year for which production figures were reported, the quantity produced was 520 thousand kg; since that year there have been only two producers in the US (US Tariff Commission, 1969).

Coumarin is used as a fixative and enhancing agent for the odour of essential oils in perfumes in quantities of about 1-4 g per gallon of perfume. Some toilet soaps, toothpastes and hair preparations contain small amounts. It is used in tobacco products to enhance and fix the natural taste, flavour and aroma. It is sometimes used in industrial products to mask disagreeable odours; its use in the electroplating of nickel has been reported (DeGarmo & Raizman, 1967).

2.2 Occurrence

Coumarin occurs naturally in woodruff (*Asperula odorat* L.) which is used as a flavouring in wine made from may flowers (hawthorn). Of 10 samples examined, only two samples contained coumarin at levels not greater than 5 mg/l (Dyer *et al.*, 1975). It also occurs in plants and essential oils such as Tonka bean (seed of *Dipteryx odorata*), cassia (*Cinnamonum cassia*), melilot (*Melilotus officinalus*), Orchidaceae, lavender (*Lavandum officinalus*) and balsam of Peru (*Myroxylon Pereirae*) (Hawley, 1971; Opdyke, 1974).

2.3 Analysis

A method for the determination of coumarin by gas chromatography has been described; the limit of detection was 0.4 mg/l (Dyer *et al.*, 1975).

3. Biological Data Relevant to the Evaluation of Carcinogenic Risk to Man

3.1 Carcinogenicity and related studies in animals

Oral administration

Rat: Groups of 12 Osborne-Mendel rats of both sexes were fed diets containing 1000, 2500 or 5000 mg coumarin per kg of diet for 2 years (food grade material, purity not specified); 3% corn oil was also added to the diet. Two groups of controls received the untreated diet or a basal diet containing 3% corn oil. Bile-duct proliferation, cholangiofibrosis and focal necrosis were observed in rats fed the two highest dose levels, but no tumours were described; exact survival rates were not reported (Hagan *et al.*, 1967).

Groups of 40 albino rats of both sexes were fed diets containing 1000, 2500 or 5000 mg coumarin per kg of diet for 2 years (food grade material, purity not specified). Of 24 rats fed 5000 mg/kg of diet and surviving 18 or more months, 11 males and 1 female developed bile-duct carcinomas. In a subsidiary experiment in which 82 rats were used, bile-duct carcinomas occurred in 4/25 males and in 1/8 females surviving 18 or more months and fed an average of 3500 mg/kg of diet. In rats fed 1000 and 2500 mg/kg of diet, a few adenomas of the bile-ducts were reported to have occurred.

No bile-duct carcinomas occurred in two separate groups of 40 and 50 controls (Bär & Griepentrog, 1967; Griepentrog, 1973).

3.2 Other relevant biological data

The LD_{50}'s in mice were 196 mg/kg bw following oral administration and 310 mg/kg bw following s.c. injection (Kitagawa & Iwaki, 1963). The oral LD_{50} in rats fed a 5% solution in corn oil was 680 mg/kg bw; that in guinea-pigs fed a 10% solution in propylene glycol was 200 mg/kg bw (Jenner et al., 1964).

The metabolism of orally administered [3-^{14}C]-coumarin has been studied in rats, rabbits and man. The compound was rapidly absorbed in rats and widely distributed in serum, liver and kidney within 5 minutes, serum levels reaching a maximum after about 30 minutes (Feuer et al., 1966). Rats excreted up to 80% in the urine, mainly as 2-hydroxyphenylacetic acid (19%), 2-hydroxyphenyllactic acid, 3-, 4-, 7- and 8-hydroxy coumarins, ortho-coumaric acid and only small amounts of 2-hydroxyphenylpropionic acid (Feuer et al., 1966; Kaighen & Williams, 1961). In rabbits, up to 90% was excreted in the urine, mainly as 2-hydroxyphenylacetic acid (20%), 3- and 7-hydroxy coumarins and 2-hydroxyphenyllactic acid (Kaighen & Williams, 1961). In man, 68-92% of an oral dose of coumarin was excreted in the urine as 7-hydroxy coumarin and 1-6% as 2-hydroxyphenylacetic acid (Shilling et al., 1969).

Coumarin and some of its metabolites have been shown to inhibit glucose-6-phosphatase in the liver and in liver microsomal preparations (Feuer et al., 1965a,b). It interferes with excision repair processes in ultra-violet-damaged DNA and with host cell reactivation of ultra-violet-irradiated phage T1 in *Escherichia coli* WP2 (Grigg, 1972).

3.3 Observations in man

No data were available to the Working Group.

4. Comments on Data Reported and Evaluation[1]

4.1 Animal data

Coumarin is carcinogenic in rats following its oral administration, the only species and route of administration tested; it produced bile-duct carcinomas.

4.2 Human data

No case reports or epidemiological studies were available to the Working Group.

---

[1] See also the section "Animal Data in Relation to the Evaluation of Risk to Man" in the introduction to this volume, p. 15.

5. References

Bär, von F. & Griepentrog, F. (1967) Die Situation in der gesundheitlichen Beurteilung der Aromatisierungsmittel für Lebensmittel. Med. Ernähr., 8, 244-251

DeGarmo, O. & Raizman, P. (1967) Coumarin. In: Kirk, R.E. & Othmer, D.F., eds, Encyclopedia of Chemical Technology, 2nd ed., Vol. 12, New York, John Wiley and Sons, pp. 425-433

Dyer, R.H., Martin, G.E. & Butts, B.B. (1975) Gas-liquid chromatographic determination of coumarin (1,2-benzopyrone) in may wine. J. Ass. off. analyt. Chem., 58, 140-142

Feuer, G., Goldberg, L. & Gibson, K.I. (1965a) Additional evidence of the identity of rat liver microsomal glucose-6-phosphatase and inorganic pyrophosphatase. Biochem. J., 97, 29-30

Feuer, G., Goldberg, L. & Le Pelley, J.R. (1965b) Liver response test. I. Exploratory studies on glucose-6-phosphatase and other liver enzymes. Fd Cosmet. Toxicol., 3, 235-249

Feuer, G., Goldberg, L. & Gibson, K.I. (1966) Liver response tests. VII. Coumarin metabolism in relation to the inhibition of rat-liver glucose-6-phosphatase. Fd Cosmet. Toxicol., 4, 157-167

Griepentrog, F. (1973) Pathologisch-anatomische Befunde zur karzinogenen Wirkung von Cumarin im Tierversuch. Toxicology, 1, 93-102

Grigg, G.W. (1972) Effects of coumarin, pyronin Y, 6,9-dimethyl 2-methyl-thiopurine and caffeine on excision repair and recombination repair in *Escherichia coli*. J. gen. Microbiol., 70, 221-230

Hagan, E.C., Hansen, W.H., Fitzhugh, O.G., Jenner, P.M., Jones, W.I., Taylor, J.M., Long, E.L., Nelson, A.A. & Brouwer, J.B. (1967) Food flavourings and compounds of related structure. II. Subacute and chronic toxicity. Fd Cosmet. Toxicol., 5, 141-157

Hawley, G., ed. (1971) The Condensed Chemical Dictionary, New York, Van Nostrand Reinhold, p. 241

Jenner, P.M., Hagan, E.C., Taylor, J.M., Cook, E.L. & Fitzhugh, O.G. (1964) Food flavourings and compounds of related structure. I. Acute oral toxicity. Fd Cosmet. Toxicol., 2, 327-343

Kaighen, M. & Williams, R.T. (1961) The metabolism of [3-^{14}C]coumarin. J. med. pharm. Chem., 3, 25-43

Kitagawa, H. & Iwaki, R. (1963) Coumarin derivatives for medicinal purposes. XVII. Pharmacological studies on coumarin derivatives having biological activity. Yakugaku Zasshi, 83, 1124-1128

Opdyke, D.L.J. (1974) Monographs on fragrance raw materials. Coumarin. Fd Cosmet. Toxicol., 12, 385-387

Schepartz, A.I., Fleischman, R.A. & Cisle, J.H. (1972) Thin-layer chromatographic and spectral properties of certain lactones and related compounds. J. Chromat., 69, 411-415

Shilling, W.H., Crampton, R.F. & Longland, R.C. (1969) Metabolism of coumarin in man. Nature (Lond.), 221, 664-665

US Tariff Commission (1969) Synthetic Organic Chemicals, US Production and Sales, 1967, TC Publication 295, Washington DC, US Government Printing Office, p. 35

CYCASIN

This substance was previously considered by an IARC Working Group in December 1971 (IARC, 1972). Since that time new data have become available, and these have been incorporated into the monograph and taken into account in the present evaluation.

The biologically active part of cycasin is its aglycone methylazoxymethanol; data on this metabolite are given in section 3.2. The chemically related methylazoxymethanol acetate has been synthesized and tested for carcinogenicity; data are given in an Appendix to this monograph.

1. Chemical and Physical Data

1.1 Synonyms and trade names

Chem. Abstr. Reg. Serial No.: 14901-08-7

Chem. Abstr. Name: (Methyl-*ONN*)azoxymethyl-β-D-glucopyranoside

β-D-Glucosyloxyazoxymethane; β-D-glucosyloxyazoxymethase; methylazoxymethanol-β-D-glucoside

1.2 Chemical formula and molecular weight

$$H_3C-N=N-CH_2OC_6H_{11}O_5$$
$$|$$
$$O$$

$C_8H_{16}N_2O_7$ Mol. wt: 252.2

1.3 Chemical and physical properties of the pure substance

(a) Description: Colourless, long needles

(b) Melting-point: 144-145°C (decomposition) (Nishida *et al.*, 1955); 154°C (decomposition) (Riggs, 1956)

(c) Optical rotation: $[\alpha]_D^{18}$ -44° (0.62% in water) (Riggs, 1956)

(d) Spectroscopy data: λ_{max} 218 nm; E_1^1 = 287.5 (Riggs, 1956)

(e) **Solubility**: Readily soluble in water and dilute ethanol; sparingly soluble in absolute ethanol; insoluble in benzene, acetone, chloroform and ethyl acetate (Nishida et al., 1955)

(f) **Chemical reactivity**: Easily hydrolysed, especially under alkaline conditions, to yield nitrogen, formaldehyde and methanol, among other products

1.4 Technical products and impurities

No data were available to the Working Group.

2. Production, Use, Occurrence and Analysis

2.1 Production and use

Cycasin is not produced or used commercially.

2.2 Occurrence

Cycasin occurs in the seeds, roots and leaves of cycad plants (family Cycadaceae), which are found in the tropical and subtropical regions of the world. It was identified by Nishida et al. (1955) in the seeds of the Japanese cycad *Cycas revoluta* Thunb. and by Riggs (1956) in the seeds of *Cycas circinalis* L., a cycad indigenous to Guam (Mariana Islands).

The amount of cycasin present in cycad nuts depends on the species of cycad. In ground and dried nuts of *Cycas circinalis* L., 0.02% cycasin was found after air drying of nuts prepared in Guam (leaching with water then sun-drying) (Matsumoto & Strong, 1963). A 2.3% level was found in unwashed, vacuum-dried nuts (Campbell et al., 1966). Using different extraction methods, 1% was detected after boiling with water for 20 minutes and 0.6% by washing for 8 days prior to boiling for 20 minutes. No cycasin was detected in chips of dried kernels of cycad nuts prepared in Guam and used as food by Guamanians; the sensitivity of the method used was of the order of 100 µg/kg (Palekar & Dastur, 1965). The wide range of levels found is due to the fact that boiling during the extraction procedure diminishes levels of the cycasin-destroying enzyme (emulsin) and results in a higher cycasin yield; washing and soaking, on the other hand, activate the enzyme (Dastur & Palekar, 1966).

The making of starch from cycad nuts is both a home and a commercial industry. Cycad starch from nuts of *Cycas circinalis* and *Cycas revoluta* is used in the Mariana Islands, on Ryukyu Island (Japan) and in Indochina, India and Africa. In these same areas the seeds are also prepared for use both as external and internal medicines (Whiting, 1963).

The biologically active part of cycasin is its aglycone, methylazoxymethanol; this compound is also the aglycone of macrozamin (β'-verosyloxyazoxymethane), which was isolated by Cooper (1941) from the seeds of an Australian cycad, *Macrozamia spiralis*. Macrozamin occurs in the seeds of other Australian cycads (Riggs, 1954) and also in *Encephalartos barkeri* and *E. hildebrandtii*, which grow in East Africa, and in *E. transvenosus* and *E. lanatus*, which grow in South Africa (Tustin, 1974).

2.3 Analysis

A method for the quantitative determination of cycasin by gas-liquid chromatography after silylation was described by Wells *et al.* (1968). An alternative method is based on determination of the formaldehyde released after hydrolysis with chromotropic acid (Matsumoto & Strong, 1963).

3. Biological Data Relevant to the Evaluation of Carcinogenic Risk to Man

This section includes tests carried out with cycasin, its aglycone (methyazoxymethanol) or food products in which it is probably present.

3.1 Carcinogenicity and related studies in animals

(a) Oral administration

Mouse: Adult male C57BL/6 mice received single doses of 0.3, 0.5 and 1.0 mg/g bw cycasin by stomach tube. Of 35 mice that survived more than 4 months, 4 developed 5 tumours (2 hepatomas, 1 lung adenoma, 1 kidney adenoma and 1 fibroma of the back); no controls were used (Hirono *et al.*, 1969).

Rat: Long-term feeding of 1-3% cycad meal in the diet to male Osborne-Mendel rats for 100-250 days induced benign and malignant tumours of the liver (hepatocellular carcinomas and reticulo-endothelial tumours) and kidney (adenomas and sarcomas) in the 21 rats reported. One lung adenoma and 2 adenocarcinomas of the large intestine were also observed (Laqueur et al., 1963). In Sprague-Dawley and Osborne-Mendel rats, feeding of 200 and 400 mg pure cycasin per kg of diet or 1-2.5% cycad meal (containing 2.3% cycasin) in the diet for 6-9 months produced tumours in the same organs. Intestinal carcinomas were also produced by short-term exposure (2-21 days) to cycad meal (Laqueur, 1965). In groups of 10 male and 10 female Sprague-Dawley rats, feeding of 0.5% and 1% unprocessed dry cycad husk in the diet produced kidney tumours, hepatomas and liver carcinomas (Yang et al., 1968). Higher concentrations (5% and 10%) of fresh and dried cycad husk in the diet for 10-250 days produced carcinomas, sarcomas and Wilms' tumours of the kidney and cholangiomas and hepatomas of the liver (Hoch-Ligeti et al., 1968). In 3 groups of 15 Osborne-Mendel rats, continuous feeding of a home-made cycad flour from Guam, intended for human consumption, at concentrations of 1.5%, 5% or 10% of flour in the diet did not induce a significant increase in tumour incidences after 715 days as compared with those in 15 untreated controls; 34 treated rats survived at the end of the experiment (Yang et al., 1966).

A high incidence of liver tumours (described as hepatomas and sarcomas) was observed in 62/73 Sprague-Dawley rats of both sexes administered cycasin in the drinking-water for life (average intake, 10 mg/kg bw/day). Lung metastases of the hepatomas were observed in 9/35 cases; 16 kidney tumours (9 nephroblastomas and 7 adenocarcinomas) were also observed (Fukunishi et al., 1972).

In single-dose experiments in weanling Osborne-Mendel rats given cycasin by stomach tube, tumours of the kidney, intestine, liver, lung and brain (in that order of frequency) were found in animals that survived 6 months or more. Tumour incidences were: 4/13 at 100 mg/kg bw; 13/13 at 250 mg/kg bw; 6/6 at 500 mg/kg bw; 0/1 at 750 mg/kg bw; and 2/3 at 1000 mg/kg bw (Hirono et al., 1968). The morphology of cycasin-induced kidney tumours has been described (Gusek & Mestwerdt, 1969; Gusek et al., 1966; 1967).

Forty-one germ-free, male Sprague-Dawley rats received a sterile diet containing 200 mg cycasin per 100 g of diet for 20 days, after which they were fed the basal diet. Among 26 animals surviving for more than 1 year, the oldest being 772 days old at autopsy, 7 animals developed tumours;

according to the authors, the tumours were typical of those occurring in old, untreated rats of this strain and were not related to the treatment. No parallel control animals were kept (Laqueur et al., 1967).

Feeding of a lipid-soluble fraction of dried cycad nuts, reported to contain methylazoxymethanol, to 3 rats for 9 months produced hepatomas in 2 of the animals (Matsumoto & Strong, 1963).

Flour prepared from nuts of *Encephalartos hildebrandtii*, a plant of the family Cycadaceae, produced liver, kidney and lung tumours in rats to which it was fed. The carcinogenic activity observed was very similar to that produced by cycasin (Mugera, 1969; Mugera & Nderito, 1968a,b).

Hamster: Two-month-old hamsters were given single doses of 0.15 or 0.1 mg/g bw cycasin by stomach tube. Among 41 animals that survived more than 150 days, 23 tumours developed, including 2 liver-cell adenomas, 7 bile-duct carcinomas, 1 haemangioendothelial sarcoma, 5 lung adenomas, 4 intestinal tumours, 1 kidney carcinoma and 3 malignant lymphomas. Animals receiving the larger single dose had about twice as many tumours. Administration of 2-4 doses of 0.1 mg/g bw at 1-month intervals produced 19 tumours in 37 animals surviving 150 days or more. No difference in tumour frequency or tumour type was seen in the groups receiving single and repeated administrations. Two tumours (1 lung adenoma and 1 carcinoma of the colon) occurred in 13 control animals (Hirono et al., 1971).

Guinea-pig: Repeated feeding of 5% cycad meal in the diet for two to three 5-day periods produced hepatocellular carcinomas and bile-duct tumours in 9/27 animals killed between 44 and 62 weeks. No such tumours occurred in 90 controls (Spatz, 1964).

Rabbit: A group of 15 rabbits received weekly oral doses of 16.6 mg/animal cycasin by stomach tube for 27-33 weeks. Of 9 rabbits surviving 200 or more days, 7 developed haemangioendotheliomas of the liver. No controls were reported (Watanabe et al., 1975).

Fish: Feeding with cycad meal, or addition of cycasin to tank water, produced malignant neoplasms of the liver in the aquarium fish, *Brachydanio rerio* (Stanton, 1966).

Chicken: Feeding of 0.5% or 1% cycad kernel and husk for 28 and 68 weeks did not produce tumours attributable to the treatment (Sanger et al., 1969).

(b) Skin application

Mouse: C57BL mice were given 3-17 applications of an aqueous extract of cycad nut to skin artificially ulcerated by croton oil injection; tumours of the liver (1 haemangioendothelioma and 1 hepatoma) and kidney (3 adenomas) and one subcutaneous haemangioma at the site of application developed in 3/11 mice surviving 12-14 months. Fourteen croton oil-treated controls killed at the same time had not developed tumours of the liver or kidney (O'Gara et al., 1964).

(c) Subcutaneous and/or intramuscular administration

Newborn and suckling mice: Groups of C57BL/6 mice less than 24-hours-old (94 animals), or 2 (51), 4 (45), 7 (29) or 14 (35) days of age, were given single s.c. injections of 0.5 mg/g bw cycasin and observed for life. Of mice surviving 180 or more days, 3/19 mice injected at 14 days of age developed only reticulum-cell sarcomas after 403-480 days; no liver tumours were seen. In all other groups reticulum-cell sarcomas and liver tumours (described as liver-cell adenomas and hepatomas) were observed, the incidences of liver tumours being 10/12, 13/16, 7/11 and 11/26 in animals injected at less than 24 hours, at 2 days, at 4 days and at 7 days of age, respectively. One lung adenoma occurred among an unstated number of controls (Shibuya & Hirono, 1973).

S.c. administration of single doses of 0.5 mg/g bw cycasin to newborn C57Bl/6 mice and of 0.5 and 1.0 mg/g bw to newborn dd mice produced liver tumours in 50% of C57Bl/6 mice surviving more than 50 days and lung tumours in more than 80% and liver tumours in 40-60% of the dd mice that survived longer than 150 days (Hirono & Shibuya, 1970; Hirono et al., 1969).

Newborn rat: S.c. injection of a single dose of 2.5 mg cycasin per animal into newborn Fischer rats produced tumours of the kidney, liver, intestine, lung and brain in 46/55 animals surviving 6 months or more (Hirono et al., 1968).

Newborn hamster: Newborn hamsters received single s.c. injections of 0.2, 0.4 and 0.6 mg/g bw cycasin. Of 73 animals that survived longer than 150 days, 24 developed tumours, which were almost exclusively confined to the liver (Hirono et al., 1971).

(d) *Intraperitoneal injection*

Rat: Female Fischer rats given weekly i.p. injections of 2, 4 or 6 mg/animal methylazoxymethanol for 1-12 weeks developed a variety of tumours, principally of the liver, kidney and intestinal tract, within 371 days (Laqueur & Matsumoto, 1966). Similar results were obtained in germ-free and conventional male Sprague-Dawley rats (Laqueur et al., 1967).

Hamster: Repeated i.p. injections of 20 mg/kg bw methylazoxymethanol produced adenocarcinomas of the gall bladder and multiple carcinomas of the colon in 2/5 animals (Spatz et al., 1969).

(e) *Intravenous administration*

Hamster: A single i.v. injection of 20 mg/kg bw methylazoxymethanol produced multiple cystadenomas and other tumours of the liver in 28 animals reported and adenomas and adenocarcinomas of the colon in 22 animals (Spatz et al., 1969).

(f) *Other experimental systems*

Prenatal exposure: Crude cycad meal containing 1,3 or 5% cycasin was fed to pregnant Sprague-Dawley rats during the 1st, 2nd and 3rd week of gestation or throughout pregnancy. The overall tumour incidence in offspring surviving 6 months was 18.5% (15/81); frequent sites of neoplasia were the brain (gliomas) and jejunum. Five out of 9 mothers that survived 10-15 months developed tumours, mainly of the kidney, but also of the liver, colon, ovary, thymus and retroperitoneum (Spatz & Laquer, 1967).

Following i.p. or i.v. injections of 20 mg/kg bw methylazoxymethanol to Fischer rats on days 14-16 or 20-21 of pregnancy, gliomas, pulmonary adenomas, benign tumours of the jejunum, colon and rectum, sarcomas of the kidney and a transitional-cell carcinoma of the kidney were observed in offspring. The lung tumours occurred in offspring whose mothers were treated on day 21 of pregnancy. Colon-rectal, intestinal and kidney tumours also occurred in treated mothers (Laqueur & Spatz, 1973).

3.2 Other relevant biological data

The biological effects of cycasin and its aglycone, methylazoxymethanol, have been reviewed (Magee *et al.*, 1976).

The oral LD_{50} for cycasin in rats is 562 mg/kg bw (Spatz, 1969). With large doses of cycasin, centrilobular liver-cell necrosis accompanied by loss in RNA and phospholipids occurs (Williams & Laqueur, 1965). Hind-leg paralysis was observed after single s.c. injections of 0.5 mg/g bw cycasin in newborn C57Bl/6 mice (Hirono & Shibuya, 1967).

Following oral administration of cycasin to conventional and germ-free rats, only 24% was recovered in the urine and faeces of conventional rats compared with 100% in that of germ-free rats (Spatz *et al.*, 1966). In rats given 45-50 mg/animal by stomach tube, 30-63% of the administered dose was recovered in the urine. Following i.p. injection of 139 mg cycasin in rats, 95-100% of the injected dose was recovered from the urine within 24 hours (Kobayashi & Matsumoto, 1965). Following its oral administration to rats, cycasin is split by β-D-glucosidase of the bacterial flora to form methylazoxymethanol (Kobayashi & Matsumoto, 1965; Laqueur & Spatz, 1968). Enzymatic hydrolysis to methylazoxymethanol also occurs in the subcutaneous tissues of newborn mice and rats, which in the early postnatal period contain a glucosidase that disappears after the 14th-25th day of life (Shibuya & Hirono, 1973; Spatz, 1968).

Alkylation of nucleic acid by methylazoxymethanol *in vitro* and by cycasin *in vivo* were described by Matsumoto & Higa (1966) and Shank & Magee (1967).

Cycasin and methylazoxymethanol cross the placenta in rats and hamsters (Spatz & Laqueur, 1968; Spatz *et al.*, 1967). Malformations of the nervous system were observed in the foetuses of female hamsters injected with 20-23 mg/kg bw methylazoxymethanol on the 8th day of pregnancy. The females were sacrificed at the 12th day of pregnancy for examination of the foetuses (Spatz *et al.*, 1967).

Methylazoxymethanol, prepared by treating cycasin with β-glucosidase, was found to induce sex-linked recessive lethals when fed to *Drosophila melanogaster* males of the Canton S strain. Strong mutagenic effects were observed after uptake of 0.09 or 0.1 µg methylazoxymethanol per fly, but uptakes of 0.76 or 9.3 µg cycasin per fly were not mutagenic (Teas & Dyson, 1967).

Methylazoxymethanol derived from crystalline cycasin induced reverse mutations in *Salmonella typhimurium*, although the parent compound was inactive (Smith, 1966). Gabridge *et al.* (1969) showed that intestinal bacteria are involved in the formation of methylazoxymethanol from cycasin; they found, using a host-mediated assay, that prior treatment of Swiss mice with ampicillin, which reduces the enteric bacteria population, abolished the mutagenicity to *Salmonella typhimurium* G-46.

3.3 Observations in man

During 1959 the natives of Miyako Islands, Okinawa, subsisted mainly on cycads. Cancer mortality, and specifically hepatoma mortality, in these islands between 1961 and 1966 did not differ significantly from that in the interior of Japan and did not increase appreciably over that period. Mortality from cirrhosis was higher than that in mainland Japan, but this did not correlate positively with estimated levels of cycad intake within districts of the islands in 1959 (Hirono *et al.*, 1970).

4. Comments on Data Reported and Evaluation[1]

4.1 Animal data

Cycasin is carcinogenic in mice, rats, hamsters, guinea-pigs, rabbits and fish; it produced a variety of malignant tumours, mainly in the liver, kidney and intestine. It is carcinogenic in rats, hamsters, guinea-pigs, rabbits and fish following its oral administration. It is active in newborn and suckling mice and newborn rats and hamsters after its subcutaneous injection both in single doses and following prenatal exposure. The carcinogenicity of its aglycone, methylazoxymethanol, has been demonstrated in rats following its intraperitoneal administration and in hamsters

---

[1] See also the section "Animal Data in Relation to the Evaluation of Risk to Man" in the introduction to this volume, p. 15.

following its intraperitoneal or intravenous administration. The closely-related synthetic substance, methylazoxymethanol acetate, is carcinogenic in rats by various routes of administration (see Appendix).

4.2 Human data

The one epidemiological study reported showed no appreciable increase in cancer mortality 2 to 7 years after heavy intake of cycads. This negative result is insufficient to exclude a possible carcinogenic effect of cycasin in man. No case reports or other epidemiological studies of cancer in relation to exposure to cycasin or methylazoxymethanol were available to the Working Group.

APPENDIX

METHYLAZOXYMETHANOL ACETATE

A. Chemical and Physical Data

A.1 Synonyms and trade names

Chem. Abstr. Reg. Serial No.: 592-62-1

Chem. Abstr. Name: (Methyl-*ONN*-azoxy)methanol, acetate ester

MAM acetate

A.2 Chemical formula and molecular weight

$$CH_3-N=N-CH_2OCOCH_3$$
$$\quad\quad\;|$$
$$\quad\quad O$$

$C_4H_8N_2O_3$ Mol. wt: 132.1

A.3 Chemical and physical properties of the pure substance

(a) Description: Colourless liquid

(b) Boiling-point: 191°C

(c) Spectroscopy data: λ_{max} 215 nm; E_1^1 = 643 (Kobayashi & Matsumoto, 1965)

(d) Chemical reactivity: Easily hydrolysed, especially under alkaline conditions, to yield nitrogen, formaldehyde and methanol, among other products

B. Biological Data

(a) Oral administration

Rat: In 26 germ-free rats fed 100 mg methylazoxymethanol acetate per kg of diet for 2 weeks, with a cumulative dose of 13.4-13.7 mg/animal, 3 carcinomas of the colon, 8 bile-duct adenomas, 4 liver-cell adenomas, 1 hepatoma and 31 kidney tumours (adenomas, nephroblastomas, interstitial tumours) were observed within 201-475 days. A total dose of 12.5 mg/rat given as 4 administrations by stomach tube over 21 days to 5 rats produced 3 carcinomas of the colon or rectum and 1 bile-duct adenoma (Laqueur et al., 1967).

(b) Subcutaneous and/or intramuscular administration

Rat: A total dose of 12.5 mg/animal of methylazoxymethanol acetate given as 4 s.c. injections over 21 days produced 5 malignant tumours of the intestine and 1 bile-duct adenoma in 5 germ-free rats; no subcutaneous tumours were reported (Laqueur et al., 1967).

(c) Intraperitoneal administration

Rat: Four i.p. injections given over a period of 21 days (total dose, 12.5 mg/animal) produced 8 tumours of the intestine and 2 bile-duct adenomas in 4 germ-free rats (Laqueur et al., 1967).

(d) Intravenous administration

Mouse: No tumours were observed within 14 months in 19 CD1 male mice given single i.v. injections of 1-25 mg/kg bw methylazoxymethanol acetate (Zedeck et al., 1972).

Rat: Single i.v. injections of 35 mg/kg bw methylazoxymethanol acetate to rats produced intestinal, kidney and liver tumours after 6-7 months. Tumours of the small and large intestine were adenocarcinomas (Zedeck & Sternberg, 1974; Zedeck et al., 1970; 1972).

(e) Other experimental systems

Prenatal exposure: In the offspring of female Fischer rats treated with 20 mg/kg bw by i.p. or i.v. injection on days 5, 6, 13, 15 or 16 of pregnancy, 2 neurilemmomas, 1 pulmonary adenoma, 1 jejunal polyp, 2 lipomas of the kidney and 2 reticulum-cell sarcomas developed within 356-637 days after birth. Such tumours were not common in the offspring of untreated Fischer rats (Laqueur & Spatz, 1973).

Intrarectal administration: Daily infusion of 1 mg methylazoxymethanol acetate in water into the lumen of the large intestine in 27 male Donryu rats for 7-26 days produced a total of 59 adenocarcinomas of the large intestine, from the caecum to the rectum, in 22/24 rats surviving 25-54 weeks. Nephroblastomas were found in 7 rats (Narisawa & Nakano, 1973).

(f) Other relevant biological data

The i.p. LD_{50} in rats was 90 mg/kg bw (Spatz, 1969). In rats injected with ^{3}H-methylazoxymethanol acetate on day 14 of pregnancy, 4% of the injected radioactivity was found in the foetuses; radioactivity was also found in the liver and kidney of treated mothers. DNA and RNA from the foetal brain contained guanine methylated in the 7-position (Nagata & Matsumoto, 1969). Microencephaly was observed in 14- and 35-day-old offspring of female Long Evans rats injected i.p. on days 13, 14, 15, 16, 17 or 18 of pregnancy; this was most severe when injections were given on days 14 or 15 of gestation (Fischer *et al.*, 1972).

Methylazoxymethanol acetate reduced DNA synthesis in rat liver and kidney (Zedeck *et al.*, 1970) and inhibited nucleolar RNA synthesis in the liver (Zedeck *et al.*, 1972). Single strand breaks in the DNA from livers of treated rats were not repaired after 14 days (Damjanov *et al.*, 1973).

Doses of 0.047 and 0.054 μg methylazoxymethanol acetate were mutagenic in *Drosophila melanogaster* (Teas & Dyson, 1967).

5. References

Campbell, M.E., Mickelsen, O., Yang, M.G., Laqueur, G.L. & Keresztesy, J.C. (1966) Effects of strain, age and diet on the response of rats to the ingestion of *Cycas circinalis*. J. Nutr., 88, 115-124

Cooper, J.M. (1941) Isolation of a toxic principle from the seeds of *Macrozamia spiralis*. Proc. roy. Soc. N.S.W., 74, 450-454

Damjanov, I., Cox, R., Sarma, D.S.R. & Faber, E. (1973) Patterns of damage and repair of liver DNA induced by carcinogenic methylating agents *in vivo*. Cancer Res., 33, 2122-2128

Dastur, D.K. & Palekar, R.S. (1966) Effect of boiling and storing on cycasin content of *Cycas circinalis* L. Nature (Lond.), 210, 841-843

Fischer, M.H., Welker, C. & Waisman, H.A. (1972) Generalized growth retardation in rats induced by prenatal exposure to methylazoxymethanol acetate. Teratology, 5, 223-232

Fukunishi, R., Terashi, S.-I., Watanabe, K. & Kawaji, K. (1972) High yield of hepatic tumours in rats by cycasin. Gann, 63, 575-578

Gabridge, M.G., Denunzio, A. & Legator, M.S. (1969) Cycasin: detection of associated mutagenic activity *in vivo*. Science, 163, 689-691

Gusek, W. & Mestwerdt, W. (1969) Cycasin-induzierte Nierentumoren bei der Wistarratte unter besonderer Berücksichtigung der Adenome. Beitr. path. Anat., 139, 199-218

Gusek, W., Buss, H. & Krüger, C.H. (1966) Morphologische und histochemische Befunde an experimentellen Nierentumoren der Ratte. Verh. dtsch. Ges. Path., 50, 337-344

Gusek, W., Buss, H. & Laqueur, G.L. (1967) Histologisch-histochemische Untersuchungen am 'Interstitiellen Cycasin-Tumor' der Rattenniere. Beitr. path. Anat., 135, 53-74

Hirono, I. & Shibuya, C. (1967) Induction of a neurological disorder by cycasin in mice. Nature (Lond.), 216, 1311-1312

Hirono, I. & Shibuya, C. (1970) High incidence of pulmonary tumours in dd mice by a single injection of cycasin. Gann, 61, 403-407

Hirono, I., Laqueur, G.L. & Spatz, M. (1968) Tumor induction in Fischer and Osborne-Mendel rats by a single administration of cycasin. J. nat. Cancer Inst., 40, 1003-1010

Hirono, I., Shibuya, C. & Fushimi, K. (1969) Tumor induction in C57BL/6 mice by a single administration of cycasin. Cancer Res., 29, 1658-1662

Hirono, I., Kachi, H. & Kato, T. (1970) A survey of acute toxicity of cycads and mortality rate from cancer in the Miyako Islands, Okinawa. Acta path. jap., 20, 327-337

Hirono, I., Hayashi, K., Mori, H. & Miwa, T. (1971) Carcinogenic effects of cycasin in Syrian golden hamsters and the transplantability of induced tumors. Cancer Res., 31, 283-287

Hoch-Ligeti, C., Stutzman, E. & Arvin, J.M. (1968) Cellular composition during tumor induction in rats by cycad husk. J. nat. Cancer Inst., 41, 605-614

IARC (1972) IARC Monograph on the Evaluation of Carcinogenic Risk of Chemicals to Man, 1, Lyon, pp. 145-156

Kobayashi, A. & Matsumoto, H. (1965) Studies on methylazoxymethanol, the aglycone of cycasin. Arch. Biochem., 110, 373-380

Laqueur, G.L. (1965) The induction of intestinal neoplasms in rats with the glycoside cycasin and its aglycone. Virchows Arch. path. Anat., 340, 151-163

Laqueur, G.L. & Matsumoto, H. (1966) Neoplasms in female Fischer rats following intraperitoneal injection of methylazoxymethanol. J. nat. Cancer Inst., 37, 217-232

Laqueur, G.L. & Spatz, M. (1968) Toxicology of cycasin. Cancer Res., 28, 2262-2267

Laqueur, G.L. & Spatz, M. (1973) Transplacental induction of tumours and malformations in rats with cycasin and methylazoxymethanol. In: Tomatis, L. & Mohr, U., eds, Transplacental Carcinogenesis, IARC Scientific Publications, No. 4, Lyon, IARC

Laqueur, G.L., Mickelsen, O., Whiting, M.G. & Kurland, L.T. (1963) Carcinogenic properties of nuts from *Cycas circinalis* L. indigenous to Guam. J. nat. Cancer Inst., 31, 919-933

Laqueur, G.L., McDaniel, E.G. & Matsumoto, H. (1967) Tumor induction in germ-free rats with methylazoxymethanol (MAM) and synthetic MAM acetate. J. nat. Cancer Inst., 39, 355-371

Magee, P.N., Montesano, R. & Preussmann, R. (1976) N-Nitroso compounds and related carcinogens. In: Searle, C.E., ed. Chemical Carcinogens, Washington DC, American Chemical Society (in press)

Matsumoto, H. & Higa, H.H. (1966) Studies on methylazoxymethanol, the aglycone of cycasin: methylation of nucleic acids *in vitro*. Biochem. J., 98, 20C-22C

Matsumoto, H. & Strong, F.M. (1963) The occurrence of methylazoxymethanol in *Cycas circinalis* L. Arch. Biochem. Biophys., 101, 299-310

Mugera, G.M. (1969) Induction of kidney tumours in rats by feeding *Encephalartos hildebrandtii* for short periods. Brit. J. Cancer, 23, 755-756

Mugera, G.M. & Nderito, P. (1968a) Toxic properties of *Encephalartos hildebrandtii*. E. Afr. med. J., 45, 732-741

Mugera, G.M. & Nderito, P. (1968b) Tumours of the liver, kidney and lungs in rats fed *Encephalartos hildebrandtii*. Brit. J. Cancer, 22, 563-568

Nagata, Y. & Matsumoto, H. (1969) Studies on methylazoxymethanol: methylation of nucleic acids in the fetal rat brain. Proc. Soc. exp. Biol. (N.Y.), 132, 383-385

Narisawa, T. & Nakano, H. (1973) Carcinoma of the large intestine of rats induced by rectal infusion of methylazoxymethanol. Gann, 64, 93-95

Nishida, K., Kobayashi, A. & Nagahama, T. (1955) Studies on cycasin, a new toxic glycoside of *Cycas revoluta* Thunb. I. Isolation and the structure of cycasin. Bull. agric. chem. Soc. Japan, 19, 77-84

O'Gara, R.W., Brown, J.M. & Whiting, M.G. (1964) Induction of hepatic and renal tumours by topical application of aqueous extract of cycad nut to artificial skin ulcers in mice. Fed. Proc., 23, 1383

Palekar, R.S. & Dastur, D.K. (1965) Cycasin content of *Cycas circinalis*. Nature (Lond.), 206, 1363-1365

Riggs, N.V. (1954) The occurrence of macrozamin in the seeds of cycads. Austr. J. Chem., 7, 123-124

Riggs, N.V. (1956) Glucosyloxyazoxymethane, a constituent of the seeds of *Cycas circinalis* L. Chemistry & Industry, September 8, p. 926

Sanger, V.L., Yang, M.G. & Mickelsen, O. (1969) Cycad toxicosis in chickens. J. nat. Cancer Inst., 43, 391-395

Shank, R.C. & Magee, P.N. (1967) Similarities between the biochemical actions of cycasin and dimethylnitrosamine. Biochem. J., 105, 521-527

Shibuya, C. & Hirono, I. (1973) Relations between postnatal days of mice and carcinogenic effect of cycasin. Gann, 64, 109-110

Smith, D.W.E. (1966) Mutagenicity of cycasin aglycone (methylazoxymethanol), a naturally occurring carcinogen. Science, 152, 1273-1274

Spatz, M. (1964) Carcinogenic effect of cycad meal in guinea pigs. Fed. Proc., 23, 1384-1385

Spatz, M. (1968) Hydrolysis of cycasin by β-D-glucosidase in skin of newborn rats. Proc. Soc. exp. Biol. (N.Y.), 128, 1005-1008

Spatz, M. (1969) Toxic and carcinogenic alkylating agents from cycads. Ann. N.Y. Acad. Sci., 163, 848-859

Spatz, M. & Laqueur, G.L. (1967) Transplacental induction of tumors in Sprague-Dawley rats with crude cycad material. J. nat. Cancer Inst., 38, 233-245

Spatz, M. & Laqueur, G.L. (1968) Transplacental chemical induction of microencephaly in two strains of rats. Proc. Soc. exp. Biol. (N.Y.), 129, 705-710

Spatz, M., McDaniel, E.G. & Laqueur, G.L. (1966) Cycasin excretion in conventional and germ free rats. Proc. Soc. exp. Biol. (N.Y.), 121, 417-422

Spatz, M., Dougherty, W.J. & Smith, D.W.E. (1967) Teratogenic effects of methylazoxymethanol. Proc. Soc. exp. Biol. (N.Y.), 124, 476-478

Spatz, M., Laqueur, G.L. & Holmes, J.M. (1969) Carcinogenic effects of methylazoxymethanol (MAM) in hamsters. Proc. Amer. Ass. Cancer Res., 10, 86

Stanton, M.F. (1966) Hepatic neoplasms of aquarium fish exposed to *Cycas circinalis*. Fed. Proc., 25, 661

Teas, H.J. & Dyson, J.G. (1967) Mutation in *Drosophila* by methylazoxymethanol, the aglycone of cycasin. Proc. Soc. exp. Biol. (N.Y.), 125, 988-990

Tustin, R.C. (1974) Toxicity and carcinogenicity of some South African cycad (*Encephalartos*) species. S. Afr. med. J., 48, 2369-2373

Watanabe, K., Iwashita, H., Muta, K., Hamada, Y. & Hamada, K. (1975) Hepatic tumors of rabbits induced by cycad extract. Gann, 66, 335-339

Wells, W.W., Yang, M.G., Bolzer, W. & Mickelsen, O. (1968) Gas-liquid chromatographic analysis of cycasin in cycad flour. Analyt. Biochem., 25, 325-329

Whiting, M.G. (1963) Toxicity of cycads. Econ. Bot., 17, 271-302

Williams, J.N., Jr & Laqueur, G.L. (1965) Response of liver nucleic acids and lipids in rats fed *Cycas circinalis* L. endosperm or cycasin. Proc. Soc. exp. Biol. (N.Y.), 118, 1-4

Yang, M.G., Mickelsen, O., Campbell, M.E., Laqueur, G.L. & Keresztesy, J.C. (1966) Cycad flour used by Guamanians: effects produced in rats by long-term feeding. J. Nutr., 90, 153-156

Yang, M.G., Sanger, V.L., Mickelsen, O. & Laqueur, G.L. (1968) Carcinogenicity of long-term feeding of cycad husk to rats. Proc. Soc. exp. Biol. (N.Y.), 127, 1171-1175

Zedeck, M.S. & Sternberg, S.S. (1974) A model system for studies of colon carcinogenesis: tumour induction by a single injection of methylazoxymethanol acetate. J. nat. Cancer Inst., 53, 1419-1421

Zedeck, M.S., Sternberg, S.S., Poynter, R.W. & McGowan, J. (1970) Biochemical and pathological effects of methylazoxymethanol acetate, a potent carcinogen. Cancer Res., 30, 801-812

Zedeck, M.S., Sternberg, S.S., McGowan, J. & Poynter, R.W. (1972) Methylazoxymethanol acetate; induction of tumours and early effects on RNA synthesis. Fed. Proc., 31, 1485-1492

CYCLOCHLOROTINE

The chemical and biological properties of this substance have been reviewed recently (Enomoto & Ueno, 1974).

1. Chemical and Physical Data

1.1 Synonyms and trade names

Chem. Abstr. Reg. Serial No.: 12663-46-6

Chem. Abstr. Name: Cyclochlorotine

Chlorine-containing cyclic penta-peptide of *Penicillium islandicum*; islanditoxin

1.2 Chemical formula and molecular weight

$C_{24}H_{31}N_5O_7Cl_2$ Mol. wt: 572.5

1.3 Chemical and physical properties of the pure substance

(a) Description: White needles

(b) Melting-point: 251°C (decomposition)

(c) Optical rotation: $[\alpha]_D^{16}$ -92.9° (in ethanol)

(d) Spectroscopy data: λ_{max} 257 nm (E_1^1 = 9.81)
Ammonolysis causes a characteristic increase in ultra-violet absorption at 268 nm (Ishikawa et al., 1970); for infra-red spectral data see Enomoto & Ueno (1974).

(e) <u>Solubility</u>: Soluble in water and *n*-butanol

(f) <u>Reactivity</u>: The compound shows a positive biuret reaction, but is negative in the Sakaguchi test, the ninhydrin reaction or with Millon's reagent (Enomoto & Ueno, 1974).

1.4 Technical products and impurities

No data were available to the Working Group.

2. Production, Use, Occurrence and Analysis

2.1 Production and use

Cyclochlorotine is not produced commercially.

2.2 Occurrence

Cyclochlorotine and several other mycotoxins are produced in culture by *Penicillium islandicum* Sopp. (Uraguchi *et al.*, 1961). Although there are no data based upon direct chemical analysis concerning the occurrence of cyclochlorotine in foods, *P. islandicum* has occasionally been reported as one of the major isolates from various grains in Japan (Miyaki *et al.*, 1970; Tsunoda, 1968), from the staple diet in Ethiopia (Pavlica & Samuel, 1970), from barley (Carnaghan, 1966/67) and from prepared foodstuffs in South Africa (Martin *et al.*, 1971).

2.3 Analysis

A method of isolation and subsequent determination by spectrophotometry from the ammonolysis reaction products has been described (Ishikawa *et al.*, 1970).

3. Biological Data Relevant to the Evaluation of Carcinogenic Risk to Man

3.1 Carcinogenicity and related studies in animals

Oral administration

<u>Mouse</u>: Groups of 20 male ddNi mice were fed 40 or 60 µg cyclochlorotine/animal/day for life. No liver-cell tumours were observed in mice given 40 µg; but of 14 mice surviving the higher dose for 200-700 days,

1 developed a liver carcinoma of a differentiated type and 2 developed liver-cell adenomas. Reticuloendotheliomas were found in 1 mouse given 40 µg and in 2 mice given 60 µg. No liver-cell tumours or reticuloendotheliomas were observed in 19 male controls, 10 of which survived 400 days and 2 of which survived at 700 days (Uraguchi et al., 1972).

3.2 Other relevant biological data

The LD_{50}'s of cyclochlorotine in male mice were 0.33 mg/kg bw following i.v. injection, 0.47 mg/kg bw following s.c. injection and 6.55 mg/kg bw following oral administration. Signs of cyclochlorotine intoxication in mice and rats were respiratory and circulatory disturbances, followed by convulsions; death occurred in less than 24 hours in most cases (Uraguchi et al., 1961; 1972). Mice intoxicated with cyclochlorotine developed initial hyperglycaemia, a rapid fall of liver glycogen, decreased levels of succinic dehydrogenase and inhibition of oxidative phosphorylation (Hara, 1964).

Cyclochlorotine causes peripheral damage to the liver lobule; the endothelial (Kupffer) cells of the sinusoids are also sensitive, and vacuolation, degeneration and nuclear damage are observed in these cells (Saito, 1959). Cyclochlorotine is a cirrhogenic agent, producing fibrosis or cirrhosis of the periportal type (Enomoto & Saito, 1973; Uraguchi et al., 1972).

Orally administered tritium-labelled cyclochlorotine appeared rapidly in the liver, and 73% of the dose was excreted in the urine (Uraguchi, 1971).

3.3 Observations in man

No data were available to the Working Group.

4. Comments on Data Reported and Evaluation[1]

4.1 Animal data

Cyclochlorotine is carcinogenic in male mice following its oral administration, the only species, sex and route of administration tested; it produced liver tumours and reticuloendotheliomas.

4.2 Human data

No case reports or epidemiological studies were available to the Working Group.

---

[1]See also section "Animal Data in Relation to the Evaluation of Risk to Man" in the introduction to this volume, p. 15.

5. References

Carnaghan, R.B.A. (1966/67) Mycotoxicoses. In: Pool, W.A., ed., The Veterinary Annual, 8th year, Bristol, John Wright & Sons, pp. 84-93

Enomoto, M. & Saito, M. (1973) Experimentally induced chronic liver injuries by the metabolites of *Penicillium islandicum* Sopp. Acta path. jap., 23, 655-666

Enomoto, M. & Ueno, I. (1974) *Penicillium islandicum* (toxic yellowed rice) - luteoskyrin - islanditoxin - cyclochlorotine. In: Purchase, I.F.H., ed., Mycotoxins, Amsterdam, Elsevier, pp. 302-326

Hara, M. (1964) Mechanism of the toxic effects of chlorine-containing peptide (Islanditoxin) produced by *Penicillium islandicum* Sopp. grown on yellow rice. Part II. Alterations of permeability of the sinusoidal wall and the liver cell membrane in the acute liver injury. Tokyo Igaku Zasshi, 72, 136, 165

Ishikawa, I., Ueno, Y. & Tsunoda, J. (1970) Chemical determination of the chlorine-containing peptide, a hepatotoxic mycotoxin of *Penicillium islandicum* Sopp. J. Biochem., 67, 753-758

Martin, P.M.D., Gilman, G.A. & Keen, P. (1971) The incidence of fungi in foodstuffs and their significance, based on a survey in the eastern Transvaal and Swaziland. In: Purchase, I.F.H., ed., Mycotoxins in Human Health, London, Basingstoke, Macmillan, pp. 281-290

Miyaki, K., Yamazaki, M., Horie, Y. & Udagawa, S. (1970) Toxigenic fungi growing on stored rice. J. Fd Hyg. Soc. Japan., 11, 373-380

Pavlica, D. & Samuel, I. (1970) Primary carcinoma of the liver in Ethiopia. Brit. J. Cancer, 24, 22-29

Saito, M. (1959) Liver cirrhosis induced by metabolites of *Penicillium islandicum* Sopp. Acta path. jap., 9, 785-790

Tsunoda, H. (1968) Micro-organisms which deteriorate stored cereals and grains. In: Herzberg, M., ed., Proceedings of the First US-Japan Conference on Toxic Microorganisms, Mycotoxins, Botulism, Washington DC, US Department of Interior, p. 143

Uraguchi K. (1971) Pharmacology of mycotoxins. In: Raskova, H., ed., International Encyclopedia of Pharmacology and Therapeutics, Oxford, Pergamon, pp. 143-298

Uraguchi, K., Tatsuno, T., Sakai, F., Tsukioka, M., Sakai, Y., Yonemitsu, O., Ito, H., Miyake, M., Saito, M., Enomoto, M., Shikata, T. & Ishiko, T. (1961) Isolation of two toxic agents, luteoskyrin and chlorine-containing peptide, from the metabolites of *Penicillium islandicum* Sopp., with some properties thereof. Japan. J. exp. Med., 31, 19-46

Uraguchi, K., Saito, M., Noguchi, Y., Takahasi, K., Enomoto, M. & Tatsuno, T. (1972) Chronic toxicity and carcinogenicity in mice of the purified mycotoxins, luteoskyrin and cyclochlorotine. Fd Cosmet. Toxicol., 10, 193-207

DAUNOMYCIN

See also monograph on adriamycin, a closely related compound.

1. Chemical and Physical Data

1.1 Synonyms and trade names

Chem. Abstr. Reg. Serial No.: 20830-81-3

Chem. Abstr. Name: (8S-*cis*)-8-Acetyl-10-[(3-amino-2,3,6-trideoxy-α-L-lyxohexapyranosyl)oxy]-7,8,9,10-tetrahydro-6,8,11-trihydroxy-1-methoxy-5,12-naphthacenedione

8-Acetyl-10-[(3-amino-2,3,6-trideoxy-α-L-lyxohexapyranosyl)oxy]-7,8,9,10-tetrahydro-6,8,11-trihydroxy-1-methoxy-(8S,10S)-5,12-naphthacenedione; 3-acetyl-1,2,3,4,6,11-hexahydro-3,5,12-trihydroxy-10-methoxy-6,11-dioxo-1-naphthacenyl-3-amino-2,3,6-trideoxy-α-L-lyxohexapyranoside(1S,3S); NSC 82151*; RP 13057; rubidomycin

Cerubidine (as the hydrochloride); Daunorubicin; Daunorubicine; Rubomycin C; Rubomycin C$_1$

1.2 Chemical formula and molecular weight

$C_{27}H_{29}NO_{10}$ Mol. wt: 527.5

1.3 Chemical and physical properties of the pure substance

(a) Description: Thin, red needles

---

* Cancer Chemotherapy National Service Centre Number, NCI, NIH, USA

(b) <u>Melting-point</u>: 188-190°C (decomposition)

(c) <u>Spectroscopy data</u>: λ_{max} 234 nm; E^1_1 = 711
    252   494
    290   163
    480   227
    495   214
    532   119

(d) <u>Identity and purity test</u>: The characteristic ultra-violet spectrum and a colour change from pink at acid pH to blue at alkaline pH can be used for identification purposes. Mild acid hydrolysis yields the red aglycone, daunomycinone, and an amino sugar, daunosamine.

(e) <u>Solubility</u>: The hydrochloride is soluble in water, methanol and aqueous alcohols; practically insoluble in chloroform, ether and benzene

(f) <u>Stability</u>: Aqueous solutions are stable for one month at 5°C; unstable at higher temperatures or at acid or alkaline pH's

(g) <u>Reactivity</u>: The aglycone can be reduced by sodium borohydride; subsequent periodate oxidation yields benzaldehyde.

1.4 Technical products and impurities

Daunomycin is available either in lyophilized form or in vials ready for injection (Bernard *et al.*, 1969).

2. Production, Use, Occurrence and Analysis

For important background information on this section, see preamble, p. 17. A review on daunomycin has been published (Bernard *et al.*, 1969).

2.1 Production and use

Daunomycin was isolated in the early 1960's independently in two industrial research laboratories in France and Italy. Both of these companies produce the drug by fermentation processes (Perlman, 1974). It is produced by *Streptomyces caeruleorubidus* obtained from soil samples from various sources by the classic procedures of submerged fermentation (Bernard et al., 1969).

Daunomycin was produced in Japan in quantities of 487 g in 1973 and 588 g in 1972 (Japan Antibiotics Research Association, 1974; 1975). Commercial sales in Japan began in 1970 (Fukai, 1974). It is also produced and used in the USSR.

The first clinical trials were carried out in France in 1965. Initially, only refractory cases of acute leukaemia were treated, but 800 patients were treated between 1965 and 1968. The first clinical trials on solid tumours were made in the US (Bernard et al., 1969). The average dose is 0.5-3 mg/kg bw daily, administered intravenously. The total cumulative dose is limited to 25-30 mg/kg bw administered over a period of six months (Bernard et al., 1969).

2.2 Occurrence

Daunomycin is obtained from cultures of *Streptomyces caeruleorubidus* and *Streptomyces peucetius*, which occur in soil. The extent of its natural occurrence from these organisms is not known.

2.3 Analysis

Details of thin-layer chromatographic procedures are to be found in the monograph on adriamycin (see p. 45). A radioimmunoassay for its determination in blood and tissues of experimental animals has been described (Van Vunakis et al., 1974).

Daunomycin has been estimated by fluorimetric techniques in serum and urine by Finkel et al. (1969), with a detection limit of 0.05 µg, and in animal tissues by Schwartz (1973), at a range of 0.2-10 µg.

3. Biological Data Relevant to the Evaluation of Carcinogenic Risk to Man

3.1 Carcinogenicity and related studies in animals

(a) Oral administration

Mouse: A group of 20 male and 20 female C57Bl/Rho mice received weekly oral doses of 12.5 mg/kg bw daunomycin for 22 weeks; 20 male and

20 female controls were used. In mice surviving 16-22 months after the start of the experiment, the incidence of reticulosarcomas or leukaemia was 4/19 in treated mice, compared with 12/35 in controls. The incidences of other tumours were reported to be similar in treated and control animals (Bernard et al., 1969).

(b) Subcutaneous and/or intramuscular administration

Mouse: A group of 20 male and 20 female XVII/Rho mice received weekly s.c. injections of 1.25 mg/kg bw daunomycin in distilled water for 12 weeks; a group of 20 male and 20 female controls received distilled water. All surviving mice were killed 22 months after the start of the experiment, and local sarcomas were found in 5 males and 5 females, but none in controls. The incidences of other tumours were not increased (Bernard et al., 1969).

(c) Intravenous administration

Rat: A group of 25 female Sprague-Dawley rats was given single i.v. injections of 12.5 mg/kg bw daunomycin. During the following year 14 rats died, 2 with malignant tumours. All rats killed at 12 months had tumours, including 11 mammary adenocarcinomas and 2 fibroadenomas (1 rhabdomyosarcoma of the thigh and 1 uterine polyp). The mean induction time was 121 days. None of the 25 control rats developed tumours within the 12-month period (Bertazzoli et al., 1971).

Groups of 20 female Sprague-Dawley rats were given single i.v. injections of 5, 10 or 20 mg/kg bw daunomycin or saline (controls) and observed for up to 12 months. All rats which received the highest dose died or were killed before 52 days due to chronic glomerulonephritis. In the group given 10 mg/kg bw, 9 rats were killed after 6 months, 2 after 10 months and 3 after 1 year; in the group given 5 mg/kg bw, 1 rat was killed after 7 months, 3 after 10 months and 15 at 1 year; all control rats were killed between 10-12 months. Of the treated rats 16/33 developed a total of 27 tumours, compared with 5/20 controls. Five tubular adenomas and two clear-cell carcinomas of the kidney were found in treated rats between 189-365 days; no such tumours were found in controls (Sternberg et al., 1972).

3.2 Other relevant biological data

The LD_{50}'s of daunomycin in GS mice were 5.6 mg/kg bw following i.p. injection and 47.0 mg/kg bw by s.c. injection. There appears to be considerable species variation with regard to the toxicity of daunomycin. The maximum tolerated i.v. dose in mice given 5 treatments on successive days with an observation period of 1 month was 8.7 mg/kg bw (Dubost et al., 1963). After 15 treatments consisting of daily i.v. doses of 2 mg/kg bw for 3 days and 3 days without treatment, all of 4 treated monkeys died after 9, 9, 7 and 6 doses. All monkeys given 0.5 or 1 mg/kg bw in the same way as above survived the 15 treatments (Prieur et al., 1972). In dogs, 1 mg/kg bw caused severe bone-marrow aplasia followed by death (Di Marco, 1967).

Doses of 12-50 mg/kg bw caused bradycardia, hypotension, ventricular arrhythmias and respiratory depression in hamsters and rhesus monkeys (Herman et al., 1971). The drug has immunosuppressive activity in mice (Gericke & Chandra, 1973).

In male Sprague-Dawley rats given 10 mg/kg daunomycin hydrochloride by i.v. injection, 16% was excreted in the bile and approximately 6% in the urine within 8 hours. Daunorubicinol was the major metabolite detected in the bile (8.8% of the injected dose); the remaining fluorescent biliary substances consisted of daunomycin (5.3%), polar metabolites (2.5%) and aglycones or non-polar metabolites (0.2%). Eight hours after administration, the spleen contained the highest concentration of total daunomycin fluorescence, while the brain had the lowest. Aglycone levels were highest in liver, spleen and small intestine (Craddock et al., 1973). In Syrian golden hamsters, daunomycin hydrochloride is metabolized primarily in the liver to deoxydaunorubicinol aglycone (Bachur et al., 1973).

Daunomycin complexes strongly with DNA, maximal binding being in the region of 0.013 molecules/DNA nucleotide, and the drug inhibits both DNA and RNA polymerases in *in vitro* systems. Incorporation of nucleic acid precursors into RNA and DNA of leukaemia L-1210 cells is inhibited by 5 μmols daunomycin (Tatsumi et al., 1974; Zunino et al., 1975).

Daunomycin hydrochloride induces high frequencies of reverse mutations in *Salmonella typhimurium* (McCann et al., 1975).

In man, nausea and vomiting together with leucopenia occur after administration of 70 mg/m^2 daunomycin (Serpik & Henderson, 1967) Daunomycin therapy is associated with cardiac toxicity, and fatal disturbances of cardiac function have been reported (Bonadonna & Monfordini, 1969).

Metabolites identified in human urine are daunorubicinol, daunorubicinol aglycone, deoxydaunorubicinol aglycone, deoxydaunomycin aglycone, desmethyldeoxydaunorubicinol aglycone, desmethyldeoxyrubicinol aglycone-4-O-sulphate, desmethyldeoxydaunorubicinol aglycone-4-O-glucuronide and deoxydaunorubicinol aglycone glucuronide (Takanashi & Bachur, 1974). Daunomycin can be converted to daunorubicinol by lymphocyte cytoplasm in a NADPH-dependent reaction (Huffman & Bachur, 1972).

Daunomycin did not induce unscheduled DNA synthesis in cultured human fibroblasts (San & Stich, 1975). At a concentration of 0.01 µg/ml it induced high frequencies of chromosome and chromatid breaks and translocations in cultures of human peripheral leucocytes (Vig et al., 1968).

3.3 Observations in man

No data were available to the Working Group.

4. Comments on Data Reported and Evaluation[1]

4.1 Animal data

Daunomycin is carcinogenic in rats following intravenous injection of single doses and in mice following its repeated subcutaneous injection; it produced mammary and kidney tumours in rats and local sarcomas in mice. No carcinogenic effect was observed in one oral study in mice.

4.2 Human data

No case reports or epidemiological studies were available to the Working Group.

---

[1] See also the section "Animal Data in Relation to the Evaluation of Risk to Man" in the introduction to this volume, p. 15.

5. References

Bachur, N.R., Egorin, M.J. & Hildebrand, R.C. (1973) Daunorubicin and adriamycin metabolism in the golden Syrian hamster. Biochem. Med., 8, 352-361

Bernard, J., Paul, R., Boiron, M., Jacquillat, C. & Maral, R. (1969) Rubidomycin. A new agent against cancer. Recent Results Cancer Res., 20, 1-178

Bertazzoli, C., Chieli, T. & Solcia, E. (1971) Different incidence of breast carcinomas or fibroadenomas in daunomycin or adriamycin treated rats. Experientia, 27, 1209-1210

Bonadonna, G. & Monfordini, S. (1969) Cardiac toxicity of dauncrubicin. Lancet, i, 837-838

Craddock, J.C., Egorin, M.J. & Bachur, N.R. (1973) Daunorubicin biliary excretion and metabolism in the rat. Arch. int. Pharmacodyn., 202, 48-61

Di Marco, A. (1967) Daunomycin and related antibiotics. In: Gottlieb, D. & Shaw, P.D., eds, Antibiotics, Vol. 1, Mechanism of Action, Berlin, Springer-Verlag, pp. 190-210

Dubost, M., Ganter, P., Maral, R., Ninet, L., Pinnert, S., Preud'homme, J. & Werner, G.H. (1963) Un nouvel antibiotique à propriétés cytostatiques; la rubidomycine. C.R. Acad. Sci. (Paris), 257, 1813-1815

Finkel, J.M., Knapp, K.T. & Mulligan, L.T. (1969) Fluorometric determination of serum levels and urinary excretion of daunomycin (NSC 82151) in mice and rats. Cancer Chemother. Rep., 53, 159-164

Fukai, S. (1974) Today's new medicinals, Tokyo, Yakuji Daily News, January 20, p. 654

Gericke, D. & Chandra, P. (1973) Immunosuppressive activity of some new cytostatic agents. Z. Krebsforsch., 79, 277-282

Herman, E., Mhatre, R., Lee, I.P., Vick, J. & Waravdekar, V.S. (1971) A comparison of the cardiovascular actions of daunomycin, adriamycin and N-acetyldaunomycin in hamster and monkeys. Pharmacology, 6, 230-241

Huffman, D.H. & Bachur, N.R. (1972) Daunorubicin metabolism by human haematological components. Cancer Res., 32, 600-605

Japan Antibiotics Research Association (1974) The Japanese Journal of Antibiotics, Vol. 27, p. 252

Japan Antibiotics Research Association (1975) The Japanese Journal of Antibiotics, Vol. 28, p. 100

McCann, J., Choi, E., Yamasaki, E. & Ames, B.N. (1975) Detection of carcinogens as mutagens in the *Salmonella*/microsome test: assay of 300 chemicals. Proc. nat. Acad. Sci. (Wash.), 72, 5135-5139

Perlman, D. (1974) Prospects for the fermentation industries, 1974-1983, Chemtech, April, pp. 211, 216

Prieur, D.J., Young, D.M. & Davis, R.D. (1972) Daunomycin (NSC 82151): pre-clinical toxicological evaluation of single daily intravenous injections in monkeys for 3 days followed by a 3-day no-treatment period. US nat. techn. Inform. Serv. PB Rep., No. 211673, Washington DC, US Government Printing Office

San, R.H.C. & Stich, H.F. (1975) DNA repair synthesis of cultured human cells as a rapid bioassay for chemical carcinogens. Int. J. Cancer, 16, 284-291

Schwartz, H.S. (1973) A fluorometric assay for daunomycin and adriamycin in animal tissues. Biochem. Med., 7, 396-404

Serpik, A. & Henderson, E.S. (1967) Observations on toxicity and clinical trials with daunomycin. Path. Biol., 15, 909-912

Sternberg, S.S., Philips, F.S. & Cronin, A.P. (1972) Renal tumours and other lesions in rats following a single intravenous injection of daunomycin. Cancer Res., 32, 1029-1036

Takanashi, S. & Bachur, N.R. (1974) New adriamycin and daunorubicin metabolites in human urine. Proc. Amer. Ass. Cancer Res., 15, 76

Tatsumi, K., Nakamura, T. & Wakisaka, G. (1974) Comparative effects of daunomycin and adriamycin on nucleic acid metabolism in leukemic cells *in vitro*. Gann, 65, 237-247

Van Vunakis, H., Langone, J.J., Riceberg, L.J. & Levine, L. (1974) Radio-immunoassays for adriamycin and daunomycin. Cancer Res., 34, 2546-2552

Vig, B.K., Kontras, S.B., Paddock, E.F. & Samuels, L.D. (1968) Daunomycin-induced chromosome aberrations and the influence of arginine in modifying the effect of the drug. Mutation Res., 5, 278

Zunino, H., Gambetta, R. & Di Marco, A. (1975) The inhibition *in vitro* of DNA polymerase and RNA polymerases by daunomycin and adriamycin. Biochem. Pharmacol., 24, 309-311

GRISEOFULVIN

1. Chemical and Physical Data

1.1 Synonyms and trade names

Chem. Abstr. Reg. Serial No.: 126-07-8

Chem. Abstr. Name: (2-S-*trans*)-7-Chloro-2',4,6-trimethoxy-6'-methylspiro[benzofuran-2(3*H*),1'-(2)-cyclohexene]-3,4'-dione

7-Chloro-4,6-dimethoxycoumaran-3-one-2-spiro-1'-(2'-methoxy-6'-methyl-cyclohex-2'-en-4'-one); 7-chloro-2',4,6-trimethoxy-6'β-methylspiro[benzofuran-2(3*H*),1'-(2)-cyclohexene]-3,4'-dione; 7-chloro-2',4,6-trimethoxy-6'-methyl-(2S-*trans*)-spiro[benzofuran-2*H*(3*H*),1'-(2)-cyclohexene]-3,4'-dione; curling factor; griscofulvin; (+)-griseofulvin; grisofulvin

Amudane; Biogrisin-FP; Delmofulvina; Fulcin; Fulcine; Fulvicin; Fulvina; Fungivin; Fulvistatin; Greosin; Gricin; Grifulvin; Grisactin; Grisefuline; Griseo; Grisetin; Grisovin; Grysio; Guservin; Lamoryl; Likuden; Neo-Fulcin; NSC 34533*; Poncyl; Spirofulvin; Sporostatin

1.2 Chemical formula and molecular weight

$C_{17}H_{17}ClO_6$ Mol. wt: 352.8

1.3 Chemical and physical properties of the pure substance

(a) Description: Colourless crystals

(b) Melting-point: 220°C

---

* Cancer Chemotherapy National Service Centre Number, NCI, NIH, USA

(c) Optical rotation: $[\alpha]_D^{21}$ +337° (1% in acetone)

(d) Spectroscopy data: λ_{max} 286, 325 nm (Stecher, 1968)

(e) Identity test: 5 mg in 1 ml sulphuric acid with 5 mg potassium dichromate give a wine-red colour

(f) Solubility: Very slightly soluble in water; soluble at 20°C in 300 parts dehydrated ethanol, in 25 parts chloroform, in 20 parts acetone, in 250 parts methanol and in tetrachloroethane

1.4 Technical products and impurities

Anhydrous USP grade griseofulvin contains a minimum of 90% active ingredient. Griseofulvin capsules contain 90-110% of the labelled amount of active ingredient; tablets contain 90-115% of the labelled amount of active ingredient (US Pharmacopeial Convention, Inc., 1970).

All batches of griseofulvin for use in the US must conform to certain standards, including a specific surface area particle size of 1.3-1.7 m^2/g (US Code of Federal Regulations, 1974).

2. Production, Use, Occurrence and Analysis

For important background information on this section, see preamble, p. 17.

A review on griseofulvin has been published (Grove, 1963).

2.1 Production and use

Griseofulvin is an antifungal antibiotic substance produced by the growth of *Penicillium griseofulvum* or by other means (US Pharmacopeial Convention, Inc., 1970). Griseofulvin was first isolated in 1938 by Oxford *et al.* (1939); its total synthesis was accomplished in 1960 and following years in four different laboratories (Brossi *et al.*, 1960; Grove, 1963). Mutant strains of *P. patulum* are used for the commercial production of the antibiotic by fermentation (Grove, 1963).

Perlman (1974) reported that griseofulvin is produced only in the UK and in Japan, by two fermentation plants in each country. However, another source has reported seven manufacturers in Japan (Anon., 1974).

Sales of griseofulvin began in Japan in 1959 (Fukai, 1974). The quantity of griseofulvin produced in Japan in 1973 was 5700 kg, an amount somewhat less than the average annual rate for the period 1969-1973 (Ministry of Health and Welfare, 1969; 1970; 1971; 1972; 1973).

Griseofulvin is used for the treatment and prophylaxis of human mycotic diseases due to *Microsporum*, *Trichophyton* and *Epidermophyton* (Blacow, 1972). The daily oral dose recommended for infants is 10 mg/kg bw. This is gradually increased with age to a level of 0.5 to 1.0 g/kg bw for adults (Goodman & Gilman, 1970).

Total US sales of griseofulvin in its various forms for use in human medicine are estimated to be in the order of 25,000 kg annually, either in tablet or capsule form for oral ingestion.

Griseofulvin is also used in veterinary medicine for the treatment of ringworm (Stecher, 1968).

2.2 Occurrence

Griseofulvin is a metabolic product of many species of *Penicillium*, but the extent to which it occurs in nature is not known. It was not detected in samples of fermented soyabean paste in Japan (Uchiyama *et al.*, 1972).

2.3 Analysis

The gas chromatographic analysis of griseofulvin has been reported (Margosis, 1972); and griseofulvin and dechlorogriseofulvin have been determined in crude extracts of *Penicillium urticae* by thin-layer and gas-liquid chromatography (limit of detection, 50 ng) (Cole *et al.*, 1970). Analysis of griseofulvin and griseofulvin-4'-ol in plasma using a thin-layer chromatography-fluorometric assay detected concentrations of 0.25-2 µg/ml (Fischer & Riegelman, 1966).

Griseofulvin has also been analysed by time-resolved phosphorimetry (McDuffie & Neely, 1973). The method was employed for concentrations in the range of 5×10^{-4} to 1×10^{-6} M. Methods of assay for the pure drug are given in the British Pharmacopeia (British Pharmacopoeia Commission, 1973), European Pharmacopoeia (Council of Europe, 1971) and The US Pharmacopeia (US Pharmacopeial Convention, Inc., 1975). A simple ultra-violet spectrophotometric method for the determination of the metabolite 6-demethylgriseofulvin in urine, with a limit of detection of 1 µg/ml, is described by Rowland & Riegelman (1973).

3. Biological Data Relevant to the Evaluation of Carcinogenic Risk to Man

3.1 Carcinogenicity and related studies in animals

(a) Oral administration

Mouse: Groups of AP stock mice were fed diets containing 0.5 or 1% griseofulvin for 400-435 days; 10/13 mice fed the 1% diet and 5/20 mice fed 0.5% for 435 days had hepatomas. A hepatoma was reported to have occurred in one mouse fed a diet containing 2.5% griseofulvin for 140 days. No mention was made of controls (Weston Hurst & Paget, 1963).

Groups of 8 male and 8 female Charles River mice, 5-6 weeks old, were fed 1% griseofulvin in the diet for 12-16 months; griseofulvin of 3 particle sizes was used: regular, microcrystalline or milled, with surface areas of 0.41, 1.3 or 1.52 m^2/g, respectively. Among mice fed regular size griseofulvin, 8/12 males and 0/13 females developed hepatomas; of those fed the two other sizes of particles, 11/11 males and 7/14 females developed hepatomas. No tumours occurred in 4 male or in 4 female controls (De Matteis et al., 1966).

(b) Intraperitoneal administration

Rat: A group of 10 male and 10 female Wistar rats received twice weekly i.p. injections of 200 mg/kg bw of a finely milled suspension of griseofulvin in aqueous 'Dispersol OG & LN' for 93 weeks. Eleven rats survived 78-93 weeks, and an adenocarcinoma of the cervix was observed in one female (Paget & Alcock, 1960). [The small number of animals and short duration of the experiment should be noted.]

(c) Subcutaneous and/or intramuscular administration

Infant mouse: Among male mice given s.c. injections of 0.5, 0.5, 1 or 1 mg griseofulvin (total dose, 3 mg/animal) on days 1, 7, 14 and 21 of age, respectively, 7/16 animals surviving 49 weeks developed hepatomas, compared with 4/48 control animals [P<0.02] (Epstein et al., 1967). Similarly, when infant Swiss mice were injected with a total of 3 mg griseofulvin on days 1, 7, 14 and 21 after birth, 24% of the males had developed hepatomas after one year, compared to less than 5% in the control group (Fujii & Epstein, 1969).

3.2 Other relevant biological data

Toxic liver necrosis was observed in mice fed 1-1.5 g/kg bw/day griseofulvin for 82 days (Barich et al., 1961). In rats and dogs, 1-2 g/kg bw/day griseofulvin administered orally for 8 weeks caused no acute toxicity (Paget & Walpole, 1960). It induces porphyria in mice and rats (De Matteis, 1966), and in guinea-pigs it is localized in the pre-keratin cells of the skin and hair follicles (Gentles et al., 1959).

In rats given oral doses of 100 mg/kg bw ^{36}Cl-griseofulvin, 10% of the activity was found in the urine after 24 hours and 4% during 24-48 hours. Of the activity found in the urine, 65% was identified as 6-desmethyl griseofulvin (Barnes & Boothroyd, 1961). In another study, within a 24-hour period only 0.14% of similar oral doses in rats was found in the urine, and 16% was recovered in the faeces. Following its i.v. injection griseofulvin was distributed evenly throughout the tissues, although higher levels were found in skin and lung (Bedford et al., 1960). Of oral doses of 10 mg/rat, 38% was recovered in the faeces after 24 hours (Davis et al., 1961). In mice, griseofulvin metabolites are excreted in urine (Linn et al., 1972); in rats, 77% of an i.v. dose was excreted in the bile and 12% in the urine, the main biliary metabolite being 4-desmethyl griseofulvin (Symchowicz et al., 1967).

Griseofulvin acted as a cocarcinogen with skin applications of 3-methylcholanthrene in mice (Barich et al., 1962; Linnik, 1972); however, Vesselinovitch & Mihailovich (1968) were unable to demonstrate any co-carcinogenic action with benzo[a]pyrene.

When female rats were administered oral doses of 1250 and 1500 mg/kg bw/day griseofulvin (microsize particles) from days 6 to 15 of pregnancy, malformations were observed in the offspring, and survival was decreased. The malformations included tail anomalies, no eyes, anal atresia and exencephaly (Klein & Beall, 1972). Slonitskaya (1969) made similar observations in rats administered oral doses of 50 or 500 mg/kg bw/day.

Griseofulvin was dissolved in N,N-dimethylformamide and tested in human tissue-culture cells (EUE heteroploid line and a hybrid line derived from it) and in phytohaemagglutinin-stimulated human lymphocytes. With concentrations of between 20 and 60 µg/ml, cells showed increased chromosome numbers distributed about tetraploidy relative to the initial karyotype (Larizza *et al.*, 1974).

3.3 Observations in man

No data were available to the Working Group.

4. Comments on Data Reported and Evaluation[1]

4.1 Animal data

Griseofulvin is hepatocarcinogenic following its oral administration to adult mice or its subcutaneous administration to male infant mice.

4.2 Human data

No case reports or epidemiological studies were available to the Working Group.

---

[1] See also the section "Animal Data in Relation to the Evaluation of Risk to Man" in the introduction to this volume, p. 15.

5. References

Anon. (1974) *Essentials for Pharmaceuticals, 1971*, Tokyo, Yakugyo News Co., p. 1080

Barich, L.L., Schwarz, J., Barich, D.J. & Horowitz, M.G. (1961) Toxic liver damage after prolonged intake of elevated doses of griseofulvin. Antibiot. Chemother., 11, 566-571

Barich, L.L., Schwarz, J. & Barich, D. (1962) Oral griseofulvin: a co-carcinogenic agent to methylcholanthrene-induced cutaneous tumors. Cancer Res., 22, 53-55

Barnes, M.J. & Boothroyd, B. (1961) The metabolism of griseofulvin in mammals. Biochem. J., 78, 41-43

Bedford, C., Bushfield, D., Child, K.J., MacGregor, I., Sutherland, P. & Tomich, E.G. (1960) Studies on the biological disposition of griseofulvin, an oral antifungal agent. A.M.A. Arch. Dermatol., 81, 735-745

Blacow, N.W., ed. (1972) *Martindale, The Extra Pharmacopoeia*, 26th ed., London, The Pharmaceutical Press, p. 763

British Pharmacopeia Commission (1973) *British Pharmacopoeia*, London, HMSO, p. 221

Brossi, A., Baumann, M., Gerecke, M. & Kyburz, E. (1960) Totalsynthese von Griseofulvin. Helv. chim. acta, 43, 1444-1447

Cole, R.J., Kirksey, J.W. & Holaday, C.E. (1970) Detection of griseofulvin and dechlorogriseofulvin by thin-layer chromatography and gas-liquid chromatography. Appl. Microbiol., 19, 106-108

Council of Europe (1971) *European Pharmacopoeia*, European Treaty Series No. 50, Vol. 2, Paris, Maisonneuve, pp. 233-235

Davis, B., Child, K.J. & Tomich, E.G. (1961) Absorption and elimination of griseofulvin from the alimentary tract of the rat. J. Pharm. Pharmacol., 13, 166-171

De Matteis, F. (1966) Hypercholesterolaemia and liver enlargement in experimental porphyria. Biochem. J., 98, 23C-25C

De Matteis, F., Donnelly, A.J. & Runge, W.J. (1966) The effect of prolonged administration of griseofulvin in mice with reference to sex differences. Cancer Res., 26, 721-726

Epstein, S.S., Andrea, J., Joshi, S. & Mantel, N. (1967) Hepatocarcinogenicity of griseofulvin following parenteral administration to infant mice. Cancer Res., 27, 1900-1906

Fischer, L.J. & Riegelman, S. (1966) Quantitative determination of griseofulvin and griseofulvin-4'-alcohol in plasma by fluorimetry on thin-layer chromatograms. J. Chromat., 21, 268-274

Fujii, K. & Epstein, S.S. (1969) Carcinogenicity of food additives, pesticides, and drugs after parenteral administration in infant mice (abstract). Toxicol. appl. Pharmacol., 14, 613-614

Fukai, S. (1974) Today's new medicinals, Tokyo, Yakuji Daily News, January 20, p. 653

Gentles, J.C., Barnes, M.J. & Fantes, K.H. (1959) Presence of griseofulvin in hair of guinea pigs after oral administration. Nature (Lond.), 183, 256-257

Goodman, L.S. & Gilman, A., eds (1970) The Pharmacological Basis of Therapeutics, 4th ed., London, Toronto, MacMillan, pp. 1302-1304

Grove, J.F. (1963) Griseofulvin. Q. Rev., 17, 1-19

Gull, K. & Trinci, A.P.J. (1973) Griseofulvin inhibits fungal mitosis. Nature (Lond.), 244, 292-294

Klein, M.F. & Beall, J.R. (1972) Griseofulvin: a teratogenic study. Science, 175, 1483-1484

Larizza, L., Simoni, G., Tredici, F. & de Carli, L. (1974) Griseofulvin: a potential agent of chromosomal segregation in cultured cells. Mutation Res., 25, 123-130

Linn, C., Chang, R., Magat, J. & Symchowicz, S. (1972) Metabolism of [^{14}C]-griseofulvin in the mouse. J. Pharm. Pharmacol., 24, 911-913

Linnik, A.B. (1972) Experimental study of the possible role of griseofulvin in carcinogenesis. Vestn. Derm. Vener., 46, 49-51

Margosis, M. (1972) Analysis of antibiotics by gas chromatography. III. Griseofulvin. J. Chromat., 70, 73-80

McDuffie, J.R. & Neely, W.C. (1973) Determination of griseofulvin by time-resolved phosphorimetry. Analyt. Biochem., 54, 507-512

Ministry of Health & Welfare (1969) Annual Statistical Report of Production in the Pharmaceutical Industry, Tokyo, Medical Department, p. 33

Ministry of Health & Welfare (1970) Annual Statistical Report of Production in the Pharmaceutical Industry, Tokyo, Medical Department, p. 34

Ministry of Health & Welfare (1971) Annual Statistical Report of Production in the Pharmaceutical Industry, Tokyo, Medical Department, p. 64

Ministry of Health & Welfare (1972) Annual Statistical Report of Production in the Pharmaceutical Industry, Tokyo, Medical Department, p. 65

Ministry of Health & Welfare (1973) *Annual Statistical Report of Production in the Pharmaceutical Industry*, Tokyo, Medical Department, p. 81

Oxford, A.E., Raistrick, H. & Simonart, P. (1939) Griseofulvin, $C_{17}H_{19}O_6Cl$, a metabolic product of *Penicillium griseofulvum* Dierckx. *Biochem. J.*, 33, 240-248

Paget, G.E. & Alcock, S.J. (1960) Griseofulvin and colchicine: lack of carcinogenic effect. *Nature (Lond.)*, 188, 867

Paget, G.E. & Walpole, A.L. (1960) The experimental toxicology of griseofulvin. *A.M.A. Arch. Dermatol.*, 81, 750-757

Perlman, D. (1974) Prospects for the fermentation industries, 1974-1983, *Chemtech*, April, pp. 210-216

Rowland, M. & Riegelman, S. (1973) Determination of 6-demethylgriseofulvin in urine. *J. pharm. Sci.*, 62, 2030-2032

Slonitskaya, N.N. (1969) Teratogenic effect of griseofulvin-forte on rat foetus. *Antibiotiki*, 14, 44-48

Stecher, P.G., ed. (1968) *The Merck Index*, 8th ed., Rahway, NJ, Merck & Co., p. 508

Symchowicz, S., Staub, M.S. & Wong, K.K. (1967) A comparative study of griseofulvin-^{14}C metabolism in the rat and rabbit. *Biochem. Pharmacol.*, 16, 2405-2411

Uchiyama, S., Nozu, K., Hayashida, N., Kondo, T. & Tanabe, H. (1972) Chemical analysis of mycotoxin. III. Examination of griseofulvin in fermented food, especially in miso. *Shokukin Eiseigaku Zasshi*, 13, 115-119

US Code of Federal Regulations (1974) *Food and Drugs*, Title 21, part 449.20, Washington DC, US Government Printing Office

US Pharmacopeial Convention, Inc. (1970) *The US Pharmacopeia*, 18th rev., Easton, Pa, Mack, pp. 291-292

US Pharmacopeial Convention, Inc. (1975) *The US Pharmacopeia*, 19th rev., Easton, Pa, Mack, pp. 225-226

Vesselinovitch, S.D. & Mihailovich, N. (1968) The inhibitory effect of griseofulvin on the 'promotion' of skin carcinogenesis. *Cancer Res.*, 28, 2463-2465

Weston Hurst, E. & Paget, G.E. (1963) Protoporphyrin, cirrhosis and hepatomata in the livers of mice given griseofulvin. *Brit. J. Dermatol.*, 73, 105-112

LUTEOSKYRIN

The chemical and biological properties of this substance have been reviewed recently (Enomoto & Ueno, 1974).

1. Chemical and Physical Data

1.1 Synonyms and trade names

Chem. Abstr. Reg. Serial No.: 21884-44-6

Chem. Abstr. Name: (1β, 1'β, 3β, 3'β) 8,8'-Dihydroxy-rugulosin

Flavomycelin; stereoisomer of 1,4,7,9,12,15,17,20-octahydroxy-3,11-dimethyl-5H,6H-6,13α,5α,14-1,2,3,4-butanetetraylcycloocta[1,2-b:5,6-b'] dinaphthalene-5,8,13,16(14H)-tetrone; 2,2',3,3'-tetrahydro-2,2', 4,4', 5,5',8,8'-octahydroxy-7,7'-dimethyl-(1,1'-bianthracene)-9,9', 10,10'-tetrone

1.2 Chemical formula and molecular weight

$C_{30}H_{22}O_{12}$ Mol. wt: 574.5

1.3 Chemical and physical properties of the pure substance

(a) Description: Yellow, rectangular crystals

(b) Melting-point: 287°C (decomposition)

(c) Optical rotation: $[\alpha]_D^{25}$ -880° (0.1% in acetone)

(d) <u>Spectroscopy data</u>: λ_{max} 280.5, 436, 457 nm (E_1^1 = 446, 562 and 559, respectively) in chloroform; λ_{max} 433, 448 nm (E_1^1 = 597, 599) in ethanol; λ_{max} 350, 353 (E_1^1 = 458, 390) in 0.1 M potassium phosphate buffer (pH 7.4). The nuclear magnetic resonance spectra of luteoskyrin are described by Sankawa *et al.* (1968) and those for X-ray diffraction by Kobayashi *et al.* (1968). For infra-red spectral data see Enomoto & Ueno (1974).

(e) <u>Identity and purity test</u>: Luteoskyrin splits into islandicin (a red compound, m.p. 218°C) when treated with sodium hyposulphite; treatment of luteoskyrin with 60% sulphuric acid yields islandicin and iridoskyrin (an orange compound, m.p. 360°C)

(f) <u>Solubility</u>: Practically insoluble in water; soluble in aqueous sodium bicarbonate; soluble in most organic solvents

(g) <u>Stability</u>: The compound is known to convert to a brownish-red quinoid substance, lumiluteoskyrin, when exposed to sunlight (Saito *et al.*, 1971).

1.4 Technical products and impurities

No data were available to the Working Group.

2. Production, Use, Occurrence and Analysis

2.1 Production and use

Luteoskyrin is not produced commercially.

2.2 Occurrence

Luteoskyrin and several other mycotoxins are produced in culture by *Penicillum islandicum* Sopp. and by *Mycelia sterilia* (Shibata *et al.*, 1957). Although there are no data based upon direct chemical analysis concerning the occurrence of luteoskyrin in foodstuffs, *P. islandicum* has occasionally been reported as one of the major isolates from various grains, including domestic and imported rice in Japan (Miyaki *et al.*, 1970; Tsunoda, 1968), the staple diet 'teff' in Ethiopia (Pavlica & Samuel, 1970) and barley (Carnaghan, 1966/67), and as a prevalent infection in prepared foodstuffs in South Africa (Martin *et al.*, 1971).

2.3 Analysis

Shibata *et al.* (1955) describe the use of paper and thin-layer chromatography for the separation and identification of luteoskyrin; a modified thin-layer chromatographic method was recommended by Ueno & Ishikawa (1969). Tatsuno *et al.* (1957) devised a method described as 'one grain culture chromatography'.

Luteoskyrin can be extracted from powdered mouldy rice with phenol (Uraguchi, 1971), from dried mycelium of *P. islandicum* (Ueno & Ishikawa, 1969) and from liver tissue (Ueno, 1975). Analytical methods are summarized by Enomoto & Ueno (1974).

3. Biological Data Relevant to the Evaluation of Carcinogenic Risk to Man

3.1 Carcinogenicity and related studies in animals

Oral administration

Mouse: Groups of 10-30 male ddNi mice received daily doses of 0, 50, 150 or 500 µg/animal purified luteoskyrin in a basal diet containing rice and/or barley; various dosing schedules were used, and the treatment was continued as long as possible. Five liver-cell adenomas and 1 liver-cell carcinoma of a differentiated type were observed in 29 mice fed 150 µg/mouse/day in a diet containing 2.25 g rice and 2.25 g barley. Liver-cell adenomas occurred in 8/29 mice fed 150 µg/mouse/day luteoskyrin in a diet containing 4.5 g rice, and 1 liver-cell adenoma occurred in 1/30 mice fed 150 µg/mouse/day in a diet containing 4.5 g barley. Six liver-cell adenomas and 2 liver-cell carcinomas of a differentiated type appeared in 30 mice fed 500 µg luteoskyrin daily in a rice and barley basal diet. Two liver-cell adenomas, 1 liver-cell carcinoma of a differentiated type and 1 liver-cell carcinoma of an undifferentiated type developed in 4/20 mice fed 500 µg luteoskyrin/mouse intermittently every other 4-5 weeks, mixed with a rice and barley diet. The minimum period for tumour development was 216 days. No liver-cell tumours developed in 33 control mice nor in 19 mice fed 50 µg luteoskyrin/mouse/day. Of 30 female mice fed 150 µg luteoskyrin/mouse in a rice and barley diet, 2 developed liver-cell adenomas and 1 a liver-cell carcinoma of a differentiated type. No tumours were observed in 8 female control mice. Hepatic reticuloendotheliomas were seen in a few mice (3 in male mice given 150 µg, 1 in a male mouse given 500 µg and 1 in a female mouse given 150 µg/day) (Uraguchi et al., 1972a).

Of 26 male DDD mice fed 160 µg/animal/day luteoskyrin (total doses, 30-52 mg), 12 developed liver-cell adenomas, 4, liver-cell carcinomas of a differentiated type and 1, a liver-cell carcinoma of an undifferentiated type. One hepatic reticuloendothelioma and 1 lymphosarcoma were also observed. No tumours developed in 18 control mice during the 328 days of the experiment (Ueno et al., 1973).

3.2 Other relevant biological data

The LD_{50}'s of luteoskyrin in male mice were reported to be 145 mg/kg bw when given by s.c. injection, 221 mg/kg bw orally and 6.65 mg/kg bw by i.v. injection. The most prominent toxic signs are centrolobular necrosis and fatty degeneration of the liver (Enomoto & Saito, 1973; Morooka et al., 1966; Saito et al., 1971; Uraguchi et al., 1961). Luteoskyrin also causes heptatotoxic effects in rats (Saito, 1959), rabbits and monkeys (Itano, 1959). Rabbits and mice were more susceptible to luteoskyrin than rats, and mice showed marked sex differences in susceptibility to luteoskyrin: females were less susceptible than males (s.c. LD_{50}, 2 g/kg bw for males versus 154 mg/kg bw for females). The toxicity of luteoskyrin was higher in younger mice: the s.c. LD_{50} values in newborn mice were 7.2 mg/kg bw in males and 6.3 mg/kg bw in females. Dietary effects and strain differences in relation to the toxicity of luteoskyrin are described by Enomoto & Ueno (1974).

Studies with ^{3}H-luteoskyrin showed that the compound is absorbed slowly following its s.c. (3 daily injections of 5 µg/g) or oral administration (9 µg/animal). Radioactivity was extremely high in the liver when compared with that in other organs, e.g., kidney, heart, spleen, lung, brain and muscle (Uraguchi et al., 1972b). Luteoskyrin was excreted via the bile and kidneys, as shown by chemical identification of luteoskyrin in the faeces and urine (Ueno, 1975).

Luteoskyrin in the presence or absence of a rat liver-microsome system did not induce 'unscheduled DNA-repair synthesis' in cultured human fibroblasts (San & Stich, 1975). Luteoskyrin was lethal to the M-45 recessive strain of *Bacillus subtilis* (Enomoto & Ueno, 1974).

3.3 Observations in man

No data were available to the Working Group.

4. Comments on Data Reported and Evaluation[1]

4.1 Animal data

Luteoskyrin is carcinogenic in mice following its oral administration, the only species and route of administration tested; it produced benign and malignant tumours of the liver.

4.2 Human data

No case reports or epidemiological studies were available to the Working Group.

---

[1]See also the section "Animal Data in Relation to the Evaluation of Risk to Man" in the introduction to this volume, p. 15.

5. References

Carnaghan, R.B.A. (1966/67) Mycotoxicoses. In: Pool, W.A., ed., The Veterinary Annual, 8th year, Bristol, John Wright & Sons, pp. 84-93

Enomoto, M. & Saito, M. (1973) Experimentally induced chronic liver injuries by the metabolites of *Penicillium islandicum* Sopp. Acta path. jap., 23, 655-666

Enomoto, M. & Ueno, I. (1974) *Penicillium islandicum* (toxic yellowed rice) - luteoskyrin - islanditoxin - cyclochlorotine. In: Purchase, I.F.H., ed., Mycotoxins, Amsterdam, Elsevier, pp. 302-326

Itano, T. (1959) Pathological studies on the toxicity of the *Penicillium islandicum* Sopp. J. Nara med. Ass., 10, 1

Kobayashi, N., Iitaka, Y., Sankawa, U., Ogihara, Y. & Shibata, S. (1968) The crystal and molecular structure of a bromination product of tetrahydrorugulosin. Tetrahedron Lett., 6135-6138

Martin, P.M.D., Gilman, G.A. & Keen, P. (1971) The incidence of fungi in foodstuffs and their significance based on a survey in the eastern Transvaal and Swaziland. In: Purchase, I.F.H., ed., Mycotoxins in Human Health, London, Basingstoke, Macmillan, pp. 281-290

Miyaki, K., Yamazaki, M., Horie, Y. & Udagawa, S. (1970) Toxigenic fungi growing on stored rice. J. Fd Hyg. Soc. Japan, 11, 373-380

Morooka, N., Nakano, N. & Uchida, N. (1966) Biochemical and histopathological studies on the tumor-developing livers of mice fed on the diets containing luteoskyrin. Japan. J. med. Sci. Biol., 20, 293-303

Pavlica, D. & Samuel, I. (1970) Primary carcinoma of the liver in Ethiopia. Brit. J. Cancer, 24, 22-29

Saito, M. (1959) Liver cirrhosis induced by metabolites of *Penicillium islandicum* Sopp. Acta path. jap., 9, 785-790

Saito, M., Enomoto, M., Tatsuno, T. & Uraguchi, K. (1971) Yellowed rice toxins. In: Ciegler, A., Kadis, S. & Ajl, S.J., eds, Microbial Toxins, Vol. 6, New York, London, Academic Press, pp. 299-380

San, R.H.C. & Stich, H.F. (1975) DNA repair synthesis of cultured human cells as a rapid bioassay for chemical carcinogens. Int. J. Cancer, 16, 284-291

Sankawa, U., Seo, S., Kobayashi, N., Ogihara, Y. & Shibata, S. (1968) Further studies on the structure of luteoskyrin, rubroskyrin and rugulosin. Tetrahedron Lett., 5557-5560

Shibata, S., Takido, M. & Nakajima, T. (1955) Metabolic products of fungi. VII. Paper chromatography of the colouring matters of *Penicillium islandicum* Sopp. Pharm. Bull. (Tokyo), 3, 286-290

Shibata, S., Kitagawa, I. & Nishikawa, H. (1957) Metabolic products of fungi. XII. The identification of flavomycelin and luteoskyrin. Pharm. Bull. (Tokyo), 5, 383-385

Tatsuno, T., Wakamatsu, H., Kanazawa, Y., Sato, T. & Tsunoda, H. (1957) On a method for detection of yellowish rice infected by *Penicillium islandicum*. I. J. pharm. Soc. Japan, 77, 689-691

Tsunoda, H. (1968) Micro-organisms which deteriorate stored cereals and grains. In: Herzberg, M., ed., Proceedings of the First US-Japan Conference on Toxic Microorganisms, Mycotoxins, Botulism, Washington DC, US Department of Interior, p. 143

Ueno, I. (1975) Pharmacokinetic studies on the hepatotoxicity of luteoskyrin. II. Extraction and identification of ^{3}H-luteoskyrin from the liver and excreta in mice. Japan. J. Pharmacol., 25, 171-179

Ueno, Y. & Ishikawa, I. (1969) Production of luteoskyrin, a hepatotoxic pigment, by *Penicillium islandicum* Sopp. Appl. Microbiol., 18, 406-409

Ueno, I., Saito, M., Enomoto, M. & Uraguchi, K. (1973) Relationship between the acute toxic dosis and carcinogenic dosis of carcinogen - study on luteoskyrin, a hepatocarcinogenic mycotoxin. Proc. Japan. Cancer Ass., 32nd Ann. Meet., 187

Uraguchi, K. (1971) Pharmacology of mycotoxins. In: Raskova, H., ed., International Encyclopedia of Pharmacology and Therapeutics, Oxford, Pergamon, pp. 143-298

Uraguchi, K., Tatsuno, T., Sakai, F., Tsukioka, M., Sakai, Y., Yonemitsu, O., Ito, H., Miyake, M., Saito, M., Enomoto, M., Shikata, T. & Ishiko, T. (1961) Isolation of two toxic agents, luteoskyrin and chlorine-containing peptide, from the metabolites of *Penicillium islandicum* Sopp., with some properties thereof. Japan. J. exp. Med., 31, 19-46

Uraguchi, K., Saito, M., Noguchi, Y., Takahasi, K., Enomoto, M. & Tatsuno, T. (1972a) Chronic toxicity and carcinogenicity in mice of the purified mycotoxins, luteoskyrin and cyclochlorotine. Fd Cosmet. Toxicol., 10, 193-207

Uraguchi, K., Ueno, I., Ueno, Y. & Komai, T. (1972b) Absorption, distribution and excretion of luteoskyrin with special reference to the selective action on the liver. Toxicol. appl. Pharmacol., 21, 335-347

MITOMYCIN C

1. Chemical and Physical Data

1.1 Synonyms and trade names

Chem. Abstr. Reg. Serial No.: 50-07-7

Chem. Abstr. Name: [1aR-(1aα,8β,8aα,8bα)]-6-Amino-8-{[(aminocarbonyl)oxy]methyl}-1,1a,2,8,8a,8b-hexahydro-8a-methoxy-5-methylazirino[2',3':3,4]pyrrolo[1,2-a]indole-4,7-dione

6-Amino-8-{([aminocarbonyl]oxy)methyl}-1,1a,2,8,8a,8b-hexahydro-8-methoxy-5-methyl[1aR-(1aα,8β,8aα,8bα)]azirino(2',3':3,4)pyrrolo-(1,2-α)indole-4,7-dione; 6-amino-1,1a,2,8,8a,8b-hexahydro-8-(hydroxymethyl)-8a-methoxy-5-methylazirino(2',3':3,4)pyrrolo(1,2-a)-indole-4,7-dione, carbamate ester; MIT-C; mitomycin; mitomycinum; NSC 2798*

Ametycin; Mutamycin (Mitomycin for injection); Mytomycin

1.2 Chemical formula and molecular weight

$C_{15}H_{18}N_4O_5$ Mol. wt: 334.3

1.3 Chemical and physical properties of the pure substance

(a) Description: Blue-violet crystals

(b) Melting-point: Above 360°C

---

* Cancer Chemotherapy National Service Centre Number, NCI, NIH, USA

(c) <u>Spectroscopy data</u>: λ_{max} 216, 360, 560 nm; E_1^1 = 742 (0.06% in methanol)

(d) <u>Solubility</u>: Soluble in water, methanol, acetone, butyl acetate and cyclohexanone; slightly soluble in benzene, carbon tetrachloride and ether

(e) <u>Stability</u>: Solutions in water at pH 6-9 are stable for seven days when protected from light and stored at <5°C.

1.4 Technical products and impurities

Mitomycin C is supplied in the United States in vials containing 5 mg mitomycin C and 10 mg mannitol. In Japan, it has been supplied for export to the Peoples' Republic of China in vials containing about 2 mg mitomycin C (Anon, 1972). It is also available in tablet form in Japan.

2. Production, Use, Occurrence and Analysis

For important background information on this section, see preamble, p. 17.

2.1 Production and use

Mitomycin C is formed by *Streptomyces caespitosus*, and its commercial production is by fermentation (Perlman, 1974).

Marketing of this antibiotic began in Japan in 1959 (Fukai, 1974); the only known manufacturers are two companies in that country (Anon., 1974). Japanese production of mitomycin C for injection in 1973 was 3.9 kg; an average of 3.2 kg was produced annually in the preceding four years (Ministry of Health and Welfare, 1969; 1970; 1971; 1972; 1973). Exports to the Peoples' Republic of China were about 30 g per year prior to 1972, when an order for 200 g was placed (Anon., 1972).

In the US, studies on the use of mitomycin C began in 1958. Commercial marketing began in August 1974 following approval by the Food & Drug Administration. Mitomycin C is imported into the United States from Japan and formulated into solutions suitable for injection.

It has been used in the treatment of advanced carcinomas at dose levels of 0.05 mg/kg bw/day for five days i.v., followed by two free days; the schedule is then repeated for five days.

As of 1973, clinical investigators at 50 hospitals and research centres in the US had treated more than 1300 patients. On the basis of an average total dose per patient of 50 mg, it can be calculated that a total quantity of about 65 g had been administered up to that time.

2.2 Occurrence

Mitomycins were first isolated from a strain of the fungus *Streptomyces caespitosus* found in a soil sample in the Tokyo area (Hata *et al.*, 1956; Wakaki *et al.*, 1958), but the extent to which mitomycin C may occur in nature is not known.

2.3 Analysis

Mitomycin may be assayed microbiologically (Hata *et al.*, 1956).

3. Biological Data Relevant to the Evaluation of Carcinogenic Risk to Man

3.1 Carcinogenicity and related studies in animals

(a) *Subcutaneous and/or intramuscular administration*

Mouse: Groups of 7 btK, 10 C57BL, 10 C3H and 10 ddO mice were given 35 twice weekly s.c. injections of 0.2 µg mitomycin C in saline and observed for a further 31 weeks, when the experiment was terminated. All btK mice and 2/10 C57Bl mice developed local sarcomas within 39-54 weeks. No tumours developed in treated C3H or ddO mice nor in respective groups of 10-11 controls of each strain given saline alone (Ikegami *et al.*, 1967).

(b) *Intraperitoneal administration*

Rat: Two groups of 25 male and 25 female Charles River CD rats were given i.p. injections of 0.038 or 0.15 mg/kg bw thrice weekly for 6 months followed by observation for a further 12 months, at which time the animals were killed. Peritoneal sarcomas developed in 27/29 males and 30/31 females (Weisburger *et al.*, 1976).

(c) Intravenous administration

Rat: A group of 96 BR46 male rats was given five i.v. injections of 0.52 mg/kg bw mitomycin C (17% of the LD_{50}) within two weeks (total dose, 2.6 mg/kg bw) and were observed for lifespan. Of 79 rats surviving at the appearance of the first tumour, 27 (34%) developed malignant tumours and 3 developed benign tumours. Malignant tumours included 2 lymphosarcomas, 4 abdominal polymorphic-cell sarcomas, 5 mammary carcinomas or sarcomas, 4 subcutaneous fibrosarcomas, 3 squamous-cell carcinomas of the lung, 1 carcinoma and 1 sarcoma of the bladder, 1 phaeochromocytoma, 1 reticulum-cell sarcoma of the liver, 1 carcinosarcoma of the oesophagus, 1 adenocarcinoma of the pyloric mucosa, 1 sarcoma of the salivary gland, 1 abdominal haemangioendothelioma and 1 haemangiosarcoma in the paw. Malignant tumours were observed in 4/65 controls surviving at the appearance of the first tumour. The average time of observation of the tumours was 18 months in treated rats and 23 months in controls (Schmähl & Osswald, 1970) [$P<0.001$].

3.2 Other relevant biological data

The LD_{50}'s of single i.p. doses (14 days of observation) were 8.5 mg/kg bw in mice and 2.5 mg/kg bw in rats. The oral LD_{50}'s of an aqueous solution were 23 mg/kg bw in mice and 30 mg/kg bw in rats. The i.v. LD_{50}'s were 5 mg/kg bw in mice (Stecher, 1968) and 1-2.5 mg/kg bw in cats, dogs and monkeys. Anorexia, weight loss, diarrhoea and dehydration were the main signs prior to death. The main pathological changes were petechial haemorrhages in the colon and other organs and depression of the haematopoietic tissues (Phillips *et al.*, 1960).

Following i.v. injection of 2 mg/kg bw mitomycin C in Wistar rats, 18% was recovered unchanged in the urine within 24 hours. At higher doses (8 mg/kg bw), 35% was recovered in the urine, but none in the faeces or tissues. Homogenates of rat liver, brain, kidney and spleen inactivated mitomycin C rapidly (Schwartz & Phillips, 1961). Thirty minutes after i.v. injection of 8 mg/kg bw to mice traces remained in the blood. In guinea-pigs the drug was concentrated in the kidneys and not in the liver, spleen or brain and was excreted in the urine (Fujita, 1971).

Mitomycin C reacts with bacterial DNA (Iyer & Szybalski, 1963) but not with isolated DNA, unless a chemical or enzymic reducing system is added (Iyer & Szybalski, 1964). The cross-linking efficiency of mitomycin C was increased in isolated bacterial DNA containing increasing amounts of cytosine and guanosine (Tomasz, 1970).

In rats given single doses of 3 mg methylcholanthrene by s.c. injection the incidence of local sarcomas after 120 days was reduced when weekly i.p. injections of mitomycin C were also given (Matsuyama, 1961). In mice which were administered 0.2 ml of a 1% solution of methylcholanthrene in benzene on the skin daily for 5-10 days, the incidence of skin papillomas was greatly increased when mitomycin C was given daily by 20 i.p. injections at a maximum tolerated dose (Southam et al., 1969). In rats given 40 µg/kg bw mitomycin C intraperitoneally and an oral dose of DMBA, the incidence of mammary tumours after 120 days was similar to that in rats given DMBA alone (Tominaga et al., 1973).

Mitomycin C induced reverse mutations in *Salmonella typhimurium* (McCann et al., 1975). It induced mitotic crossing over in the yeast *Saccharomyces cerevisiae*, in the smut fungus *Ustilago maydis* (Holliday, 1964) and in the soyabean *Glycine max*. L. (Vig & Paddock, 1968) and induced mitotic as well as meiotic crossing over in *Drosophila melanogaster* (Schewe et al., 1971a,b). It induced chromosomal aberrations in *Drosophila* oocytes (Walker & Williamson, 1975) and dominant and recessive mutations in the wasp *Habrobracon* (Smith, 1969).

Mitomycin C of unspecified origin and purity injected into male (101 x C3H)F_1 hybrid mice as a single dose of 5.25 mg/kg bw induced specific locus mutations in spermatogonia (Ehling, 1973). It induced chromosomal breaks and rearrangements in cultures of human peripheral leucocytes (Cohen & Shaw, 1964).

3.3 <u>Observations in man</u>

No data were available to the Working Group.

4. Comments on Data Reported and Evaluation[1]

4.1 Animal data

Mitomycin C is carcinogenic in mice following its subcutaneous injection and in rats following its intraperitoneal or intravenous injection. In rats it produced both local and distant tumours.

4.2 Human data

No case reports or epidemiological studies were available to the Working Group.

---

[1] See also the section "Animal Data in Relation to the Evaluation of Risk to Man" in the introduction to this volume, p. 15.

5. References

Anon. (1972) Kyowa providing China with antibiotics. Japan Chemical Week, December 28, p. 6

Anon. (1974) Essentials for Pharmaceuticals, 1971, Tokyo, Yakugyo News Co., p. 1012

Cohen, M.M. & Shaw, M.W. (1964) Effects of mitomycin C on human chromosomes. J. cell. Biol., 23, 386-395

Ehling, U.H. (1973) Mutagenitätsprüfung von Fremdstoffen. In: Meinck, F., ed., Hygienisch-toxikologische Bewertung von Trinkwasser in Haltsstoffen. Schriftenreihe des Vereins für Wasser-, Boden- und Lufthyciene, Berlin-Dahlem, H. 40, Stuttgart, Gustav Fischer Verlag, pp. 21-37

Fujita, H. (1971) Comparative studies on the blood level, tissue distribution, excretion and inactivation of anticancer drugs. Jap. J. clin. Oncol., 12, 151-162

Fukai, S. (1974) Today's new medicinals, Tokyo, Yakuji Daily News, January 20, p. 654

Hata, T., Sano, Y., Sugawara, R., Matsumae, A., Kanamari, K., Shuma, T. & Hoshi, T. (1956) Mitomycin, a new antibiotic from Streptomyces. I. J. Antibiotics, 9, 141-146

Holliday, R. (1964) The induction of mitotic recombination by mitomycin C in Ustilago and Saccharomyces. Genetics, 50, 323-335

Ikegami, R., Akamatsu, Y. & Haruta, M. (1967) Subcutaneous sarcomas induced by mitomycin C in mice. Acta path. jap., 17, 495-501

Iyer, V.N. & Szybalski, W. (1963) A molecular mechanism of mitomycin action : linking of complementary DNA strands. Microbiology, 50, 355-362

Iyer, V.N. & Szybalski, W. (1964) Mitomycins and porfiromycin : chemical mechanism of action and cross-linking of DNA. Science, 164, 55-58

Matsuyama, M. (1961) The influences of mitomycin C and carzinophilin upon methylcholanthrene sarcoma in rats. A preliminary report. Nagoya med. J., 7, 71-74

McCann, J., Spingarn, N.E., Kobori, J. & Ames, B.N. (1975) Detection of carcinogens as mutagens : bacterial tester strains with R factor plasmids. Proc. nat. Acad. Sci. (Wash.), 72, 979-983

Ministry of Health and Welfare (1969) Annual Statistical Report of Production in the Pharmaceutical Industry, Tokyo, Medical Department, p. 39

Ministry of Health and Welfare (1970) *Annual Statistical Report of Production in the Pharmaceutical Industry*, Tokyo, Medical Department, p. 40

Ministry of Health and Welfare (1971) *Annual Statistical Report of Production in the Pharmaceutical Industry*, Tokyo, Medical Department, p. 69

Ministry of Health and Welfare (1972) *Annual Statistical Report of Production in the Pharmaceutical Industry*, Tokyo, Medical Department, p. 70

Ministry of Health and Welfare (1973) *Annual Statistical Report of Production in the Pharmaceutical Industry*, Tokyo, Medical Department, p. 82

Perlman (1974) Prospects for the fermentation industries, 1974-1983, *Chemtech*, April, p. 212

Philips, F.S., Schwartz, H.S. & Sternberg, S.S. (1960) Pharmacology of mitomycin C. I. Toxicity and pathologic effects. *Cancer Res.*, 20, 1354-1361

Schewe, M.J., Suzuki, D.T. & Erasmus, U. (1971a) The genetic effects of mitomycin C in *Drosophila melanogaster*. I. Induced mutations and X-Y chromosomal inter-changes. *Mutation Res.*, 12, 255-268

Schewe, M.J., Suzuki, D.T. & Erasmus, U. (1971b) The genetic effects of mitomycin C in *Drosophila melanogaster*. II. Induced meiotic recombination. *Mutation Res.*, 12, 269-279

Schmähl, D. & Osswald, H. (1970) Experimentelle Untersuchungen über carcinogene Wirkingen von Krebs-Chemotherapeutica und Immunosuppressiva. *Arzneimittel.-Forsch.*, 20, 1461-1467

Schwartz, H.S. & Phillips, F.S. (1961) Pharmacology of mitomycin C. II. Renal excretion and metabolism by tissue homogenates. *J. Pharm. exp. Ther.*, 133, 335-342

Smith, R.H. (1969) Induction of mutations in *Habrobracon* sperm with mitomycin C. *Mutation Res.*, 7, 231-234

Southam, C.M., Tanaka, S., Arata, T., Simkovic, D., Miura, M. & Petropulos, S.F. (1969) Enhancement of response to chemical carcinogens by nononcogenic viruses and antimetabolites. *Progr. exp. Tumor Res. (Basel)*, 11, 194-212

Stecher, P.G., ed. (1968) *The Merck Index*, 8th ed., Rahway, NJ, Merck & Co., 697-698

Tomasz, M. (1970) Novel assay of 7-alkylation of guanine residues in DNA. Application to nitrogen mustard, triethylenemelamine and mitomycin C. *Biochim. biophys. acta*, 213, 288-295

Tominaga, T., Taguchi, T. & Shiba, S. (1973) Effect of actinomycin-D and mitomycin-C on induction of rat mammary cancer with 7,12-dimethylbenz[a]anthracene. *Gann*, 64, 301-303

Vig, B.K. & Paddock, E.F. (1968) Alteration by mitomycin C of spot frequencies in soybean leaves. J. Hered., 59, 225-229

Wakaki, S., Marumo, H., Tomioka, K., Schimizu, G., Kato, E., Kamada, H., Kudo, S. & Fujimoto, Y. (1958) Isolation of new fractions of anti-tumour mitomycins. Antibiot. Chemother., 8, 228-241

Walker, V.K. & Williamson, J.H. (1975) Genetic analysis of mitomycin C-induced interchange in *Drosophila melanogaster* females. Mutation Res., 28, 227-237

Weisburger, J.H., Griswold, D.P., Jr, Prejean, J.D., Casey, A.E., Wood, H.B., Jr & Weisburger, E.K. (1976) The carcinogenic properties of some of the principal drugs used in cancer chemotherapy. Recent Results Cancer Res. (in press)

NATIVE CARRAGEENANS

1. Chemical and Physical Data

A review article has been written by Towle (1973).

1.1 Synonyms and trade names

Chem. Abstr. Reg. Serial No.: 9000-07-1

Chem. Abstr. Name: Carrageenan

3,6-Anhydro-D-galactan; carrageenan gum; carrageenin; carragheen; carragheenin; chondrus; chondrus extract; gum carrageenan; gum chon 2; gum chrond; Irish moss gelose; killeen; pearlpuss; pigwrack; self rock moss

Burtonite V-40-E; Galozone; Pellugel; Viscarin

1.2 Chemical formula and molecular weight

κ-carrageenan
Chem. Abstr. Reg.
Serial No.: 11114-20-8

λ-carrageenan
Chem. Abstr. Reg.
Serial No.: 9064-57-7

ι-carrageenan
Chem. Abstr. Reg.
Serial No.: 9062-07-1

Carrageenan is a sulphated polysaccharide which can be fractionated with potassium chloride into two separate components. One fraction, which gels under the action of potassium ion, was designated κ-carrageenan; the other, which is insensitive to potassium ion, was named λ-carrageenan. κ- and λ-carrageenan represent, respectively, about 40 and 60% of the unfractionated extract (Smith & Cook, 1953).

κ-Carrageenan is composed of sulphated D-galactose and 3,6-anhydro-D-galactose residues in approximately equimolar amounts and possesses a branched structure; it has a molecular weight of between 1.8 and 3.2×10^5. Using immunological methods, Di Rosa (1972) estimated a molecular weight of 2.8×10^5.

λ-Carrageenan is composed almost entirely of sulphated D-galactose and has a molecular weight of between 4 and 7×10^5. Di Rosa (1972) calculated a molecular weight of 3.5×10^5 by immunological methods.

ι-Carrageenan is the major component of extracts of *Euchema cottonii* and *E. spinosum*.

Degraded carrageenan is prepared commercially by acid hydrolysis and peroxide oxidation, resulting in severe break-down of the polymeric molecules. It has a molecular weight of 20,000-30,000 and dissolves readily (Anderson, 1967; Anderson & Soman, 1966).

1.3 <u>Chemical and physical properties of the commercially available substance</u>

(a) <u>Description</u>: Yellowish to colourless, coarse to fine powder; practically odourless; mucilaginous texture. It is a polyanionic colloid with three components which are associated with ammonium, calcium, potassium or sodium ions or with combinations of these four occurring in varying proportions.

(b) <u>Identity and purity test</u>: Instructions for identification and purity determinations are given by FAO/WHO (1970).

(c) <u>Solubility</u>: One g dissolves in 100 ml water at about $80°C$, forming a viscous, clear or slightly opalescent solution which flows readily. It disperses in water more readily if first moistened with ethanol, glycerol or a saturated solution of sucrose in water or if the water contains salts that induce gelation. Insoluble in ethanol

(d) <u>Reactivity</u>: Reacts with large molecular weight cationic molecules with hydrophilic components, such as cetyl pyridinium chloride, to form insoluble reaction products

(e) _Stability_: While some degradation of native carrageenan may take place during processing of acid food at relatively high temperatures, the extent seems to be very limited (Nilson & Wagner, 1959).

(f) _Viscosity_: Potassium, caesium, rubidium and ammonium salts increase the viscosity of carrageenan solutions and enhance their gelling properties. The potassium sensitivity resides only in part of the carrageenan, and this fraction, 40% of the carrageenan, is precipitated with potassium salts when the solution is too dilute to gel. The precipitate can be removed from solution by centrifugation, and λ-carrageenan, which does not gel, remains in solution. In the presence of specific metal cations, such as potassium, κ-carrageenan solutions form short, inelastic, thermally reversible gels on heating and cooling; ι-carrageenan forms elastic gels with calcium salts.

1.4 Technical products and impurities

Standardization procedures have been developed for particular uses, and these are not the same for all companies. Product specifications agreed upon by producer and purchaser are useful only specifically and are of little value in comparing or establishing grades among producers (Towle, 1973).

When carrageenan is isolated by alcohol precipitation, a relatively small amount of soluble salt impurities remain in it, due to occlusion and absorption. When it is isolated by a drum-drying procedure, larger amounts of soluble salt impurities are found in the product (Towle, 1973).

2. Production, Use, Occurrence and Analysis

For important background information on this section, see preamble, p. 17.

2.1 Production and use

Carrageenan is obtained by extraction with water from members of the Gigartinaceae and Solieriaceae families of the class Rhodophyceae (red seaweed), including _Chondrus crispus, C. ocellatus, Eucheuma cottonii,_

E. spinosum, Gigartina acicularis, G. pistillata, G. radula and *G. stellata*. *C. crispus* and *G. stellata* are the chief sources.

The seaweed is harvested by various methods and then dried. The dried weed is first washed in cold water to remove soluble impurities; it may subsequently be subjected to ion exchange if monovalent salts are desired. Extraction of carrageenan is then carried out in hot water with materials blended to achieve the desired composition: usually, one part of weed is extracted with 50 parts of dilute alkaline solution for one to four hours at approximately 80°C. The crude extract, containing about 1% solids, is treated with adsorbents to remove soluble impurities then vacuum filtered and concentrated to 2-3% solids. Drum-drying or alcohol precipitation is used to recover the carrageenan from the concentrated extract. The drum-dried material contains whatever impurities remained in the extract; the alcohol precipitation method leaves most of these impurities behind in solution, but the stringy precipitate which is recovered must be further dried to remove residual water and solvent (Towle, 1973).

The ability of κ-carrageenan to form gels with potassium ions is the basis for its use in many foods. A level of 0.2% potassium chloride is often used. The temperature of gel formation is determined by the concentration and type of ions in solution but is usually 45-55°C; the gels can be melted at approximately 10°C above setting temperature. Carrageenan solutions and gels are fairly stable over a wide pH range at room temperature or lower but are rapidly degraded under conditions of low pH and high temperature.

Since the 1930's, commercial production of carrageenans in the US has grown steadily, and current production is approximately equivalent to that in Europe and Asia combined. World production in 1971 was approximately 4500 tons; of this, about 2300 tons were produced in the US; most of the remainder was produced in Denmark and France and some in Japan, Spain and the UK (Towle, 1973).

The **unique property of carrageenan as a hydrocolloid is** its high degree of reactivity with certain proteins; its reactivity with milk protein, in particular, is the basis for its use in a number of foods.

This reaction between casein and carrageenan, called 'milk reactivity', makes it possible to suspend cocoa or other particles in milk with the use of a very small amount of carrageenan (0.025%); a thixotropic system is created, forming a weak gel, but the viscosity of the milk is only slightly increased. If more carrageenan is used (0.15%), strong gels with the consistency of custards or flans are formed.

Approximately 80% of the present production of carrageenan is used by food industries, as a gelling agent, a viscosity builder or an emulsifying agent. It is used as a thickening agent and stabilizer in beverages (0.03%), baked goods (0.01-0.1%), jellies (0.1-1.2%), syrups (0.1-0.3%), puddings (0.2-1%), ice-creams (0.01-0.05%), iced lollies (3-4%), beer, soups, sauces, soft drinks and toppings (0.03-0.05%) (Klose & Glicksman, 1968; NAS-NRC, 1963; Towle, 1973). Carrageenans are also used in meat products and tooth pastes and powders (Towle, 1973).

2.3 Analysis

Analytical methods to quantitate carrageenans in milk products involve digestion of the isolated fraction and analysis of the carbohydrate moiety by a phenol-sulphuric acid method (Graham, 1968), or methanolysis and tri-methylsilylation, followed by identification of the specific gas chromatographic peak of 2,4,5-tri-O-trimethylsilyl-3,6-anhydrogalactosedimethylacetal (Schmolck & Mergenthaler, 1973).

Spectrophotometric methods specific for the sulphate part of the κ- and ι-carrageenan molecules entail reaction with barium chloranilate (Graham, 1966) or with o-tolidine and sodium hypochlorite (Graham, 1972).

3. Biological Data Relevant to the Evaluation of Carcinogenic Risk to Man

3.1 Carcinogenicity and related studies in animals

(a) Oral administration

Mouse: Groups of 5 male and 5 female mice of two unidentified strains were maintained throughout their lifespan on diets containing 1, 5, 15 or 25% food-grade native carrageenan added to the diet at the expense of equal weights of ground yellow corn and other cereals. No effect was noted with regard to mortality, but food consumption increased in proportion to the increase in carrageenan. There were no apparent pathological effects on the gastrointestinal tract, liver or kidneys (Nilson & Wagner, 1959).

<u>Rat</u>: The same authors also studied the effect of food-grade native carrageenan on groups of 5 male and 5 female rats of two unspecified strains at the same dose levels as used for mice. The same lack of effect was noted regarding mortality, and the same effect was seen on food consumption; however, in animals fed 25% there were some cases of hepatic cirrhosis, although no changes occurred in the intestinal tract, kidneys or liver in animals fed the lower dose levels (Nilson & Wagner, 1959).

(b) <u>Subcutaneous and/or intramuscular administration</u>

<u>Rat</u>: Female Wistar rats, 60 days old, received s.c. injections of 5 ml 1% w/v carrageenan in 0.9% saline solution in the left flank. These animals served as controls for another experiment in which it had been established that 7 days after such injections a mass of new fibrous tissue containing many young fibroblasts was formed at the injection site. The animals were thus given s.c. injections of saline into both flanks on the 7th day. Of 39 rats surviving 400 days 11 developed sarcomas on the left side and none on the right, within 825 days. In all other experiments in which carrageenan was injected into the left flank, sarcomas were found only at that site; secondary treatment with alkylating agents seemed to have no effect (Cater, 1961).

3.2 <u>Other relevant biological data</u>

In guinea-pigs, the native form of carrageenan was not absorbed; degraded carrageenan could be detected in the urine of the animals at levels of about 0.3 mg/ml after 1.85 g had been administered in drinking-water or at levels of between 0.03 and 0.3 mg/ml when 4-15 mg/kg bw of the degraded carrageenan had been administered intravenously (Anderson & Soman, 1966). Native carrageenan fed to young rats at levels of 2-20% in the diet was found to be excreted quantitatively in the faeces (Hawkins & Yaphe, 1965).

No storage of carrageenan was found in rhesus monkeys given 1% native carrageenan in drinking-water over 7-11 weeks, followed by a 24-week recovery period. In contrast, degraded carrageenan, which was retained after absorption in the reticuloendothelial tissue, could still be found in Kupffer cells six months after administration (Abraham *et al.*, 1972).

Administration to rhesus monkeys of 1% native carrageenan in drinking-water, providing an intake of 1.3 g/kg bw/day for 7-14 weeks, produced no adverse effect. Administration of degraded carrageenan at the same dose level resulted in weight loss, haemorrhages in the intestinal tract and anaemia; lesions included mucosal erosion leading to ulceration, formation of granulation tissue in the lamina propria and multiple crypt abscesses (Benitz *et al.*, 1973).

When a 5% solution of native or a 1% solution of degraded carrageenan was administered as drinking-water to guinea-pigs and rats, with or without the addition of neomycin, ulceration of the large intestine was produced only in guinea-pigs, whether or not neomycin was present, while the rats showed slight diarrhoea with faecal softening but no ulceration (Grasso *et al.*, 1973). With 5% solutions of degraded carrageenan severe diarrhoea was observed in rats (Grasso *et al.*, 1975).

Watt & Marcus (1969) also observed ulcerative colitis in guinea-pigs given 1% native carrageenan or 5% degraded carrageenan in drinking-water. In those on native carrageenan, multiple ulcerative lesions in the caecum were observed in 2/4 animals after 20 days; 6 animals were killed after 30 days, and these also had lesions in the caecum, extending into the colon in 2 animals; the overall incidence of ulceration was 80%. Similar results were seen in the group given degraded carrageenan, the incidence of ulceration being 100%.

3.3 Observations in man

No case reports of cancer or epidemiological studies were available to the Working Group.

4. Comments on Data Reported and Evaluation

4.1 Animal data

One type of carrageenan was tested in rats by subcutaneous injection and produced local sarcomas (see also preamble, p. 21). In mice and rats administered food-grade native carrageenan orally, the incidence of tumours was greater than that in controls; however, this negative experiment is inadequate in terms of the number of animals used.

4.2 Human data

No case reports or epidemiological studies were available to the Working Group.

5. References

Abraham, R., Goldberg, L. & Coulston, F. (1972) Uptake and storage of degraded carrageenan in lysosomes of reticuloendothelial cells of the rhesus monkey, *Macaca mulatta*. Exp. mol. Path., 17, 77-93

Anderson, W. (1967) Carrageenan - structure and biological activity. Canad. J. pharm. Sci., 2, 81-90

Anderson, W. & Soman, P.D. (1966) The absorption of carrageenans. J. Pharm. Pharmacol., 18, 825-827

Benitz, K.-F., Goldberg, L. & Coulston, F. (1973) Intestinal effects of carrageenans in the rhesus monkey (*Macaca mulatta*). Fd Cosmet. Toxicol., 11, 565-575

Cater, D.B. (1961) The carcinogenic action of carrageenin in rats. Brit. J. Cancer, 15, 607-614

Di Rosa, M. (1972) Biological properties of carrageenan. J. Pharm. Pharmacol., 24, 89-102

FAO/WHO (1970) Specifications for the identity and purity of some food colours, emulsifiers, stabilizers, anti-caking agents and certain other food additives. FAO Nutr. Mtgs Rep. Ser. No. 46B; WHO/Food Add./70.37, pp. 38-40

Graham, H.D. (1966) Spectrophotometric determination of carrageenan ester sulfate in milk and milk products with barium chloranilate. J. Dairy Sci., 49, 1102-1108

Graham, H.D. (1968) Quantitative determination of carrageenan in milk and milk products using papain and cetyl pyridinium chloride. J. Fd Sci., 33, 390-394

Graham, H.D. (1972) *Ortho*-tolidine and sodium hypochlorite for the determination of carrageenan and other ester sulfates. J. Dairy Sci., 55, 1675-1682

Grasso, P., Sharratt, M., Carpanini, F.M.B. & Gangolli, S.D. (1973) Studies on carrageenan and large-bowel ulceration in mammals. Fd Cosmet. Toxicol., 11, 555-564

Grasso, P., Gangolli, S.D., Butterworth, K.R. & Wright, M.G. (1975) Studies on degraded carrageenan in rats and guinea pigs. Fd Cosmet. Toxicol., 13, 195-201

Hawkins, W.W. & Yaphe, W. (1965) Carrageenan as a dietary constituent for the rat: faecal excretion, nitrogen absorption, and growth. Canad. J. Biochem., 43, 479-484

Klose, R.E. & Glicksman, M. (1968) Gums. In: Furia, T.E., ed., Handbook of Food Additives, Cleveland, Ohio, The Chemical Rubber Company, pp. 325-327

NAS-NRC (National Academy of Sciences - National Research Council) (1963) Food Chemicals Codex, Publ. 1143, Washington DC, pp. 422-424

Nilson, H.W. & Wagner, J.S. (1959) Feeding test with carrageenin. Fd Res., 24, 235-239

Schmolck, W. & Mergenthaler, E. (1973) Beiträge zur Analytik von Polysacchariden, die als Lebensmittelzusatzstoffe verwendet werden. II. Gaschromatographischer Nachweis nach Methanolyse und Trimethylsilylierung. Z. Lebensmittel. Untersuch., 152, 263-273

Smith, D.B. & Cook, W.H. (1953) Fractionation of carrageenin. Arch. Biochem. Biophys., 45, 232-233

Towle, G.A. (1973) Carrageenan. In: Whistler, R.L. & BeMiller, J.N., eds, Industrial Gums: Polysaccharides and their Derivatives, 2nd ed., New York, London, Academic Press, pp. 83-114

Watt, J. & Marcus, R. (1969) Ulcerative colitis in the guinea-pig caused by seaweed extract. J. Pharm. Pharmacol., 21, 187S-188S

OCHRATOXIN A

The chemical and biological properties of this substance have been reviewed recently (Harwig, 1974).

1. Chemical and Physical Data

1.1 Synonyms and trade names

Chem. Abstr. Reg. Serial No.: 303-47-9

Chem. Abstr. Name: (R)N-[(5-chloro-3,4-dihydro-8-hydroxy-3-methyl-1-oxo-1H-2-benzopyran-7-yl)carbonyl](-L-)phenylalanine

[R]-N-[(5-Chloro-8-hydroxy-3-methyl-1-oxo-7-isochromanyl)carbonyl]-1-3-phenyl(-)alanine

1.2 Chemical formula and molecular weight

$C_{20}H_{18}ClNO_6$ Mol. wt: 403.8

1.3 Chemical and physical properties of the pure substance

(a) <u>Description</u>: Colourless crystals; fluorescent in ultraviolet light, emitting green and blue fluorescence in acid and alkaline solutions, respectively

(b) <u>Melting-point</u>: 169°C

(c) <u>Spectroscopy data</u>: λ_{max} 215 nm and 333 nm (E_1^1 = 910 and 150, respectively) at pH 4; above pH 9 λ_{max} are 333 nm and 380 nm (E_1^1 = 150 and 189) (in ethanol); in ethanol, fluorescence emission max 465 nm (Chu, 1974)

(d) _Identity and purity test_: Purity can be determined by visual examination of fluorescence on chromatograms under ultra-violet light; microgram quantities can be discerned under optimum conditions (Nesheim et al., 1973).

(e) _Solubility_: The sodium salt is soluble in water; as an acid, it is moderately soluble in polar organic solvents (e.g., chloroform and methanol).

(f) _Stability_: Relatively unstable to light and air; fading and degradation products appear upon brief exposure of chromatograms to light, especially at high humidity. Ethanol solutions are stable for more than a year if kept in dark and cold. The toxin is fairly stable in cereal products, and an appreciable percentage (up to 35%) survives autoclaving for up to three hours.

(g) _Chemical reactivity_: Acid and enzymic hydrolysis of ochratoxin A yield L-β-phenylalanine and the isocoumarin acid (ochratoxin α).

1.4 Technical products and impurities

No data were available to the Working Group.

2. Production, Use, Occurrence and Analysis

2.1 Production and use

While ochratoxin A is not produced commercially, it is offered for sale in small quantities by one firm in Israel.

2.2 Occurrence

Ochratoxin-producing fungi are encompassed in the genera *Penicillium* and *Aspergillus*; the *Penicillium* strains appear to be responsible for ochratoxin formation in colder climatic areas (Northern Europe, Canada), whereas in tropical and subtropical areas the *Aspergillus ochraceus* group may also produce it. Ochratoxin A has been detected in mouldy cereals (wheat, maize, rye, barley, oats), beans and peanuts (range, 9-27,500 µg/kg) (Krogh et al., 1973; Scott et al., 1970; 1972). It has been detected in barley intended for beer production, and, although a pronounced degradation takes place during malting and fermentation, some carryover of ochratoxin A into beer cannot be excluded (Chu et al., 1975; Krogh et al., 1974a). On the other hand, one survey failed to detect any ochratoxin A in beer and malted barley (sensitivity of the method, 10 µg/kg) (Fischbach & Rodricks, 1973).

2.3 Analysis

Chemical assay methods are available for the detection and quantification of ochratoxin A in various foodstuffs (Chu, 1974). A procedure developed for barley by Nesheim et al. (1973), but applicable to other commodities, has been tested collaboratively (Nesheim, 1973). The method has a limit of detection lower than 12 µg/kg, and with ammoniation this limit can be reduced to 3-5 µg/kg. This procedure has received the status 'Recommended method' by the International Union of Pure and Applied Chemistry.

3. Biological Data Relevant to the Evaluation of Carcinogenic Risk to Man

3.1 Carcinogenicity and related studies in animals

(a) Oral administration

Rat: Ochratoxin A was administered at doses of 100 or 300 µg/rat on 5 days a week for 50 weeks to groups of 5 male and 5 female Wistar rats; the only tumour observed was a hamartoma of the kidney in 1/10 rats receiving the highest dose (Purchase & van der Watt, 1971).

Trout: Rainbow trout fed a diet containing 20 µg ochratoxin A per kg of diet, together with sterculic acid, developed hepatomas (number unspecified). No tumours were observed when ochratoxin A was fed alone at concentrations of 16, 32, or 64 µg/kg of diet for 8 months (Doster et al., 1971).

(b) Subcutaneous and/or intramuscular administration

Mouse: Each animal of a group of 10 male and 10 female CBA mice received s.c. injections of 10 µg ochratoxin A suspended in 0.1 ml arachis oil twice weekly for 36 weeks; no tumours were observed in 7 survivors after 81 weeks (Dickens & Waynforth, 1968).

Rat: Ten female Wistar rats received s.c. injections of ochratoxin A suspended in sunflower-seed oil, at a dose of 2.5 mg/kg bw, injected twice weekly for 18 weeks. At weeks 73 and 87, 2/10 animals had developed local fibrosarcomas; 2/10 controls injected with sunflower-seed oil alone also developed local fibrosarcomas at week 87 (Purchase & van der Watt, 1971).

3.2 Other relevant biological data

The acute oral LD_{50}'s of ochratoxin A in rats were 22 mg/kg bw for males and 20 mg/kg bw for females (Purchase & Theron, 1968). Ochratoxin A-induced nephropathy has been demonstrated experimentally in pigs, dogs, rats, chickens and trout (Chu, 1974; Krogh *et al.*, 1974b), and ochratoxin A is thought to be the causative agent in field cases of nephropathy in pigs and poultry (Krogh, 1976).

Pregnant mice given a single dose of 5 mg/kg bw ochratoxin A by i.p. injection on days 7, 8, 9, 10, 11 or 12 of gestation showed increased prenatal mortality, decreased foetal weight and foetal malformations (Hayes *et al.*, 1974).

Because of striking similarities in the changes of renal function and structure seen in Balkan endemic nephropathy and in ochratoxin A-induced porcine nephropathy, surveys were initiated in those areas where the disease is prevalent in order to establish a causal relationship with food-borne ochratoxin A. Preliminary results from one village show that up to 20% of home-grown cereals (maize, barley, wheat) are contaminated with ochratoxin A; however, levels were not reported (Krogh, 1974).

3.3 Observations in man

No case reports on cancer or epidemiological studies were available to the Working Group.

4. Comments on Data Reported and Evaluation

4.1 Animal data

Ochratoxin A has been tested orally in rats and trout and by subcutaneous injection in mice and rats. All studies were inadequate in terms of the numbers of animals used and survival rates; no evaluation can be made.

4.2 Human data

No case reports on cancer or epidemiological studies were available to the Working Group.

5. References

Chu, F.S. (1974) Studies on ochratoxins. *C.R.C. Crit. Rev. Toxicol.*, 2, 499-524

Chu, F.S., Chang, C.C., Ashoor, S.H. & Prentice, N. (1975) Stability of aflatoxin B_1 and ochratoxin A in brewing. *Appl. Microbiol.*, 29, 313-316

Dickens, F. & Waynforth, H.B. (1968) Studies on carcinogenesis by lactones and related substances. *Rep. Brit. Emp. Cancer Campn*, 46, 108

Doster, R.C., Sinnshuber, R.O., Wales, J.H. & Lee, D.J. (1971) Acute toxicity and carcinogenicity of ochratoxin in rainbow trout (*Salmo gairdneri*). *Fed. Proc.*, 30, 578

Fischbach, H. & Rodricks, J.H. (1973) Current efforts of the Food and Drug Administration to control mycotoxins in food. *J. Ass. off. analyt. Chem.*, 56, 767-770

Harwig, J. (1974) *Ochratoxin A and related metabolites.* In: Purchase, I.F.H., ed., *Mycotoxins*, Amsterdam, Elsevier, pp. 345-367

Hayes, A.W., Hood, R.D. & Lee, H.L. (1974) Teratogenic effects of ochratoxin A in mice. *Teratology*, 9, 93-98

Krogh, P. (1974) *Mycotoxic porcine nephropathy: a possible model for Balkan endemic nephropathy.* In: Puchlev, A., Dinev, I.V., Milev, B. & Doichinov, D., eds, *Endemic Nephropathy*, Sofia, Bulgarian Academy of Sciences, pp. 266-270

Krogh, P. (1976) Mycotoxic nephropathy. *Advanc. vet. Sci. comp. med.* (in press)

Krogh, P., Hald, B. & Pedersen, E.J. (1973) Occurrence of ochratoxin A and citrinin in cereals associated with mycotoxic porcine nephropathy. *Acta path. microbiol. scand., Section B*, 81, 689-695

Krogh, P., Hald, B., Gjertsen, P. & Myken, F. (1974a) Fate of ochratoxin A and citrinin during malting and brewing experiments. *Appl. Microbiol.*, 28, 31-34

Krogh, P., Axelsen, N.H., Elling, F., Gyrd-Hansen, N., Hald, B., Hyldgaard-Jensen, J., Larsen, A.E., Madsen, A., Mortsensen, H.P., Møller, T., Petersen, O.K., Ravnskov, U., Rostgaard, M. & Aaland, O. (1974b) Experimental porcine nephropathy. Changes of renal function and structure induced by ochratoxin A-contaminated feed. *Acta path. microbiol. scand., Section A*, Suppl. 246, 1-21

Nesheim, S. (1973) Analysis of ochratoxins A and B and their esters in barley, using partition and thin-layer chromatography. II. Collaborative study. J. Ass. off. analyt. Chem., 56, 822-826

Nesheim, S., Hardin, N.F., Francis, O.J., Jr & Langham, W.S. (1973) Analysis of ochratoxins A and B and their esters in barley, using partition and thin-layer chromatography. I. Development of the method. J. Ass. off. analyt. Chem., 56, 817-821

Purchase, I.F.H. & Theron, J.J. (1968) The acute toxicity of ochratoxin A to rats. Fd Cosmet. Toxicol., 6, 479-483

Purchase, I.F.H. & van der Watt, J.J. (1971) The long-term toxicity of ochratoxin A to rats. Fd Cosmet. Toxicol., 9, 681-682

Scott, P.M., van Walbeek, W., Harwig, J. & Fennell, D.I. (1970) Occurrence of a mycotoxin, ochratoxin A, in wheat and isolation of ochratoxin A and citrinin producing strains of *Penicillium viridicatum*. Canad. J. Plant Sci., 50, 583-585

Scott, P.M., van Walbeek, W., Kennedy, B. & Anyeti, D. (1972) Mycotoxins (ochratoxin A, citrinin and sterigmatocystin) and toxigenic fungi in grains and other agricultural products. J. agric. Fd Chem., 20, 1103-1109

PARASORBIC ACID

1. Chemical and Physical Data

1.1 Synonyms and trade names

Chem. Abstr. Reg. Serial No.: 10048-32-5

Chem. Abstr. Name: (S)-5,6-Dihydro-6-methyl-2H-pyran-2-one

5-Hydroxy-2-hexanoic acid δ-lactone; sorbic oil (Vogelbeeröl)

1.2 Chemical formula and molecular weight

$C_6H_8O_2$ Mol. wt: 112.1

1.3 Chemical and physical properties of the pure substance

(a) Description: Oily liquid with a sweet aromatic odour; irritant vapours

(b) Boiling-point: 104-105°C at 14 mm Hg

(c) Density: d_4^{18} 1.079

(d) Optical rotation: $[\alpha]_D^{18}$ +49.3° (in water); $[\alpha]_D^{19}$ +210° (2% in ethanol)

(e) Solubility: Soluble in water; freely soluble in ethanol and diethyl ether

(f) Volatility: Volatile at room temperature (Letzig & Handschack, 1963)

(g) Stability: Aqueous solutions are neutral but become acid on storage.

(h) Reactivity: In the presence of a strong alkali and heat, 70% is converted into sorbic acid after several hours (Letzig & Handschack, 1963).

1.4 Technical products and impurities

No data were available to the Working Group.

2. Production, Use, Occurrence and Analysis

2.1 Production and use

Parasorbic acid is not produced in significant commercial quantities in the US. The naturally occurring (5S)-(+)-parasorbic acid has been isolated from ripe berries of the mountain ash (*Sorbus aucuparia* L.) since 1859. The optically inactive isomer (+) can be synthesised (Haynes & Jones, 1946), and a method of synthesis from sorbic acid was recently reported (Stafford *et al.*, 1972).

In parts of the German Democratic Republic *Sorbus aucuparia* var. *edulis* (Dieck) has been consumed as a fruit (eaten as such or as a purée), and during the 1950's it was acclaimed for its high content of ascorbic acid. Nowadays, mountain ash berries are pressed to give a crude concentrate which can be consumed as a fruit drink after the addition of sugar and water; alternatively the concentrate is thickened by vacuum drying, the volume being reduced by 3-4 times, to give a thick syrup which is used as a natural acidifying agent in place of citrus fruits in home food preparation. It is also used to acidify the milk given to babies (Letzig & Handschack, 1963).

Crude preparations of mountain ash berries have been, and may still be, used in some countries in human medicine (Dickens, 1967).

2.2 Occurrence

Concentrations of parasorbic acid in the ripe fruit of *Sorbus aucuparia* (var. *edulis*) are from 0.2-2 g/kg (Letzig & Handschack, 1963). It was not found in pears, apples, lemons, oranges, tomatoes, grapes or cranberries (Diemair & Franzen, 1959).

2.3 Analysis

Parasorbic acid may be separated from sorbic acid (which is used as a food preservative) by column chromatography, and levels as low as 20 mg/kg can be estimated quantitatively by thin-layer chromatography (Stafford *et al.*, 1972). Parasorbic acid was not detected in several grades of commercial sorbic acid by these authors, nor by Murphy & Wardleworth (1973), who developed a still more sensitive assay method involving extraction by dichloromethane followed by gas chromatography using a flame ionization detector (limit of detection, 0.5 mg/kg).

3. Biological Data Relevant to the Evaluation of Carcinogenic Risk to Man

3.1 Carcinogenicity and related studies in animals

(a) Oral administration

Rat: Pure (+)-parasorbic acid was administered in the drinking-water to 2 groups of 6 male rats (100 g bw) at concentrations of 2 and 10 mg/l for 64 weeks; on the basis of average weekly water consumption, total amounts ingested were 28 and 198 mg/animal at the two dose levels.* Three animals receiving the lower dose died of infection early in the treatment period. No tumours of the liver or other tissues were observed after 64 weeks in 3/6 survivors of the low dose level group, nor in 4/6 survivors of the high dose level group. The only tumour seen was a Leydig-cell tumour of the testis in a rat receiving the low dose which died during the 103rd week (Dickens *et al.*, 1966).

Groups of 48 male and 48 female Wistar rats were fed diets containing 12,000 mg sorbic acid per kg of diet or 12,000 mg sorbic acid containing 1000 mg synthetic parasorbic acid per kg of diet for 2 years (daily intake of parasorbic acid, 0.24 mg/day). Of the parasorbic acid/sorbic acid-treated rats, 28 males and 32 females survived 106 weeks; among 42 males and 45 females autopsied, 20 and 38 tumours were found, compared with 19 and 26 tumours in 36 males and 45 females autopsied after receiving sorbic acid alone. In males, tumours were mainly chromophobe adenomas, and in females, mammary fibroadenomas and chromophobe adenomas. Such tumours were reported to occur frequently in this strain of rat. Tumours found only in

---

*Natural (+)-parasorbic acid was replaced by synthetic acid after 31 weeks (personal communication).

rats receiving parasorbic/sorbic acid included two cyst adenomas of the thyroid, one adenoma of the pancreas, one myoma, one subcutaneous and one uterine fibrosarcoma, one squamous-cell carcinoma of the skin and two reticulum-cell neoplasms in the liver and ileum. Such tumours also occur in untreated rats, but no concurrent controls were used (Mason *et al.*, 1976).

(b) Subcutaneous and/or intramuscular administration

Rat: Pure (+)-parasorbic acid was administered by s.c. injection to 2 groups of six male rats (100 g bw) at doses of 0.2 or 2 mg/animal in oil twice weekly for 32 weeks (total doses, 12.8 and 128 mg/rat). Local sarcomas were observed in 4/6 and 4/5 rats in the 2 groups within 95-106 weeks. The first tumours appeared 61-63 weeks after the start of treatment, and 6/8 sarcomas were successfully transplanted into young rats. No tumours occurred in controls injected with arachis oil alone (Dickens & Jones, 1963). [For further control data see Appendix.]

3.2 Other relevant biological data

The i.p. LD_{50} in mice is 750 mg/kg bw (Stecher, 1968).

No data on metabolism were available to the Working Group.

3.3 Observations in man

No data were available to the Working Group.

4. Comments on Data Reported and Evaluation

4.1 Animal data

Parasorbic acid administered by subcutaneous injection to rats produced local sarcomas. Feeding experiments in rats where parasorbic acid was given in combination with sorbic acid cannot be evaluated because of the relatively low dose of parasorbic acid administered and the lack of contemporary control groups. A further oral study in rats was considered inadequate due to the small number of surviving animals (see also preamble, p. 21).

4.2 Human data

No case reports or epidemiological studies were available to the Working Group.

APPENDIX

Collected table of control experiments with rats injected subcutaneously with arachis oil

All rats received twice weekly subcutaneous injections of 0.5 ml arachis oil for the stated periods to approximately the same area on the right side.

Ref.	No. of rats	Injection period (weeks)	Termination at week	Total no. of tumours		Local tumours at weeks		No. of survivors at weeks
				local	other	52	80-85	100-104
Short-term experiments								
a	6	54	54	0	0	0/6	-	-
a	5	61	61	0	0	0/5	-	-
c	5	45	45	0	0	-	-	-
Long-term experiments								
a	5	61	107	0	1*	0/4	0/4	0/3
b	6	61	106	0	2†	0/4	0/4	0/4
c	6	65	106	0	0	0/5	0/5	0/3
d	6	65	89	1+	0	0/4	1+/3	0/2
e	12	60	108	0	0	0/9	0/5	0/3
Total of long-term experiments only								
a-e	35	60-65	89-108	1+	3	0/26	1+/21	0/15

References:

(a) Dickens & Jones (1961) (b) Dickens & Jones (1963)
(c) Dickens & Jones (1965) (d) Dickens *et al.* (1966)
(e) Dickens *et al.* (1968)

Footnotes:

* 1 thoracic tumour
† 1 thyroid carcinoma with a secondary in adrenal
+ 1 local sarcoma-like, but histologically non-malignant, tumour

5. References

Dickens, F. (1967) Drugs with lactone groups as potential carcinogens. *UICC Monogr. Ser.*, 7, 144-151

Dickens, F. & Jones, H.E.H. (1961) Carcinogenic activity of a series of reactive lactones and related substances. *Brit. J. Cancer*, 15, 85-100

Dickens, F. & Jones, H.E.H. (1963) Further studies on the carcinogenic and growth-inhibitory activity of lactones and related substances. *Brit. J. Cancer*, 17, 100-108

Dickens, F. & Jones, H.E.H. (1965) Further studies on the carcinogenic action of certain lactones and related substances in the rat and mouse. *Brit. J. Cancer*, 19, 392-403

Dickens, F., Jones, H.E.H. & Waynforth, H.B. (1966) Oral, subcutaneous and intratracheal administration of carcinogenic lactones and related substances: the intratracheal administration of cigarette tar in the rat. *Brit. J. Cancer*, 20, 134-144

Dickens, F., Jones, H.E.H. & Waynforth, H.B. (1968) Further studies on the carcinogenicity of sorbic acid in the rat. *Brit. J. Cancer*, 22, 762-768

Diemair, W. & Franzen, K. (1959) Über das Vorkommen der Parasorbinsäure und der Sorbinsäure. *Z. Lebensmittel. Untersuch.*, 109, 373-378

Haynes, L.J. & Jones, E.R.C. (1946) A new route to growth-inhibitory $\alpha\beta$-ethylenic γ- and δ-lactones. *J. chem. Soc.*, 954-960

Letzig, E. & Handschack, W. (1963) Vergleichende Untersuchunger über einige Inhaltsstoffe bitterer und süsser Ebereschenfrüchte während des Reifens. *Nahrung*, 7, 591-605

Mason, P.L., Gaunt, I.F., Hardy, J., Kiss, I.S., Butterworth, K.R. & Gangolli, S.D. (1976) Long-term toxicity of parasorbic acid in rats. *Fd Cosmet. Toxicol.*, 13 (in press)

Murphy, J.M. & Wardleworth, D.F. (1973) Improved method for the estimation of parasorbic acid in sorbic acid. *J. Sci. Fd Agric.*, 24, 253-255

Stafford, A.E., Black, D.R., Haddon, W.F. & Waiss, A.C., Jr (1972) Analysis and improved synthesis of parasorbic acid. *J. Sci. Fd Agric.*, 23, 771-776

Stecher, P.G., ed. (1968) *The Merck Index*, 8th ed., Rahway, NJ, Merck & Co., p. 783

PATULIN

The chemical and biological properties of this substance have been reviewed recently (Scott, 1974).

1. Chemical and Physical Data

1.1 Synonyms and trade names

Chem. Abstr. Reg. Serial No.: 149-29-1

Chem. Abstr. Name: 4-Hydroxy-4H-furo[3,2-c]pyran-2(6H)-one

Clairformin; clavacin; clavatin; claviform; claviformin; 2,4-dihydroxy-2H-pyran-δ3(6H),α-acetic acid-3,4-lactone; [2,4-dihydroxy-2H-pyran-3(6H)-ylidene]acetic acid-3,4-lactone; expansin; expansine; mycoin; mycoin C; mycoin C$_3$; patuline; penicidin; tercinin

1.2 Chemical formula and molecular weight

$C_7H_6O_4$ Mol. wt: 154.1

1.3 Chemical and physical properties of the pure substance

(a) Description: Colourless prisms or thick plates from ether or chloroform

(b) Melting-point: 111°C

(c) Spectroscopy data: Ultra-violet, mass and nuclear magnetic resonance spectral data are given by Scott (1974) and Scott *et al.* (1972).

(d) Solubility: Soluble in water and common organic solvents, except light petroleum

(e) Stability: Unstable in alkali solutions

(f) Reactivity: Reduces warm Fehling's solution and alkaline permanganate; forms an acetate and a trimethylsilyl derivative

1.4 Technical products and impurities

No data were available to the Working Group.

2. Production, Use, Occurrence and Analysis

For important background information on this section, see preamble, p. 17.

2.1 Production and use

Patulin is an antibiotic derived from the metabolism of a number of fungi. It was first described by Birkinshaw et al. (1943) and was first synthesized by Woodward & Singh (1950). Chain et al. (1942) reported the isolation of claviformin from *Penicillium claviforme*, and this substance was subsequently shown to be identical with patulin.

Patulin has both bacteriostatic and bactericidal effects and is effective against various Gram-negative and Gram-positive bacteria. It has been tested for treatment of the common cold (Birkinshaw et al., 1943).

Patulin is not produced commercially, but it is available from one company in the US for experimental purposes only and is also available in Israel. This chemical is not authorized for use as a drug by the US Food and Drug Administration.

2.2 Occurrence

Patulin has been identified in rotten apples contaminated by *Penicillium expansum* (Brian et al., 1956; Harwig et al., 1973); up to 18 mg/apple were detected. Scott et al. (1972) found patulin (1 mg/l) in one sample of commercial 'sweet apple cider'. Wilson & Nuovo (1973) found up to 45 mg/l in cider made in mills using rotten apples which had been stored for long periods before use. Drillean & Bohnen (1973) found 0.1-0.3 mg/l in samples of cider, and it was detected at levels ranging from 44-309 µg/l in 8 of 13 samples of commercial apple juice (Ware et al., 1974). Escoula (1974) found that 50% of silage samples were contaminated with from 1.5-40 mg/kg. It has also been found in soil (1.5 mg/kg) after stubble-mulching (Norstadt & McCalla, 1969).

2.3 Analysis

A variety of methods were used by the authors cited above. Among the more recent methods are an improved method for detection in apple juice using thin-layer chromatography (limit of detection, 20 µg/l) (Scott & Kennedy, 1973) and a thin-layer method for analysis of patulin in corn (limit of detection, 40 µg/kg) (Pohland & Allen, 1970). Pohland et al. (1970) described a gas-liquid chromatography method for determination of patulin in apple juice (limit of detection, 0.7 µg/ml). Ware et al. (1974) used high-pressure liquid chromatography also for its detection in apple juice (limit of detection, 11 µg/l), and this method has been modified for its determination in apple butter (Ware, 1975).

3. Biological Data Relevant to the Evaluation of Carcinogenic Risk to Man

3.1 Carcinogenicity and related studies in animals

Subcutaneous and/or intramuscular administration

Rat: Two groups of 5 male Wistar rats (100 g bw) were given twice weekly s.c. injections of 0.2 or 2 mg/rat patulin in 0.5 ml arachis oil. All animals given the higher dose died, but injection of the lower dose was continued for 61 weeks. All of 4 rats surviving at the appearance of the first tumour (58 weeks) developed local sarcomas before 69 weeks; no tumours were observed at other sites. In a similar experiment, 4 rats survived 62 weeks after receiving twice-weekly injections of 0.2 mg patulin; 2 developed local sarcomas between 62 and 64 weeks (end of experiment). No local tumours occurred in 14 controls injected with 0.5 ml arachis oil and surviving 54-107 weeks (Dickens & Jones, 1961). [For additional control data see Appendix to monograph on parasorbic acid, p. 203]

3.2 Other relevant biological data

The LD_{50}'s in mice were 15 mg/kg bw by s.c. injection, 25 mg/kg bw by i.v. injection, 5 mg/kg bw by i.p. injection (Stecher, 1968) and about 35 mg/kg bw by oral administration. In rats, the s.c. LD_{50} was 15 mg/kg bw. In mice and guinea-pigs given repeated doses by s.c. injection, subcutaneous oedema and necrosis were observed (Broom et al., 1944; Katzman et al., 1944); in rats, doses of 20 mg/kg bw in oil given by s.c. injection were fatal but caused less local tissue reaction (Dickens & Jones, 1961).

Patulin of unspecified purity and origin dissolved in dimethylsulphoxide at a concentration of 3.5×10^{-6} M induced a significantly increased number of chromosomal aberrations in cultures of human peripheral leucocytes (Withers, 1966). Patulin of unspecified purity and origin induced single and double strand breaks in DNA of HeLa cells (Umeda *et al.*, 1972).

3.3 Observations in man

No data were available to the Working Group.

4. Comments on Data Reported and Evaluation

4.1 Animal data

In the only study available patulin was shown to produce sarcomas in rats at the site of its subcutaneous injection (see also preamble, p. 21).

4.2 Human data

No case reports or epidemiological studies were available to the Working Group.

5. References

Birkinshaw, J.H., Michael, S.E., Bracken, A. & Raistrick, H. (1943) Patulin in the common cold. II. Biochemistry and chemistry. Lancet, ii, 625-631

Brian, P.W., Elson, G.W. & Lowe, D. (1956) Production of patulin in apple fruits by *Penicillium expansum*. Nature (Lond.), 178, 263-264

Broom, W.A., Bülbring, E., Chapman, C.J., Hampton, J.W.F., Thomson, A.M., Ungar, J., Wien, R. & Woolfe, G. (1944) The pharmacology of patulin. Brit. J. exp. Path., 25, 195-207

Chain, E., Florey, H.W. & Jennings, M.A. (1942) An antibacterial substance produced by *Penicillium claviforme*. Brit. J. exp. Path., 23, 202-205

Dickens, F. & Jones, H.E.H. (1961) Carcinogenic activity of a series of reactive lactones and related substances. Brit. J. Cancer, 15, 85-100

Drillean, J.F. & Bohnen, G. (1973) Patulin in cider products. C.R. hebd. Seanc. Acad. Agric. franç., 59, 1031-1037

Escoula, L. (1974) Moisissures toximogènes des fourrages ensilés. I. Présence de patuline dans les fronts de coupe d'ensilages. Ann. Rec. vétér., 5, 423

Harwig, J., Chen, Y.K., Kennedy, B.P.C. & Scott, P.M. (1973) Occurrence of patulin and patulin-producing strains of *P. expansum* in natural rots of apples in Canada. Canad. Inst. Fd Sci. Technol., 8, 22-25

Katzman, P.A., Hays, E.E., Cain, C.K., Van Wyk, J.J., Reithel, F.J., Thayer, S.A. & Doisy, E.A. (1944) Clavacin, an antibiotic substance from *Aspergillus clavatus*. J. biol. Chem., 154, 475-486

Norstadt, F.A. & McCalla, T.M. (1969) Microbial populations in stubble-mulched soil. Soil Sci., 107, 188-193

Pohland, A.E. & Allen, R. (1970) Analysis and chemical confirmation of patulin in grains. J. Ass. off. analyt. Chem., 53, 686-687

Pohland, A.E., Sanders, K. & Thorpe, C.W. (1970) Determination of patulin in apple juice. J. Ass. off. analyt. Chem., 53, 692-695

Scott, P.M. (1974) Patulin. In: Purchase, I.F.H., ed., Mycotoxins, Amsterdam, Elsevier, pp. 383-403

Scott, P.M. & Kennedy, B.P.C. (1973) Improved method for the thin-layer chromatographic detection of patulin in apple juice. J. Ass. off. analyt. Chem., 56, 813-816

Scott, P.M., Miles, W.F., Toft, P. & Dube, J.G. (1972) Occurrence of patulin in apple juice. J. agric. Fd Chem., 22, 450-451

Stecher, P.G., ed. (1968) The Merck Index, 8th ed., Rahway, NJ, Merck & Co., p.785

Umeda, M., Yamamoto, T. & Saito, M. (1972) DNA-strand breakage of HeLa cells induced by several mycotoxins. Japan. J. exp. Med., 42, 527-535

Ware, G.M. (1975) High-pressure liquid chromatographic method for the determination of patulin in apple butter. J. Ass. off. analyt. Chem., 58, 754-756

Ware, G.M., Thorpe, G.W. & Pohland, A.E. (1974) A liquid chromatographic method for the determination of patulin in apple juice. J. Ass. off. analyt. Chem., 57, 1111-1113

Wilson, D.M. & Nuovo, G.J. (1973) Patulin production in apples decayed by *Penicillium expansum*. Appl. Microbiol., 26, 124-125

Withers, R.F.J. (1966) The action of some lactones and related compounds on human chromosomes. In: Landa, Z., ed., Mechanisms of Mutation and Inducing Factors. Proceedings of a symposium held in Prague, 1965, Prague, Academia, pp. 359-364

Woodward, R.B. & Singh, G. (1950) The synthesis of patulin. J. Amer. chem. Soc., 72, 1428

PENICILLIC ACID

1. Chemical and Physical Data

1.1 Synonyms and trade names

Chem. Abstr. Reg. Serial No.: 90-65-3

Chem. Abstr. Name: 3-Methoxy-5-methyl-4-oxo-2,5-hexadienoic acid

γ-Keto-β-methoxy-δ-methylene-δ(α)-hexenoic acid

1.2 Chemical formula and molecular weight

(I) γ-keto acid structure   (II) γ-hydroxylactone structure

$C_8H_{10}O_4$ Mol. wt: 170.2

1.3 Chemical and physical properties of the pure substance

(a) Description: Colourless crystals from light petroleum; exists as monohydrate when crystallized from water

(b) Melting-point: 84.5°C

(c) Spectroscopy data: λ_{max} 220 nm; $E_1^1 = 735$ (in KOH)

(d) Solubility: Moderately soluble in cold water; freely soluble in hot water; soluble in ethanol, ether, benzene and chloroform; slightly soluble in hot light petroleum

(e) Reactivity: In both acid and alkaline solutions it reacts as the lactol (formula II above) (Raphael, 1947a). It reacts readily with SH compounds, e.g., cysteine (Black, 1966; Ciegler et al., 1972; Dickens & Cooke, 1965), with loss of antibiotic activity and toxicity; it also reacts with amino acids, such as in meat protein (Ciegler et al., 1972).

1.4 Technical products and impurities

No data were available to the Working Group.

2. Production, Use, Occurrence and Analysis

2.1 Production and use

Penicillic acid is a mycotoxin first isolated from *Penicillium puberulum* in 1913 by Alsberg & Black. The structure was determined by Birkinshaw *et al.* (1936), and it was first synthesized by Raphael (1947b).

Its antibiotic properties against Gram-positive bacteria are much weaker than those of penicillin, but it is more active than penicillin against Gram-negative organisms. It is only weakly fungistatic.

No evidence was found that this chemical has ever been produced commercially.

2.2 Occurrence

Penicillic acid is an antibiotic substance produced by the following fungi: *Penicillium puberulum, P. cyclopium, P. thomii, P. suaveolens, P. baarnense, Aspergillus ochraceus* and *A. melleus* (Stecher, 1968).

Penicillic acid can be produced in corn infected with *Penicillium martensii* (Ciegler & Kurtzman, 1970), in mouldy corn (Pero *et al.*, 1972) and in poultry feed (Bacon *et al.*, 1973). Storage of corn infected with *P. martensii* at low temperatures and high moisture levels may increase the amount of toxin produced (Kurtzman & Ciegler, 1970). No penicillic acid was detected in mould-fermented sausage (salami), but since it reacts readily with amino acids it may not have been detected by the method used (Ciegler *et al.*, 1972). About 3% of penicillic acid added to cigarette tobacco was recovered in the smoke condensate, and small amounts were found in mouldy tobacco (Snow *et al.*, 1972). Penicillic acid was present in 7 of 20 commercial corn samples analysed, at levels ranging from 5-230 µg/kg, and in 5 of 20 samples of commercial dried beans at levels from 11-179 µg/kg (Thorpe & Johnson, 1974).

2.3 Analysis

The earlier colorimetric methods are not sensitive enough for detection of penicillic acid in most foodstuffs (lower limit of detection, about 200 µg); however, Ciegler & Kurtzman (1970) described a fluorimetric method which is sensitive to about 1-9 µg and is suitable for this purpose.

Pero et al. (1972) developed a gas-chromatographic method of analysis enabling the simultaneous determination of very small amounts (1 µg/100 µg of extract) of both penicillic acid and patulin in similar materials. A gas-liquid chromatographic method for the detection of penicillic acid in corn, dried beans and apple juice, with a limit of detection of 4 µg/kg, was described by Thorpe & Johnson (1974).

3. Biological Data Relevant to the Evaluation of Carcinogenic Risk to Man

3.1 Carcinogenicity and related studies in animals

(a) Inhalation and/or intratracheal administration

Rat: Six male rats received doses of 0.3 mg/animal penicillic acid in 30 µl arachis oil by intratracheal intubation twice weekly for 30 weeks (total dose, 18 mg). Six further rats received 30 µl oil alone for the same period. No tumours of the lung or other organs were detected in any of these rats up to the termination of the experiment in its 92nd week. Four rats which received penicillic acid survived 72-92 weeks (Dickens et al., 1966).

(b) Subcutaneous and/or intramuscular administration

Mouse: A group of 10 male and 10 female mice (Tuck No. 1 strain) was given twice weekly s.c. injections of 0.2 mg penicillic acid in 0.1 ml arachis oil for up to 65 weeks; 20 controls were injected with arachis oil alone. Local tumours developed in 6/19 treated mice between 38-81 weeks. One control developed a mammary adenoma near the injection site after 69 weeks (Dickens & Jones, 1965).

Rat: Groups of 5-6 male rats were given twice weekly s.c. injections of 0.1 or 1 mg penicillic acid in 0.5 ml arachis oil or 2 mg in water for 61, 64 and 52 weeks respectively. Local sarcomas or fibrosarcomas developed at between 48 and 67 weeks in 4/4 rats given the higher dose in oil and in 1/4 rats given the lower dose at between 94 and 106 weeks. Of the rats given penicillic acid in water, 4/5 surviving 56-104 weeks developed local tumours. No tumours occurred in 7 controls surviving 83 or more weeks (Dickens & Jones, 1961; 1963; 1965).

3.2 Other relevant biological data

The LD_{50}'s of penicillic acid in mice were 250 mg/kg bw by i.v. injection and 600 mg/kg bw orally (Murnaghan, 1946). Application of penicillic acid to rabbit skin caused severe oedema and necrosis within 2 hours (Ciegler et al., 1972).

Penicillic acid induced single and double strand breaks in DNA of HeLa cells (Umeda et al., 1972).

3.3 Observations in man

No data were available to the Working Group.

4. Comments on Data Reported and Evaluation

4.1 Animal data

Penicillic acid was tested by subcutaneous injection in mice and rats; it produced local sarcomas (see also preamble, p. 21).

4.2 Human data

No case reports or epidemiological studies were available to the Working Group.

5. References

Bacon, C.W., Sweeney, J.G., Robbins, J.D. & Burdick, D. (1973) Production of penicillic acid and ochratoxin A on poultry feed by *Aspergillus ochraceus*: temperature and moisture requirements. Appl. Microbiol., 26, 155-160

Birkinshaw, J.H., Oxford, A.E. & Raistrick, H. (1936) Studies on the biochemistry of microorganisms. XLVIII. Penicillic acid, a metabolic product of *P. puberulum* Bainier and *P. cyclopium* Westling. Biochem. J., 30, 394-411

Black, D.K. (1966) The addition of L-cysteine to unsaturated lactones and related compounds. J. chem. Soc., 1123-1127

Ciegler, A. & Kurtzman, C.P. (1970) Fluorodensitometric assay of penicillic acid. J. Chromat., 51, 511-516

Ciegler, A., Mintzlaff, H.J., Weisleder, D. & Leistner, L. (1972) Potential production and detoxification of penicillic acid in mold-fermented sausage (salami). Appl. Microbiol., 24, 114-119

Dickens, F. & Cooke, J. (1965) Rates of hydrolysis and interaction with cysteine of some carcinogenic lactones and related substances. Brit. J. Cancer, 19, 404-410

Dickens, F. & Jones, H.E.H. (1961) Carcinogenic activity of a series of reactive lactones and related substances. Brit. J. Cancer, 15, 85-100

Dickens, F. & Jones, H.E.H. (1963) Further studies on the carcinogenic and growth-inhibitory activities of lactones and related substances. Brit. J. Cancer, 17, 100-108

Dickens, F. & Jones, H.E.H. (1965) Further studies on the carcinogenic action of certain lactones and related substances in the rat and mouse. Brit. J. Cancer, 19, 392-403

Dickens, F., Jones, H.E.H. & Waynforth, H.B. (1966) Oral, subcutaneous and intratracheal administration of reactive lactones and related substances: the intratracheal administration of cigarette tar in the rat. Brit. J. Cancer, 20, 134-144

Kurtzman, C.P. & Ciegler, A. (1970) Mycotoxin from a blue-eye mold of corn. Appl. Microbiol., 20, 204-207

Murnaghan, M.F. (1946) The pharmacology of penicillic acid. J. Pharmacol. exp. Ther., 88, 119-132

Pero, R.W., Harvan, D., Owens, R.G. & Snow, J.P. (1972) A gas-chromatographic method for the mycotoxin penicillic acid. J. Chromat., 65, 501-506

Raphael, R.A. (1947a) Compounds related to penicillic acid. II. Synthesis of dihydropenicillic acid. J. chem. Soc., 805-808

Raphael, R.A. (1947b) Synthesis of the antibiotic, penicillic acid. Nature (Lond.), 160, 261-262

Snow, J.P., Lucas, G.B., Harvan, D., Pero, R.W. & Owens, R.G. (1972) Analysis of tobacco and smoke condensate for penicillic acid. Appl. Microbiol., 24, 34-36

Stecher, P.G., ed. (1968) The Merck Index, 8th ed., Rahway, NJ, Merck & Co., p. 790

Thorpe, C.W. & Johnson, R.L. (1974) Analysis of penicillic acid by gas-liquid chromatography. J. Ass. off. analyt. Chem., 57, 861-865

Umeda, M., Yamamoto, T. & Saito, M. (1972) DNA-strand breakage of HeLa cells induced by several mycotoxins. Japan. J. exp. Med., 42, 527-535

RESERPINE

1. Chemical and Physical Data

1.1 Synonyms and trade names

Chem. Abstr. Reg. Serial No.: 50-55-5

Chem. Abstr. Name: 3β,16β,17α,18β,20α-Yohimban-16-carboxylic acid, 11,17-dimethoxy-18-[(3,4,5-trimethoxybenzoyl)oxy]methyl ester

Anquil; banisil; bioserpine; deserpine; 11,17-dimethoxy-18-[(3,-4,5-trimethoxybenzoyl)oxy]-3β,16β,17α,18β,20α-yohimban-16-carboxylic acid methyl ester; elserpine; eserpine; 18β-hydroxy-11,17α-dimethoxy-3β,20α-yohimban-16β-carboxylic acid methyl ester 3,4,5-trimethoxy benzoate (ester); kitine; lemiserp; loweserp; mayserpine; methyl-1α,2β,3α,4,4aα,5,7,8,13,13bβ,14,14aα-dodecahydro-2α,11-dimethoxy-3β-(3,4,5-trimethoxybenzoyloxy)benz[g]indolo(2,3α)quinolizine-1β-carboxylate; methylreserpate 3,4,5-trimethoxybenzoic acid; methyl reserpate 3,4,5-trimethoxybenzoic acid ester; raucap; raulen; raupasil; raurine; rausedil; rausedyl; rausingle; rauwilid; resercen; reserpamed; reserpene; resine; respital; restan; riserpa; serpaloid; serpentina; serpicon; sertabs; sertina; 3,4,5-trimethoxy benzoic acid ester with methyl 18β-hydroxy-11,17α-dimethoxy-3β,20α-yohimban-16β-carboxylate; 3,4,5-trimethoxybenzoyl methyl reserpate; t-serp; vioserpine; yohimban-16-carboxylic acid derivative of benz[g]indolo(2,3,-a)quinolizine

Alserin; Austrapine; Crystoserpine; Eskaserp; Quiescin; Rau-sed; Reserpex; Reserpoid; Rivasin; Roxinoid; Sandril; Sedaraupin; Serfin; Serolfia; Serpanray; Serpasil; Serpasol; Serpate; Serpen; Serpiloid; Serpine

Other preparations containing reserpine

Abicol; Adelphane; Hypercal B; Hypertane Compound; Hypertane Forte; Hypertensan; Mio-pressin; Raudixin; Rautrax; Rauwiloid; Rauwiloid +; Veriloid; Salupres; Seominal; Serpasil-Esidrex; Serpasil-Esidrex K; Serplex-K; Tensanyl

1.2 Chemical formula and molecular weight

$C_{33}H_{40}N_2O_9$ Mol. wt: 608.7

1.3 Chemical and physical properties of the pure substance

(a) Description: White to tan crystals

(b) Melting-point: 262-266°C (decomposition) (Hesse, 1964)

(c) Spectroscopy data: λ_{max} 216 nm; E_1^1 = 101
        267   43
        295   17

(d) Optical rotation: $[\alpha]_D^{26}$ -168° (0.624% in dimethylformamide)

(e) Identity and purity test: Identity and specification tests are given in the British Pharmacopoeia (British Pharmacopoeia Commission, 1973), and in the European Pharmacopoeia (Council of Europe, 1975)

(f) Solubility: Very sparingly soluble in water; freely soluble in chloroform, methylene chloride and glacial acetic acid; soluble in benzene and ethyl acetate; slightly soluble in acetone, methanol, ether and aqueous solutions of acetic or citric acid; 1 g dissolves in about 1800 ml ethanol or 6 ml chloroform

(g) Stability: Solutions on standing acquire a yellow colour with pronounced fluorescence, especially after addition of acid or exposure to light.

(h) Reactivity: A weak base (pKa 6.6); forms salts with acids

1.4 Technical products and impurities

Reserpine is available as USP and BP grades. These grades for injection and reserpine tablets must contain no less than 90% of the stated amount of active ingredient (British Pharmacopoeia Commission, 1973; US Pharmacopeial Convention, Inc., 1970). The European grade contains no less than 99% and no more than the equivalent of 101% total alkaloids and no less than 98% and no more than the equivalent of 102% reserpine (Council of Europe, 1975).

2. Production, Use, Occurrence and Analysis

For important background information on this section, see preamble, p. 17.

A review on reserpine has been published (Saxton, 1956).

2.1 Production and use

Reserpine was isolated from the roots of *Rauwolfia serpentina* and its structure determined in 1954 by Dorfman *et al.*; it was synthesized by Woodward *et al.* in 1956 (Stecher, 1968). There is no known commercial production of synthetic reserpine; the alkaloid is extracted from the roots with alcohols or aqueous acid and then purified.

There are six producers of reserpine in the US (Anon. 1974); however, since reserpine is not a synthetic organic chemical, its production and sales are not reported to the US International Trade Commission. There are producers of reserpine in the Federal Republic of Germany, France and Italy (Chemical Information Services, Ltd, 1975).

Extracts of *R. serpentina* have been used medicinally in India for centuries (Saxton, 1956). Reserpine is used to lower blood pressure and reduce heart rate, as a tranquilizer and as a sedative. Its use is indicated in the treatment of mild essential hypertension, and it is also used as an adjunct with other antihypertensive agents in the more severe forms of hypertension and for the relief of symptoms in agitated psychotic states.

Formulations in France, the UK and the US include drugs containing only reserpine, those with a diuretic, those containing a barbiturate and various mixtures of these and other additives. Dose levels range from 0.1-5.0 mg/day

(British Pharmacopoeia Commission, 1973; *Dictionnaire Vidal*, 1975; Goodman & Gilman, 1970).

Annual US sales of reserpine for use in human medicine are estimated to be in the order of 200 thousand kg, almost all in tablet form.

In the US reserpine is also used as a tranquilizer and sedative in animal feeds. When used in the feeds of chickens and turkeys raised for human consumption, up to 0.0002% reserpine may be used (US Code of Federal Regulations, 1972).

2.2 Occurrence

Reserpine, which is a naturally occurring alkaloid, is produced by some members of the genus *Rauwolfia*, a climbing shrub of the Apocynacea family, indigenous to India, Burma, Malaysia, Thailand and Indonesia (see also Hesse, 1964).

2.3 Analysis

Reserpine can be analysed by spectrophotometric determination of the reaction product with sodium nitrite in acid solution (British Pharmacopoeia Commission, 1973). Methods for its determination in plant material by thin-layer chromatography are described by Drost & Reith (1970) and Timmins & Court (1974).

3. Biological Data Relevant to the Evaluation of Carcinogenic Risk to Man

3.1 Carcinogenicity and related studies in animals

(a) Oral administration

Mouse: A group of 24 female C3H mice 45-50 days of age and a further group of 11 female XVII nc mice of the same age received an average of 0.24 µg reserpine per day in the food, while 22 C3H controls and 11 XVII nc controls received the basal diet only. Mammary tumour incidence in C3H mice compared with that in controls was increased by drug treatment, and tumour latent period decreased. Fifteen animals developed mammary tumours, the earliest by 216 days and the latest by 15 months. Of the C3H controls, 12 animals developed mammary tumours, the earliest appearing at 320 days and the latest at 17 months. No mammary tumours occurred in treated XVII nc mice, surviving from 200 days to 32 months, nor were any noted in the 11 controls (Lacassagne & Duplan, 1959).

Rat: A group of 92 female and 43 male Wistar rats received 100 µg reserpine per kg of diet daily in a semi-liquid diet. A group of 30 female and 20 male controls received a solid dry basal diet only. The experiment was carried on for 18 months, when both test and control animals were sacrificed. The first tumours (lymphosarcomas and hepatomas) appeared in females after 8-8½ months and in males 2 months later; 16% of the test animals, but no controls, developed tumours. In a later experiment in which 80 female and 50 male Wistar controls received a semi-liquid diet, 13% of the animals developed lymphosarcomas and hepatomas from about the 12th month onwards; animals were sacrificed at 18 months (Tuchmann-Duplessis & Mercier-Parot, 1962).

Sprague-Dawley rats fed 8 mg reserpine per kg of diet (0.08 mg/day) together with 600 mg dimethylaminoazobenzene per kg of diet (6 mg/day) developed more tumours than animals fed the azo dye alone (Hurst *et al.*, 1958).

(b) Subcutaneous and/or intramuscular administration

The incidence of mammary tumours in Sprague-Dawley rats given a single i.v. injection of dimethylbenz[*a*]anthracene was increased by subsequent daily s.c. administration of 100 µg/kg bw reserpine for 50 days after the appearance of the first tumour (Welsch & Meites, 1970b).

3.2 Other relevant biological data

In rats the i.v. LD_{50} was 15 mg/kg bw; in mice the oral LD_{50} was 500 mg/kg bw and the i.p. LD_{50} was 70 mg/kg bw (Usdin & Efron, 1972).

Reserpine induces gastric haemorrhage and erosion in mice (Blackman *et al.*, 1959) and suppresses the immune response of lymph node cells in C57Bl/6 and CBA mice (Devoino & Yeliseyeva, 1971).

In rats, after an i.v. injection of 400 µg ^{14}C-reserpine, peak radioactivity occurred in most tissues except body fat within 60 minutes, with a rapid decline for up to 6 hours (Sheppard *et al.*, 1955). In male guinea-pigs radioactivity in the brain after i.v. injection of 2 mg ^{3}H-reserpine reached a maximum within 20-30 minutes and then declined rapidly, whereas radioactivity in the liver reached similar levels but fell more slowly (Sheppard et al., 1958).

Metabolic studies showed that hydrolysis of reserpine and oxidation of the 4-methoxy group of the 3,4,5-trimethoxybenzoic acid moiety occur. Rat liver slices efficiently demethylate at this position, converting as much as 20% of the drug to carbon dioxide in 3 hours. Guinea-pig microsomes contain considerable esterase activity and can convert 80% of the drug to trimethoxybenzoic acid in 3 hours (Sheppard & Tsien, 1955).

Reserpine has been reported to inhibit the growth of leukaemia in L1210 cells in male mice (Goldin et al., 1957) and to suppress the growth of sarcoma 37 in mice (Belkin & Hardy, 1957). In both cases, doses between 30 and 50 mg/kg bw were used. In contrast, reserpine did not affect the growth of transplanted mammary adenocarcinomas in C3H mice (Cranston, 1958). It blocks the release of prolactin-inhibiting factor and thus raises serum prolactin levels (Welsch & Meites, 1970a).

Nine male Wistar rats given 16 mg reserpine per kg of diet were protected against the carcinogenic effects of nitrosodiethylamine (50 mg/l in the drinking-water) (Lacassagne et al., 1968). Fifteen daily s.c. injections of reserpine in rats from the age of 50 days, followed at the age of 55 days by a single i.v. injection of dimethylbenz[a]anthracene, resulted in an inhibitory action on mammary tumour production by dimethylbenz[a]anthracene alone (81% versus 100%) (Welsch & Meites, 1970b).

I.p. injections of 0.92 and 4.60 mg/kg bw reserpine to ICR/Ha Swiss mice did not increase early foetal deaths or preimplantation losses (Epstein et al., 1972). No chromosomal aberrations were observed in human peripheral leucocyte cultures exposed to concentrations of 2.5-25 µg/ml (Bishun et al., 1975).

In man, after oral administration of 0.25 mg ^{3}H-reserpine, tritium was rapidly absorbed into the blood, reaching a peak within 1-2 hours. Radioactivity was tightly bound to red blood cells and remained constant over a 96-hour period. Disappearance of radioactivity in plasma was biphasic:

the first component had a half-life of 4.5 hours, and the second, 271 hours. Six per cent of the dose was excreted in the urine by 24 hours, mainly as trimethoxybenzoic acid; but radioactivity was still detectable in plasma, urine and faeces 11-12 days after drug administration (Maas *et al.*, 1969).

3.3 <u>Observations in man</u>

Three papers, published concurrently, reported an association between *Rauwolfia* derivatives and breast cancer. In a multi-purpose survey carried out in 1972 in Boston, Massachusetts, a positive association was observed between a history of *Rauwolfia* derivative use, obtained by interview, and a discharge diagnosis of breast cancer (Boston Collaborative Drug Surveillance Program, 1974). This association was studied in detail in 150 newly-diagnosed cases of breast cancer and in 600 surgical and 600 medical matched control patients. Both control groups had taken part in the original survey. Among breast cancer patients 7.3% had taken *Rauwolfia* derivatives regularly during the 3 months before hospitalization, compared with 2.2% in both control groups. This gave a risk ratio for breast cancer among the drug users of 3.5, with 95% confidence limits of 1.6-8.0. In 5 of the 6 different *Rauwolfia* preparations used by patients in this study reserpine was the only *Rauwolfia* alkaloid; 1 contained standardized *Rauwolfia serpentina*. There was no evidence of an association between breast cancer and other hypotensive drugs. The survey also suggested the possibility of a positive association between use of *Rauwolfia* derivatives and malignancies of the brain, corpus uteri, pancreas, skin and kidneys.

The two other studies were initiated by the Boston survey. The first was a retrospective study of patients with newly-diagnosed neoplasms reported to the South-West Regional Cancer Records Bureau, UK, in 1971, 1972 and part of 1973 (Armstrong *et al.*, 1974). Data on drug therapy at the time of first admission to hospital for treatment of the neoplasm were obtained from medical records for 708 patients with breast cancer and for 1430 patients with other neoplasms. A positive association was found between breast cancer and the use of *Rauwolfia* derivatives (risk ratio, 2.0, with 90% confidence limits of 0.74-5.53); this association became statistically significant at the 5% level (risk ratio, 3.9) when patients with the other neoplasms which were suggested by the Boston group to be associated with *Rauwolfia* derivatives were removed from the control group. This latter group of neoplasms, when compared with the remaining neoplasms, also showed a significant positive association with *Rauwolfia* derivatives (risk ratio, 4.0). Patients in this study used reserpine alone, standardized *Rauwolfia serpentina*, methoserpidine or deserpidine. No positive association was found between breast cancer and other hypotensive drugs or other drugs known to stimulate prolactin secretion (phenothiazines or tricyclic antidepressants).

The last of these three studies was a survey of newly-diagnosed breast cancer patients in Helsinki, Finland (Heinonen et al., 1974). Of 438 women with breast cancer, 53 (12.1%) had used *Rauwolfia* derivatives at some time before admission to hospital, as had 31 (7.1%) of 438 matched control patients admitted to hospital for a variety of surgical procedures; in both groups, information on drug use came from hospital records. From these data a risk ratio of 2.0, with 95% confidence limits of 1.2-3.4 was calculated. Patients in this study used either reserpine, methyldopa or a combination of *Rauwolfia* alkaloids.

Since these three initial studies, three further case-control studies have been reported. Mack et al. (1975) studied 99 women with breast cancer, matched individually to 396 other women living in the same retirement community in Los Angeles, California. Patients with a past history of any cancer were excluded from both groups. Data on the use of *Rauwolfia* derivatives at any time before the date of diagnosis of cancer were obtained for each patient with breast cancer and for her four matched controls from records of the medical clinic serving the community. The risk ratio for breast cancer in women who had ever used *Rauwolfia* derivatives was 1.2, with 95% confidence limits of 0.7-2.2; the risk ratio for those who first used such drugs 5 or more years before diagnosis of the cancer was 1.6, with 95% confidence limits of 0.7-3.4. Altogether, 20% of women in the control group had used *Rauwolfia* derivatives at some time. Risk ratio estimates for associations between use of other hypotensive drugs, other drugs and clinic facilities with breast cancer varied from 1.1 to 2.6. Over 90% of the *Rauwolfia* preparations used by patients in this study contained reserpine alone.

O'Fallon et al. (1975) reported a study of the use of *Rauwolfia* derivatives at any time up to 6 months before diagnosis in 453 women with breast cancer diagnosed betwen 1955 and 1973 and in 475 patients with cholelithiasis diagnosed between 1955 and 1970 in Olmsted County, Minnesota. *Rauwolfia* derivatives had been used by 6.4% of breast cancer patients and by 8.0% of patients with cholelithiasis; significantly fewer breast cancer patients (37.1%) than cholelithiasis patients (47.4%) had a past history of hypertension, and, when this was taken into account, the risk ratio for breast cancer in users of *Rauwolfia* derivatives was 1.02. Of the breast cancer patients, 61% had been exposed to reserpine only, and the remainder to whole-root *Rauwolfia* or a mixture of the two.

Laska et al. (1975) studied 55 patients with breast cancer diagnosed between 1965 and 1974 among in-patients of the Rockland Psychiatric Center, New York State. A matched control group of 55 women was selected from among all patients in the centre on 1 April 1969. A complete history of use of *Rauwolfia* derivatives was obtained from hospital notes for each cancer patient, up to the time of diagnosis of the cancer, and for each of the matched controls. In all, 32 breast cancer patients and 31 controls had received reserpine; more breast cancer patients than controls had received it during the 4 years immediately before diagnosis of cancer, but this difference was not statistically significant. A diagnosis of hypertension had been made in 53% of the breast cancer patients and in 32% of the controls.

Two studies have considered the relationship of *Rauwolfia* derivatives to cancer in men. Newball & Byar (1973) compared the survival of 49 men with cancer of the prostate and hypertension and treated with reserpine to that of 49 other men with cancer of the prostate only, matched to the first group for age, stage of cancer and other relevant variables, but who had not taken reserpine. There was no significant difference in survival of the two groups.

Dyer et al. (1975) reported a positive relationship between high systolic and diastolic blood pressures at entry to hospital and cancer mortality 14 years later in 1233 men in Chicago, Illinois (risk ratios varied from 1.5-3.0, according to the method of analysis). This relationship held for lung cancer, colon cancer, and all other cancers taken together, exclusive of leukaemia, after allowing for age, smoking habits and serum cholesterol levels. There was no evidence that this association was due to the use of *Rauwolfia* derivatives or of any other type of hypotensive medication.

4. Comments on Data Reported and Evaluation

4.1 Animal data

No adequate tests to assess the carcinogenicity of reserpine in experimental animals were available to the Working Group.

4.2 Human data

Results from a number of epidemiological studies are not consistent in indicating an increased risk of cancer in patients exposed to *Rauwolfia* derivatives, and any conclusion about the existence of a risk should await further evidence.

5. References

Anon. (1974) *Chemical Week Buyers Guide*, New York, McGraw-Hill, October 30, p. 580

Armstrong, B., Stevens, N. & Doll, R. (1974) Retrospective study of the association between use of *Rauwolfia* derivatives and breast cancer in English women. *Lancet*, ii, 672-675

Belkin, M. & Hardy, W.G. (1957) Effect of reserpine and chlorpromazine on sarcoma 37. *Science*, 125, 233-234

Bishun, N., Smith, N. & Williams, D. (1975) Chromosomes, mitosis and reserpine. *Lancet*, i, 926

Blackman, J.G., Campion, D.S. & Fastier, F.N. (1959) Mechanism of action of reserpine in producing gastric haemorrhage and erosion in the mouse. *Brit. J. Pharmacol.*, 14, 112-116

Boston Collaborative Drug Surveillance Program (1974) Reserpine and breast cancer. *Lancet*, ii, 669-671

British Pharmacopoeia Commission (1973) *British Pharmacopoeia*, London HMSO, pp. 411-412

Chemical Information Services, Ltd (1975) *Directory of Western European Chemical Producers, 1975/76*, Oceanside, NY

Council of Europe (1975) *European Pharmacopoeia*, European Treaty Series No. 50, Vol. 3, Paris, Maisonneuve, pp. 339-341

Cranston, E.M. (1958) Effects of some tranquilisers on a mammary adenocarcinoma in mice. *Cancer Res.*, 18, 897-899

Devoino, L.V. & Yeliseyeva, L.S. (1971) Influence of some drugs on the immune response. III. Effect of serotonin, 5-hydroxytryptophan, reserpine, monoamine oxidase inhibitors and DOPA on the involvement of lymph node cells in the immune response. *Europ. J. Pharmacol.*, 14, 71-76

Dictionnaire Vidal (1975) 51st ed., Paris, Office de Vulgarisation Pharmaceutique, pp. 1423-1424

Drost, R.H. & Reith, J.F. (1970) Identificatie van stoffen in de toxicologische analyse met behulp van extractie met 1,2-dichloorethaan, dunnelaagchromatografie en UV spectrofotometrie. III. Neutrale Stoffen. *Pharm. Weekblad.*, 105, 1129-1138

Dyer, A.R., Stamler, J., Berkson, D.M., Lindberg, H.A. & Stevens, E. (1975) High blood-pressure: a risk factor for cancer mortality? *Lancet*, i, 1051-1056

Epstein, S.S., Arnold, E., Andrea, J., Bass, W. & Bishop, Y. (1972) Detection of chemical mutagens by the dominant lethal assay in the mouse. Toxicol. appl. Pharmacol., 23, 288-325

Goldin, A., Burton, R.M., Humphreys, S.R. & Venditti, J.M. (1957) Antileukemic action of reserpine. Science, 125, 156-157

Goodman, L.S. & Gilman, A., eds (1970) The Pharmacological Basis of Therapeutics, 4th ed., London, Toronto, MacMillan, pp. 170-173, 574-577

Heinonen, O.P., Shapiro, S., Tuominen, L. & Turunen, M.I. (1974) Reserpine use in relation to breast cancer. Lancet, ii, 675-677

Hesse, M. (1964) Indol Alkaloide in Tabellen, Heidelberg, Springer-Verlag

Hurst, L., Lacassagne, A. & Rosenberg, A.J. (1958) Action de la réserpine sur la cancérisation du foie chez le rat. C.R. Soc. Biol. (Paris), 152, 441-443

Lacassagne, A. & Duplan, J.F. (1959) Le méchanisme de la cancérisation de la mamelle chez la souris, considéré d'après les résultats d'expérience au moyen de la réserpine. C.R. Acad. Sci. (Paris), 249, 810-812

Lacassagne, A., Buu-Hoi, N.P., Giao, N.B. & Ferrando, R. (1968) Action retardrice de la réserpine sur la cancérisation du foie du rat par la diéthylnitrosamine. Bull. Cancer, 55, 87-90

Laska, E.M., Siegel, C., Meisner, M., Fischer, S. & Wanderling, J. (1975) Matched-pairs study of reserpine use and breast cancer. Lancet, ii, 296-300

Maas, A.R., Jenkins, B., Shen, Y. & Tannenbaum, P. (1966) Studies on absorption, excretion and metabolism of ^{3}H-reserpine in man. Clin. Pharmacol. Ther., 10, 366-371

Mack, T.M., Henderson, B.E., Gerkins, V.R., Arthur, M., Baptista, J. & Pike, M.C. (1975) Reserpine and breast cancer in a retirement community. New Engl. J. Med., 292, 1366-1371

Newball, H.H. & Byar, D.P. (1973) Does reserpine increase prolactin and exacerbate cancer of prostate? Case control study. Urology, 11, 525-529

O'Fallon, W.M., Labarthe, D.R. & Kurland, L.T. (1975) Rauwolfia derivatives and breast cancer. Lancet, ii, 292-296

Saxton, J.E. (1956) The indole alkaloids including harmine and strychnine. Q. Rev., 10, 108-147

Sheppard, H. & Tsien, W.H. (1955) Metabolism of reserpine-C^{14}. II. Species differences as studied *in vitro*. Proc. Soc. exp. Biol. (N.Y.), 90, 437-440

Sheppard, H., Lucas, R.C. & Tsien, W.H. (1955) The metabolism of reserpine-C^{14}. Arch. int. Pharmacol., 103, 256-269

Sheppard, H., Tsien, W.H., Plummer, A.J., Peets, E.A., Giletti, B.J. & Schubert, A.R. (1958) Brain reserpine levels following large and small doses of reserpine-H^3. Proc. Soc. exp. Biol. (N.Y.), 97, 717-721

Stecher, P.G., ed. (1968) The Merck Index, 8th ed., Rahway, NJ, Merck & Co., p. 912

Timmins, P. & Court, W.E. (1974) Root alkaloids of *Rauwolfia oreogiton*. Planta med., 26, 170-173

Tuchmann-Duplessis, H. & Mercier-Parot, L. (1962) Apparition de tumeurs malignes dans une lignée de rats Wistar. C.R. Acad. Sci. (Paris), 254, 1535-1537

US Code of Federal Regulations (1972) Food and Drugs, Title 21, part 121:205, Washington DC, US Government Printing Office, pp. 36-37

Usdin, E. & Efron, D.H. (1972) Psychotropic Drugs and Related Compounds, 2nd ed., Washington DC, US Department of Health, Education and Welfare, p. 111

US Pharmacopeial Convention, Inc. (1970) The US Pharmacopeia, 18th rev., Easton, Pa, Mack, pp. 587-590

Welsch, C.W. & Meites, J. (1970a) Effects of reserpine on development of carcinogen-induced mammary tumours in rats. In: Proceedings of the International Union of Physiological Sciences: 24th International Congress of Physiological Sciences, Washington DC, 1968, Bethesda, Md, Federation of American Societies for Experimental Biology

Welsch, C.W. & Meites, J. (1970b) Effects of reserpine on development of 7,12-dimethylbenzanthracene-induced mammary tumours in female rats. Experientia, 26, 1133-1134

SAFROLE, ISOSAFROLE AND DIHYDROSAFROLE

These substances were previously considered by an IARC Working Group in December, 1971 (IARC, 1972). Since that time new data have become available, and these have been incorporated into the monograph and taken into account in the present evaluation.

1. Chemical and Physical Data

Safrole

1.1 Synonyms and trade names

Chem. Abstr. Reg. Serial No.: 94-59-7

Chem. Abstr. Name: 5-(2-Propenyl)-1,3-benzodioxole

5-Allyl-1,3-benzodioxole; allylcatechol methylene ether; allyldioxybenzene methylene ether; 1-allyl-3,4-methylenedioxybenzene; 4-allyl-1,2-(methylenedioxy)benzene; 4-allyl-1,2-methylenedioxybenzene; allylpyrocatechin methylene ether; m-allylpyrocatechin methylene ether; 4-allylpyrocatechol, formaldehyde acetal; allylpyrocatechol methylene ether; 3,4-methylenedioxyallylbenzene

Rhyuno oil; Safrol; Safrole MF; Shikimole; Shikomol

1.2 Chemical formula and molecular weight

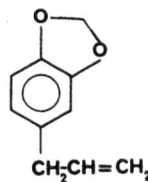

$C_{10}H_{10}O_2$ Mol. wt: 162.2

1.3 Chemical and physical properties of the pure substance

(a) Description: A colourless or slightly yellow liquid with an odour of sassafras

(b) Boiling-point: 232-234°C

(c) *Melting-point:* About 11°C

(d) *Density:* d_4^{20} 1.096

(e) *Spectroscopy data:* λ_{max} (in ethanol) 285 nm; E_1^1 = 234
236 nm; E_1^1 = 257

(f) *Refractive index:* n_D^{20} 1.5383

(g) *Solubility:* Practically insoluble in water; very soluble in ethanol; miscible with ether and chloroform

1.4 Technical products and impurities

Safrole is a constituent of several essential oils, notably oil of sassafras. In addition to safrole, oil of sassafras contains small amounts of eugenol, pinene, phellandrene, sesquiterpene and d-camphor; these are, therefore, potential impurities in technical safrole (Stecher, 1968).

Isosafrole

1.1 Synonyms and trade names

Chem. Abstr. Reg. Serial No.: 120-581

Chem. Abstr. Name: 5-(1-Propenyl)-1,3-benzodioxole

1,2-(Methylenedioxy)-4-propenylbenzene; 3,4-methylenedioxy-1-propenylbenzene; 3,4-(methylenedioxy)propenylbenzene; 1,2-methylenedioxy-4-propenylbenzene; 1,2-(methylenedioxy)-4-propenylbenzene; 5-(propen-1-yl)-1,3-benzodioxole; 4-propenyl-1,2-methylenedioxybenzene

1.2 Chemical formula and molecular weight

$C_{10}H_{10}O_2$ Mol. wt: 162.2

1.3 Chemical and physical properties of the pure substance

(a) Description: A colourless liquid with an odour of anise

(b) Boiling-point: 253°C; 127-128°C at 15 mm Hg

(c) Melting-point: 6.8°C

(d) Density: d_4^{20} 1.122

(e) Spectroscopy data: λ_{max} (in 96% ethanol) 305 nm; E_1^1 = 329
                                                                   267   716
                                                                   260   744

(f) Refractive index: n_D^{20} 1.5782

(g) Solubility: Practically insoluble in water; miscible with many organic solvents

1.4 Technical products and impurities

No data were available to the Working Group.

Dihydrosafrole

1.1 Synonyms and trade names

Chem. Abstr. Reg. Serial No.: 94-58-6

Chem. Abstr. Name: 5-Propyl-1,3-benzodioxole

Dihydroisosafrole; 1,2-(methylenedioxy)-4-propylbenzene; 3,4-methylenedioxypropylbenzene; 4-propyl-1,2-(methylenedioxy)benzene

1.2 Chemical formula and molecular weight

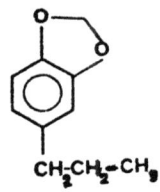

$C_{10}H_{12}O_2$ Mol. wt: 164.2

1.3 **Chemical and physical properties of the pure substance**

(a) *Description:* Oily liquid

(b) *Boiling-point:* 228°C

(c) *Density:* d_4^{20} 1.0695

(d) *Refractive index:* n_D^{25} 1.5187

(e) *Solubility:* Miscible with ethanol, ether, acetic acid and benzene

1.4 **Technical products and impurities**

No data were available to the Working Group.

2. Production, Use, Occurrence and Analysis

For important background information on this section, see preamble, p. 17.

2.1 **Production and use**

Safrole is produced by distillation of essential oils rich in this chemical (Furia & Bellanca, 1971). It was first isolated in 1908 by Knoll who also synthesized the pure chemical. Although there are two producers of safrole in the United States, current production figures are not available; the amount produced in 1969 was 117 thousand kg and in 1970, 126 thousand kg. In 1971, 22 thousand kg were reported to have been sold in the US (US Tariff Commission, 1969; 1971; 1972; 1973). Importation of 1000 kg was reported in 1972, but none was reported in 1973 (US Bureau of the Census, 1973).

Safrole is used in perfumery and soaps, as a flavouring agent in drugs and as a chemical intermediate for the manufacture of heliotropin and piperonyl butoxide (Hawley, 1971). Oil of sassafras containing safrole was formerly used as a flavouring agent in soft drinks, and up to 27 mg/l was present in root-beer (Wilson, 1959); however, this use is no longer permitted in the US (Furia & Bellanca, 1971).

Oil of sassafras, containing safrole, has been used medically as a topical antiseptic, pediculicide and carminative (Stecher, 1968).

Isosafrole was purified and separated from safrole by Balbiano in 1911, and its synthesis was first reported by Bert in 1941 (Stecher, 1968). It is produced by the isomerization of safrole with alcoholic potassium hydroxide. There is no evidence that isosafrole is produced commercially in the US at the present time, but it has been reported to be used in the manufacture of heliotropin, which is derived from isosafrole by oxidation, and in the manufacture of perfumes, flavours and pesticide synergists (Hawley, 1971).

Dihydrosafrole is produced from safrole or isosafrole by catalytic hydrogenation. Although there is no evidence that dihydrosafrole is produced commercially in the US, it is known to be produced as an intermediate in the production of piperonyl butoxide, a synergist for pyrethroid insecticides.

Until 1960, safrole, isosafrole and dihydrosafrole were all used as flavouring agents in root-beer in the US.

2.2 Occurrence

Safrole is a constituent of several essential oils. Sassafras oil contains up to 93% (Gemballa, 1958) and lesser quantities occur in essential oils from nutmeg, mace, ginger, cinnamon and black pepper, usually in the range of <1-10% of the oil (Bejnarowicz & Kirch, 1963; Furia & Bellanca, 1971; Itty & Nigam, 1966). Star anise oil obtained from the Japanese tree *Illicium anisatum* Linn. also contains about 6% safrole (Cook & Howard, 1966), whereas no safrole was detected in star anise oil obtained from the Chinese tree *Illicium verum* Hooker (Bricout, 1974).

Isosafrole occurs naturally in low quantities in essential oils of some spices. Its distribution is generally similar to that of safrole.

No data on the natural occurrence of dihydrosafrole were available to the Working Group. It has been identified in piperonyl butoxide, a synthetic pesticidal synergist (Albro *et al.*, 1972).

2.3 Analysis

Sensitive, specific analytical methods for the determination of safrole in biological materials utilize either combined liquid and gas-liquid chromatography (Russell & Jennings, 1969) or spectral properties of the compound (Wilson, 1959).

3. Biological Data Relevant to the Evaluation of Carcinogenic Risk to Man

3.1 Carcinogenicity and related studies in animals

(a) Oral administration

Mouse: Groups of 18 male and 18 female (C57BL/6 x C3H/Anf)F_1 or (C57BL/6 x AKR)F_1 mice were given 464 mg/kg bw safrole by stomach tube at 7 days of age and daily until the animals were 28 days of age. Subsequently the compound was administered in the diet at a concentration of 1112 mg/kg of diet for up to 82 weeks. Liver-cell tumours occurred in 11/17 males and 16/16 females and 3/17 males and 16/17 females of the two strains, respectively, compared with 8/79 male and 0/87 female and 5/90 male and 1/82 female controls, respectively. For each strain the difference was significantly different from that in controls (P=0.01) when the incidences in male and female were combined. Isosafrole was given at a lower dose (215 mg/kg bw then 517 mg/kg of diet); it induced liver-cell tumours in 5/18 males and 1/16 females and 2/17 males and 0/16 females of the two strains, respectively. The difference from controls was statistically significant (P=0.05) only in (C57BL/6 x C3H/Anf)F_1 males and females combined. Dihydrosafrole, given at a dose of 464 mg/kg bw and then 1400 mg/kg of diet for up to 82 weeks, induced liver-cell tumours in 10/17 males and 0/17 females and 8/17 males and 1/18 females of the two strains, respectively. The incidences were significantly different from those in controls (P=0.01) only in males of each strain. The incidence of pulmonary tumours was also significantly increased (P=0.01), but only when male and female mice of both strains were combined (Innes *et al.*, 1968; 1969).

In 3 groups of 35-40 male CD1 mice fed a diet containing 4000 or 5000 mg safrole per kg of diet for 13 months, 23/87 mice surviving 12-16 months developed hepatocellular carcinomas, compared with 7/70 controls (Borchert *et al.*, 1973a) [P<0.01].

Rat: Small groups of 5 or 9 male CFN rats were fed 0.1% or 1% safrole in a basal diet deficient in riboflavin and protein, or a protein-deficient diet containing riboflavin or casein and/or tocopherol supplements. Liver adenomas occurred in 4/5 rats fed riboflavin and/or the deficient diet plus

1% safrole. Adenomas visible at autopsy occurred in 9/9 and 9/9 rats fed 1% safrole in the basal diet with 30% casein and/or tocopherol, respectively; average survival times were about 200 days. No liver adenomas occurred in rats fed the basal diets with or without the supplements (Hamburger et al., 1961).

In groups of 25 male and 25 female Osborne-Mendel rats fed 0, 100, 500, 1000 or 5000 mg safrole per kg of diet for two years, liver tumours occurred in 19/47 autopsied rats fed the highest level. Fourteen of the liver tumours were hepatocellular and cholangiocarcinomas. Liver tumours also occurred in 3/40 controls ($P<0.001$). Of rats fed 1000 mg/kg of diet, 8 developed benign liver tumours ($P>0.05$). The incidences of liver tumours in rats fed the two lowest levels were similar to that in controls (Long et al., 1963). Similar results were reported by Hagan et al. (1965).

Of 48 male CD rats fed 5000 mg safrole per kg of diet for 8.5-10 months, followed by a control diet up to 16 months, 2 developed hepatocellular carcinomas and 1 a benign tumour described as a liver adenoma. No liver tumours occurred in 48 controls (Borchert et al., 1973a).

Groups of 10 male and 10 female Osborne-Mendel rats were fed 0, 1000, 2500 or 10,000 mg dihydrosafrole per kg of diet for 2 years. Two additional groups of 25 males and 25 females received 0 or 5000 mg/kg of diet. Among those fed the highest level, 35% of the animals survived 50 weeks, and 20% survived 75 weeks; of those fed 5000 mg/kg of diet, 66% survived at 75 weeks and 10% at 100 weeks. Tumours of the oesophagus (papillomas and epidermoid carcinomas) developed in 75% of rats fed the two upper levels and in 20% of rats fed 2500 mg/kg of diet. No oesophageal tumours occurred in rats fed 1000 mg/kg of diet, nor in controls. Very few liver tumours (number not stated) were observed in treated rats (Hagan et al., 1965; Long & Jenner, 1963).

In similar numbers of rats fed 0, 1000, 2500, 5000 or 10,000 mg isosafrole per kg of diet for 2 years, liver tumours (2 hepatic-cell adenomas and 3 hepatic-cell carcinomas) were reported to have occurred in 5 rats fed 5000 mg/kg of diet (Hagan et al., 1965; 1967) [No further details were available].

(b) Subcutaneous and/or intramuscular administration

Infant mouse: Infant Swiss albino mice were injected subcutaneously with a suspension of safrole in tricaprylin on days 1, 7, 14 and 21 after birth. Of males that received a total dose of 0.66 mg, 6/12 animals developed hepatomas within 49-53 weeks; of those that received a total dose of 6.6 mg, 18/31 males developed hepatomas. No hepatomas developed in 9 and 29 treated females; however, 13/81 treated animals also developed pulmonary adenomas or adenocarcinomas. No lung tumours were observed in controls killed after 53 weeks, but 4 hepatomas occurred in 78 solvent-injected male controls (Epstein et al., 1970) [P<0.001]. Hepatomas were also produced in male but not female infant CD1 mice given s.c. injections of safrole on the 1st, 7th, 14th and 21st day of life and observed up to 16 months. The incidences of liver tumours were 14/35 in treated males and 3/36 in male controls. No liver tumours occurred in 27 treated females or in 31 female controls (Borchert et al., 1973a).

Rat: No local tumours were observed in 23 or 25 male CD rats given 20 twice weekly s.c. injections of 3 mg/animal safrole or isosafrole and surviving 18 months (Borchert et al., 1973a).

(c) Intraperitoneal administration

Mouse: Groups of 15 male and 15 female strain A/He mice were given 12 i.p. injections of safrole in tricaprylin thrice weekly (total doses, 0.9 and 4.5 g/kg bw). All surviving mice were killed at 24 weeks, and 2/14 males and 4/13 females and 1/10 males and 2/10 females at the two dose levels, respectively, developed lung tumours, with 0.14, 0.31, 0.1 and 0.3 lung tumours per mouse. Of controls injected with tricaprylin alone, 28% of 77 males and 20% of 77 females developed lung tumours, with 0.24 and 0.2 lung tumours per mouse (Stoner et al., 1973).

3.2 Other relevant biological data

The oral LD_{50}'s of safrole in mice and rats were 3.4 and 1.95 g/kg bw, respectively. The oral LD_{50} in mice of a 50% solution in corn oil was 2.35 g/kg bw. For mice and rats, the oral LD_{50}'s of dihydrosafrole were 4.3 and 2.26 g/kg bw; the respective values for isosafrole were 2.47 and 1.34 g/kg bw (Jenner et al., 1964).

In mice given ^{14}C-labelled safrole or dihydrosafrole orally, 96 and 101% of the radioactivity were recovered; 64 and 61% were found in CO_2, 18 and 23% in urine, 6 and 5% in faeces and intestine, 2 and 2.5% in liver and 6 and 9% in carcasses (Kamienski & Casida, 1970).

Following oral or i.p. administration of safrole to rats and guinea-pigs, 3'-N,N-dimethylamino-1'-(3,4-methylenedioxyphenyl)-1'-propanone was identified as the major urinary metabolite in guinea-pigs and as a minor metabolite in rats. 3'-Pyrrolidinyl-1'-(3,4-methylenedioxyphenyl)-1'-propanone, a further minor metabolite, and 3'-piperidyl-1'-(3,4-methylenedioxyphenyl)-1'-propanone were found in the urine of rats (Oswald et al., 1971). In male Sprague-Dawley rats and male guinea-pigs given i.p. injections of safrole, the main urinary metabolites were identified as 1,2-dihydroxy-4-allylbenzene, conjugated 1'-hydroxysafrole, 1,2-methylenedioxy-4-(2',3'-dihydroxypropyl)benzene and 1,2-dihydroxy-4-(2',3'-hydroxypropyl)-benzene. The diols were probably formed through their intermediate epoxides, since administration of 2',3'-epoxy safrole to rats and guinea-pigs yielded the same compounds. 1'-Ketosafrole was not identified (Stillwell et al., 1974).

Conjugated 1'-hydroxysafrole also occurs as a urinary metabolite of safrole in mice, rats, guinea-pigs and hamsters, and treatment of urine with β-glucuronidase released 1'-hydroxysafrole. Rats, guinea-pigs and hamsters excreted 1-3.5% of an i.p. dose of safrole as 1'-hydroxysafrole; male mice excreted 33% of the injected dose as this compound and female mice, 19%. When safrole was fed to rats, 5-10% of the daily intake was excreted as 1'-hydroxysafrole during the first 18 days, and 3-4% thereafter. The urinary excretion of 1'-hydroxysafrole was increased by about 10-fold if male rats were pre-treated with phenobarbital in the drinking-water or given an i.p. injection of 3-methylcholanthrene prior to the safrole treatment. Phenobarbital treatment did not increase the percentage excretion of 1'-hydroxysafrole in safrole-treated mice. When 1'-hydroxysafrole was given orally or by i.p. injection to male rats, about 40% was excreted unchanged; this was not affected by phenobarbital or 3-methylcholanthrene administration. No 1'-hydroxysafrole was excreted in the bile. 1'-Acetoxysafrole was shown to react with methionine, guanosine, adenosine and cytidine in vitro (Borchert et al., 1973b).

1'-Hydroxysafrole and 1'-acetoxysafrole produced a greater incidence of liver tumours in male infant mice than did equimolar concentrations of safrole; 4 s.c. injections were given on days 1, 7, 14 and 21 of life. In male rats given 5500 mg 1'-hydroxysafrole per kg of diet for 8.5-10 months, the incidence of liver tumours in rats killed at 12 or 16 months was higher than that in rats receiving safrole; in addition, forestomach papillomas were produced by 1'-hydroxysafrole. When groups of 18 adult rats were given twice weekly s.c. injections of 18.6 μmol 1'-hydroxysafrole or 1'-acetoxysafrole for 10 weeks, followed by observation for 17-18 months, local tumours occurred in both groups. A high incidence (20/65) of interscapular sarcomas (mainly angiosarcomas) was observed in mice fed 1'-hydroxysafrole (Borchert et al., 1973a).

1'-Hydroxysafrole, 3'-hydroxysafrole and 3'-acetoxysafrole, but not safrole or 1'-ketosafrole, induced unscheduled DNA repair synthesis in cultured human fibroblasts (San & Stich, 1975).

1'-Acetoxysafrole caused reverse mutations in *Salmonella typhimurium* TA100 (McCann et al., 1975).

3.3 Observations in man

No data were available to the Working Group.

4. Comments on Data Reported and Evaluation[1]

4.1 Animal data

Safrole and isosafrole are carcinogenic in mice and rats; they produce liver tumours following their oral administration. Safrole also produced liver and lung tumours in male infant mice following its subcutaneous injection. Dihydrosafrole given orally is carcinogenic in rats, in which it produces tumours of the oesophagus, and in mice, in which it produces liver tumours in males and an increased incidence of lung tumours in both males and females.

---

[1] See also the section "Animal Data in Relation to the Evaluation of Risk to Man" in the introduction to this volume, p. 15.

4.2 Human data

No case reports or epidemiological studies were available to the Working Group.

5. References

Albro, P.W., Fishbein, L. & Fawkes, J. (1972) Purification and characterization of pesticidal synergists. I. Piperonyl butoxide. J. Chromat., 65, 521-532

Bejnarowicz, E.A. & Kirch, E.R. (1963) Gas chromatographic analysis of oil of nutmeg. J. pharm. Sci., 52, 988-993

Borchert, P., Miller, J.A., Miller, E.C. & Shires, T.K. (1973a) 1'-Hydroxysafrole, a proximate carcinogenic metabolite of safrole in the rat and mouse. Cancer Res., 33, 590-600

Borchert, P., Wislocki, P.G., Miller, J.A. & Miller, E.C. (1973b) The metabolism of the naturally occurring hepatocarcinogen safrole to 1'-hydroxysafrole and the electrophilic reactivity of 1'-acetoxysafrole. Cancer Res., 33, 575-589

Bricout, J. (1974) Sur la constitution de l'huile essentielle de badiane. Bull. Soc. chim. Fr., 9-10, 1901-1903

Cook, W.B. & Howard, A.S. (1966) The essential oil of *Illicium anisatum* Linn. Canad. J. Chem., 44, 2461-2464

Epstein, S.S., Fujii, K., Andrea, J. & Mantel, N. (1970) Carcinogenicity testing of selected food additives by parenteral administration to infant Swiss mice. Toxicol. appl. Pharmacol, 16, 321-334

Furia, T.E. & Bellanca, N., eds (1971) Fenaroli's Handbook of Flavor Ingredients, Cleveland, Ohio, Chemical Rubber Company, p. 610

Gemballa, G. (1958) Brasilianisches Sassafrasöl. Sci. pharm. (Wien), 26, 8-14

Hagan, E.C., Jenner, P.M., Jones, W.I., Fitzhugh, O.G., Long, E.L., Brouwer, J.G. & Webb, W.K. (1965) Toxic properties of compounds related to safrole. Toxicol. appl. Pharmacol., 7, 18-24

Hagan, E.C., Hanson, W.H., Fitzhugh, O.G., Jenner, P.M., Jones, W.I., Taylor, J.M., Long, E.L., Nelson, A.A. & Brouwer, J.B. (1967) Food flavourings and compounds of related structure. II. Subacute and chronic toxicity. Fd Cosmet. Toxicol., 5, 141-157

Hawley, G., ed. (1971) The Condensed Chemical Dictionary, New York, Van Nostrand Reinhold, p. 771

Homburger, F., Kelley, T., Jr, Friedler, G. & Russfield, A.B. (1961) Toxic and possible carcinogenic effects of 4-allyl-1,2-methylenedioxybenzene (safrole) in rats on deficient diets. Med. exp. (Basel), 4, 1-11

IARC (1972) *IARC Monographs on the Evaluation of Carcinogenic Risk of Chemicals to Man*, 1, Lyon

Innes, J.R.M., Fishbein, L., Donnelly, R.D., Petrucelli, L., Ulland, B., Valerio, M. & Cameron, D. (1968) Evaluation of carcinogenic, teratogenic and mutagenic activities of selected pesticides and industrial chemicals. In: *Carcinogenic Study*, Vol. 1, PB-223 159, Washington DC, National Technical Information Service, US Department of Commerce

Innes, J.R.M., Ulland, B.M., Valerio, M.G., Petrucelli, L., Fishbein, L., Hart, E.R., Pallotta, A.J., Bates, R.R., Falk, H.L., Gart, J.J., Klein, M., Mitchell, I. & Peters, J. (1969) Bioassay of pesticides and industrial chemicals for tumorigenicity in mice: a preliminary note. *J. nat. Cancer Inst.*, 42, 1101-1114

Itty, M.I. & Nigam, S.S. (1966) Chemische Untersuchung des aetherischen Oeles von *Myristica fragrans* Houtt. *Riechst. Aromen. Körperpflegemittel.*, 16, 399-412

Jenner, P.M., Hagan, E.C., Taylor, J.M., Cook, E.L. & Fitzhugh, O.G. (1964) Food flavourings and compounds of related structure. I. Acute oral toxicity. *Fd Cosmet. Toxicol.*, 2, 327-343

Kamienski, F.X. & Casida, J.E. (1970) Importance of demethylation in the metabolism *in vivo* and *in vitro* of methylenedioxyphenyl synergists and related compounds in mammals. *Biochem. Pharmacol.*, 19, 91-112

Long, E.L. & Jenner, P.M. (1963) Esophageal tumors produced in rats by the feeding of dihydrosafrole. *Fed. Proc.*, 22, 275

Long, E.L., Nelson, A.A., Fitzhugh, O.G. & Hansen, W.H. (1963) Liver tumors produced in rats by feeding safrole. *Arch. Path.*, 75, 595-604

McCann, J., Spingarn, N.E., Kobori, J. & Ames, B.N. (1975) Detection of carcinogens as mutagens: bacterial tester strains with R factor plasmids. *Proc. nat. Acad. Sci. (Wash.)*, 72, 979-983

Oswald, E.O., Fishbein, L., Corbett, B.J. & Walker, M.P. (1971) Identification of tertiary aminomethylenedioxypropiophenones as urinary metabolites of safrole in the rat and guinea pig. *Biochem. biophys. acta*, 230, 237-247

Russell, G.F. & Jennings, W.G. (1969) Constituents of black pepper. Some oxygenated compounds. *J. agric. Fd Chem.*, 17, 1107-1112

San, R.H.C. & Stich, H.F. (1975) DNA repair synthesis of cultured human cells as a rapid bioassay for chemical carcinogens. *Int. J. Cancer*, 16, 284-291

Stecher, P.G., ed. (1968) *The Merck Index*, 8th ed., Rahway, NJ, Merck & Co., pp. 592, 761, 928

Stillwell, W.G., Carman, M.J., Bell, L. & Horning, M.G. (1974) The metabolism of safrole and 2',3'-epoxysafrole in the rat and guinea pig. *Drug Metab. Disp.*, 12, 489-498

Stoner, G.D., Shimkin, M.B., Kniazeff, A.J., Weisburger, J.H., Weisburger, E.K. & Gari, G.B. (1973) Test for carcinogenicity of food additives and chemotherapeutic agents by the pulmonary tumour response in strain A mice. *Cancer Res.*, 33, 3069-3085

US Bureau of the Census (1973) *US Imports for Consumption, 1972*, FT 246, Washington DC, US Government Printing Office, p. 357

US Tariff Commission (1969) *Synthetic Organic Chemicals, US Production and Sales, 1967*, TC Publication 295, Washington DC, US Government Printing Office, p. 35

US Tariff Commission (1971) *Synthetic Organic Chemicals, US Production and Sales, 1969*, TC Publication 412, Washington DC, US Government Printing Office, p. 124

US Tariff Commission (1972) *Synthetic Organic Chemicals, US Production and Sales, 1970*, TC Publication 479, Washington DC, US Government Printing Office, p. 124

US Tariff Commission (1973) *Synthetic Organic Chemicals, US Production and Sales, 1971*, TC Publication 614, Washington DC, US Government Printing Office, p. 122

Wilson, J.B. (1959) Determination of safrole and methylsalicylate in soft drinks. *J. Ass. off. agric. Chem.*, 42, 696-698

STERIGMATOCYSTIN

This substance was previously considered by an IARC Working Group in December, 1971 (IARC, 1972). Since that time new data have become available, and these have been incorporated into the monograph and taken into account in the present evaluation.

1. Chemical and Physical Data

1.1 Synonyms and trade names

Chem. Abstr. Reg. Serial No.: 10048-13-2

Chem. Abstr. Name: 3a,12c-Dihydro-8-hydroxy-6-methoxy-7H-furo-[3',2':4,5]furo[2,3-c]xanthen-7-one

1.2 Chemical formula and molecular weight

$C_{18}H_{12}O_6$ Mol. wt: 324.3

1.3 Chemical and physical properties of the pure substance

(a) Description: Pale-yellow crystals

(b) Melting-point: 246°C (decomposition)

(c) Spectroscopy data: λ_{max} 205, 233, 246 and 325 nm; E_1^1 = 775, 922, 1045 and 500, respectively

(d) Solubility: Insoluble in water and strong aqueous alkali; sparingly soluble in most organic solvents; readily soluble in chloroform, pyridine and dimethylsulphoxide

(e) Reactivity: Forms deep-yellow colour with aqueous sodium hydroxide and dark green-brown colour with sulphuric acid; emits orange-red fluorescence in ultra-violet light

1.4　Technical products and impurities

No data were available to the Working Group.

2. Production, Use, Occurrence and Analysis

2.1　Production and use

Sterigmatocystin is not produced or used commercially. It has been produced in the laboratory from cultures of *Aspergillus versicolor* (Vuillemin) Tiraboshi, from *A. nidulans* (Eidam) Wint. and from an undescribed strain of *Bipolaris* (Holzapfel et al., 1966).

2.2　Occurrence

Of 16 cultures of *Aspergillus versicolor* found on country-cured hams, 10 were found to be capable of producing sterigmatocystin in culture on three types of laboratory media. When spores of the *Aspergillus* were inoculated onto slices of ham, 4-8 µg sterigmatocystin per slice were found in all except one sample after 14 days at 20°C; 6-20 µg sterigmatocystin per slice were found in all samples after 14 days at 28°C (Halls & Ayres, 1973).

Sterigmatocystin was also identified in salami inoculated with two strains of *Aspergillus versicolor*; 1-2 mg/kg were found on the casing and 0.1 mg/kg in the interior (Alperden et al., 1973). It has been found as a natural contaminant in green coffee beans (1.1 mg/kg) and in wheat (0.3 mg/kg) (Purchase & Pretorius, 1973; Scott et al., 1972).

2.3　Analysis

Vorster & Purchase (1968) described an assay for the quantitative determination of as little as 0.0025 µg sterigmatocystin in grain and oil seeds using thin-layer chromatography (TLC): sterigmatocystin is converted to the acetate, which possesses an intense light-blue colour under ultra-violet light. A TLC method in which aluminium chloride is sprayed onto the developed plate has detected 30 µg/kg sterigmatocystin in spiked wheat or other grain samples (Stack & Rodricks, 1971). A TLC method has also been developed for screening fungal extracts (Scott et al. 1970) and for the analysis of groundnuts for three mycotoxins, including sterigmatocystin, with a limit of detection of 0.01 µg (Vorster, 1969).

3. Biological Data Relevant to the Evaluation of Carcinogenic Risk to Man

3.1 Carcinogenicity and related studies in animals

(a) Oral administration

Mouse: Two groups of 28 and 69 three week-old ICR mice of both sexes were fed a diet containing 5 mg pure sterigmatocystin per kg of diet or 5 mg *Aspergillus versicolor* culture per kg of diet, respectively, for 58 weeks. The experimental diets were fed for periods of 2 weeks, alternating with a 2-week period of control diet. Pulmonary adenomas were observed in 21/25 and 33/55 treated mice, respectively, surviving 30 or more weeks, compared with 4/37 in controls. Adenocarcinomas of the lung occurred in 9/25 and 3/55 treated mice, but not in controls. No increased incidence of tumours at other sites was observed (Zwicker et al., 1974).

Rat: When sterigmatocystin was administered by stomach tube or in the diet of Wistar rats at doses of 0.15-2.25 mg/animal/day for 52 weeks, 39/50 animals that survived 42 or more weeks developed hepatocellular carcinomas within 123 weeks. No liver tumours occurred in 19 controls given sunflower oil by stomach tube and/or fed a basal diet alone (Purchase & van der Watt, 1970).

(b) Skin application

Rat: Two groups of 10 male Wistar rats received 1 mg sterigmatocystin in either 0.1 ml dimethylsulphoxide (DMSO) or 0.15 ml acetone on the shaved dorsal skin twice weekly for 70 weeks, at which time the experiment was terminated. Groups of 10 controls received one of the solvents alone or no treatment. Skin papillomas and carcinomas occurred in 4 and 6 rats given sterigmatocystin in DMSO and in 3 and 7 rats given the compound in acetone. Hepatocellular carcinomas also occurred in 5 and 7 rats given sterigmatocystin in DMSO or acetone, respectively. No liver or skin tumours occurred in 30 controls (Purchase & van der Watt, 1973).

(c) Subcutaneous and/or intramuscular administration

Rat: Twice weekly s.c. injections of 0.5 mg sterigmatocystin suspended in arachis oil were given to a group of 6 rats for 24 weeks, each rat receiving a total dose of 24 mg. Local sarcomas were observed in 3/6 animals by 65 weeks; the first tumour appeared at 47 weeks, at which time all animals were alive. One animal also developed a hepatoma, and one, a cholangioma after 50 and 62 weeks, respectively. No malignant tumours occurred in 6 control animals; 1 benign sarcoma-like tumour occurred at 81 weeks (Dickens et al., 1966).

3.2 Other relevant biological data

The oral LD_{50}'s (10 days) were 166 mg/kg bw in male rats, when the compound was dissolved in dimethylformamide, and 120 mg/kg bw in female rats, when it was dissolved in wheat-germ oil. In male rats, the i.p. LD_{50} was 60-65 mg/kg bw, depending on the solvent used (Purchase & van der Watt, 1969). In vervet monkeys, the i.p. LD_{50} was 32 mg/kg bw for sterigmatocystin dissolved in dimethylsulphoxide (DMSO); liver and kidney damage were evident in treated animals (van der Watt & Purchase, 1970). Oral dosing of monkeys with 20 mg/kg bw sterigmatocystin once each fortnight for 4-6 months resulted in chronic hepatitis; after 12 months' exposure hyperplastic liver nodules were observed (Purchase & van der Watt, 1971).

In rats given a single i.p. injection of 6.4 mg/animal ^{14}C-sterigmatocystin in DMSO, 5.6% of the activity was found in the urine, 67% in the faeces and gastro-intestinal tract and 11% in the liver after 12 hours. These levels declined slightly after 24 hours. In fasted or non-fasted rats given 1.4 mg/animal ^{3}H-sterigmatocystin orally, the highest activity after 16 hours was found in the faeces and gastrointestinal tract; lesser amounts were found in the urine, blood, expired air, liver and kidneys. I.p. injection of sterigmatocystin inhibited the incorporation of ^{14}C-orotic acid into liver RNA (Nel et al., 1971).

In vervet monkeys the major urinary metabolite was identified as sterigmatocystin-β-D-glucuronide, which accounted for 75% of the oral dose administered (Thiel & Steyn, 1973).

Sterigmatocystin was toxic to Salmonella typhimurium TA 1530 in the presence of rat liver-microsomal preparations (Garner et al., 1972) and induced frameshift mutations in Salmonella typhimurium (Ames et al., 1973; McCann et al., 1975).

3.3 *Observations in man*

Many similarities were observed between sterigmatocystin-produced lesions in rats and the pathology of hepatitis in Africans in Mozambique; however, it is difficult to attribute liver disease in the Bantu to any single agent in their environment. The authors concluded that their observations "are not incompatible with the theory that mycotoxins may be involved". They stated that it was not known whether sterigmatocystin was present in the Bantu diet (Torres *et al.*, 1970).

4. Comments on Data Reported and Evaluation[1]

4.1 *Animal data*

Sterigmatocystin is carcinogenic in mice and rats following its oral administration; it produced lung tumours in mice and liver tumours in rats. In rats, it also produced skin and liver tumours following its application to the skin and sarcomas at the site of its subcutaneous injection.

4.2 *Human data*

No case reports or epidemiological studies were available to the Working Group.

---

[1] See also the section "Animal Data in Relation to the Evaluation of Risk to Man" in the introduction to this volume, p. 15.

5. References

Alperden, I., Mintzlaff, H.-J., Tauchmann, F. & Leistner, L. (1973) Bildung von Sterigmatocystin in mikrobiologischen Nährmedien und in Rohwurst durch *Aspergillus versicolor*. Fleischwirtschaft, 53, 707-710

Ames, B.N., Durston, W.E., Yamasaki, E. & Lee, F.D. (1973) Carcinogens are mutagens: a simple test system combining liver homogenates for activation and bacteria for detection. Proc. nat. Acad. Sci. (Wash.), 70, 2281-2285

Dickens, F., Jones, H.E.H. & Waynforth, H.B. (1966) Oral, subcutaneous and intratracheal administration of carcinogenic lactones and related substances: the intratracheal administration of cigarette tar in the rat. Brit. J. Cancer, 20, 134-144

Garner, R.C., Miller, E.C. & Miller, J.A. (1972) Liver microsomal metabolism of aflatoxin B_1 to a reactive derivative toxic to *Salmonella typhimurium*. Cancer Res., 32, 2058-2066

Halls, N.A. & Ayres, J.C. (1973) Potential production of sterigmatocystin on country-cured ham. Appl. Microbiol., 26, 636-637

Holzapfel, C.W., Purchase, I.F.H., Steyn, P.S. & Gouws, L. (1966) The toxicity and chemical assay of sterigmatocystin, a carcinogenic mycotoxin, and its isolation from two new fungal sources. S. Afr. med. J., 40, 1100-1101

IARC (1972) IARC Monographs on the Evaluation of Carcinogenic Risk of Chemicals to Man, 1, Lyon

Nel, W., Kempff, P.G. & Pitout, M.J. (1971) The metabolism and some metabolic effects of sterigmatocystin. In: Purchase, I.F.H., ed., Mycotoxins in Human Health : Proceedings of a Symposium held in Pretoria, 1970, London, Macmillan, pp. 11-18

McCann, J., Spingarn, N.E., Kobori, J. & Ames, B.N. (1975) Detection of carcinogens as mutagens : bacterial tester strains with R factor plasmids. Proc. nat. Acad. Sci. (Wash.), 72, 979-983

Purchase, I.F.H. & Pretorius, M.E. (1973) Sterigmatocystin in coffee beans. J. Ass. off. analyt. Chem., 56, 225-226

Purchase, I.F.H. & van der Watt, J.J. (1969) Acute toxicity of sterigmatocystin to rats. Fd Cosmet. Toxicol., 7, 135-139

Purchase, I.F.H. & van der Watt, J.J. (1970) Carcinogenicity of sterigmatocystin. Fd Cosmet. Toxicol., 8, 289-295

Purchase, I.F.H. & van der Watt, J.J. (1971) The acute and chronic toxicity of sterigmatocystin. In: Purchase, I.F.H., ed., Mycotoxins in Human Health : Proceedings of a Symposium held in Pretoria, 1970, London, Macmillan, pp. 209-213

Purchase, I.F.H. & van der Watt (1973) Carcinogenicity of sterigmatocystin to rat skin. Toxicol. appl. Pharmacol., 26, 274-281

Scott, P.M., Lawrence, J.W. & van Walbeek, W. (1970) Detection of mycotoxins by thin-layer chromatography : application to screening of fungal extracts. Appl. Microbiol., 20, 839-842

Scott, P.M., van Walbeek, W., Kennedy, B. & Anyeti, D. (1972) Mycotoxins (ochratoxin A, citrinin and sterigmatocystin) and toxigenic fungi in grains and other agricultural products. J. agric. Fd Chem., 20, 1103-1109

Stack, M. & Rodricks, J.V. (1971) Method of analysis and chemical confirmation of sterigmatocystin. J. Ass. off. analyt. Chem., 54, 86-90

Thiel, P.G. & Steyn, M. (1973) Urinary excretion of the mycotoxin, sterigmatocystin by vervet monkeys. Biochem. Pharmacol., 22, 3267-3273

Torres, F.O., Purchase, I.F.H. & van der Watt, J.J. (1970) The aetiology of primary liver cancer in the Bantu. J. Path., 102, 163-169

Vorster, L.J. (1969) A method for the analysis of cereals and groundnuts for three mycotoxins. Analyst, 94, 136-142

Vorster, L.J. & Purchase, I.F.H. (1968) A method for the determination of sterigmatocystin in grain and oilseeds. Analyst, 93, 694-696

van der Watt, J.J. & Purchase, I.F.H. (1970) The acute toxicity of retrorsine, aflatoxin, and sterigmatocystin in vervet monkeys. Brit. J. exp. Path., 51, 183-190

Zwicker, G.M., Carlton, W.W. & Tuite, J. (1974) Long-term administration of sterigmatocystin and *Penicillium viridicatum* to mice. Fd Cosmet. Toxicol., 12, 491-497

TANNIC ACID AND TANNINS

1. Chemical and Physical Data

Tannic acid

1.1 Synonyms and trade names

Chem. Abstr. Reg. Serial No.: 1401-55-4

Chem. Abstr. Name: Tannic acid

Gallotannic acid; gallotannin; glycerite

1.2 Chemical formula and molecular weight of commercial tannic acid

The empirical formula is usually given as $C_{76}H_{52}O_{46}$; molecular weight is 1701.2. It is a pentadigalloyl glucoside.

1.3 Chemical and physical properties of reagent-grade tannic acid

(a) Description: Yellowish-white to light-brown, amorphous, bulky powder or scales; faint characteristic odour; astringent taste

(b) Solubility: One g dissolves in 0.35 ml water or in 1 ml warm glycerol; very soluble in ethanol and acetone; practically insoluble in benzene, chloroform, ether, petroleum ether, carbon disulphide and carbon tetrachloride

(c) Stability: Gradually darkens on exposure to air and light; when heated to approximately 210-215°C, it decomposes primarily into pyrogallol and carbon dioxide; aqueous solutions decompose on heating.

(d) Identity and specification test: Such tests are given in the British Pharmacopoeia (British Pharmacopoeia Commission, 1973) and The US Pharmacopeia (US Pharmacopeial Convention, Inc., 1970)

(e) Reactivity: Insoluble precipitates are formed with albumin, starch, gelatin and most alkali and metallic salts; it has been reported to catalyse the formation of nitrosodiethylamine (Walker et al., 1975)

1.4 Technical products and impurities

Specifications for a typical commercial grade are as follows: residue after ignition, 1% max; loss on drying, 8-12%; tannin, 86.1%; non-tannin, 4.5%; insoluble materials, 0.4%; water, 9.0%; total solids, 91.0%; soluble solids, 90.6%; ratio of tannin:total solids, 94.6%; tannin: soluble solids, 95.0%. Tannic acid is listed in the European Pharmacopoeia (Council of Europe, 1969).

Tannins

The term 'tannin' was introduced in 1796 by Sequin (Haworth, 1961) to denote substances with the capacity to convert animal skin to leather. Tannins of vegetable origin constitute a large group of phenolic compounds widely distributed in nature in complex mixtures. Compounds which are considered to be tannins vary from simple phenols such as gallic acid to macromolecules with molecular weights of between 500 and 3000.

Extensive studies on the chemistry of the vegetable tannins have been made by Haworth (1961), who has reviewed some problems in the chemistry of gallotannins. Tea tannins have been investigated in considerable detail, in particular by Roberts & Myers (1959; 1960). The chemistry of vegetable tannins has also been reviewed by Haslam (1966).

In 1920, the vegetable tannins were divided into two groups - the non-hydrolysable or condensed tannins and the hydrolysable tannins; the former contain little or no carbohydrate, while the latter are esters hydrolysed by acids, alkalis and enzymes into glucose or other polyhydric alcohols and phenolic acids such as gallic acid (1) and ellagic acid (2), among others. The hydrolysable tannins are sub-divided, on the basis of the phenolic acids which they contain, into the two groups, gallotannins and ellagitannins (Haworth, 1961).

Little is known concerning the structure of condensed tannins. They were once thought to be derived solely from the catechins; however, extensive work on the tea phenols, for example, has shown that this is not the case (Haslam, 1966). It is now known that anthocyanins and flavones also form the basic structures for this type of tannin.

2. Production, Use, Occurrence and Analysis

For important background information on this section, see preamble, p. 17.

2.1 Production and use

Tannic acid is the astringent or tanning principle occurring in the wood, bark, fruit, leaves and roots of a large number of plants. In recent years, tannic acid has been prepared commercially in the United States almost entirely by solvent extraction from Aleppo gall-nuts from the Eastern Mediterranean region and from tara pods from South America. Asian gall-nuts, largely a product of the Peoples' Republic of China, are used in other countries (US Tariff Commission, 1971).

There is only one producer of tannic acid in the US (US International Trade Commission, 1975). Annual imports of tannic acid through the principal US customs districts during 1965-1970 ranged between 275 thousand kg in 1965 and 400 thousand kg in 1966. National Formulary grade tannic acid accounted for the greater part of the total imports during these years. Most came from the UK; Belgium and France were other important sources of National Formulary and other grades of tannic acid; and other grades were also imported from Italy (US Tariff Commission, 1971).

Tannic acid has the following industrial uses: in textile dyeing as a mordant and for pre-treatment and after-treatment; as a treating agent in textile fibre processing; as an additive for printing inks and writing fluids; as a component of plate-desensitizing solutions and fountain solutions in lithographic printing; as a precipitating agent in pigment manufacture; as a component of industrial stains; as a deflocculating agent for clay and refractory casting slips; and as a tanning agent and dye bath component in leather and fur processing. The major industrial use of tannic acid is in combination with tartar emetic in the after-treatment of acid-dyed nylon; it is estimated that over 100 thousand kg are used annually by the textile industry in the US (Anon., 1971).

In human medicine, tannic acid has been administered orally for the symptomatic treatment of diarrhoea, topically for the management of extensive burns and rectally for the relief of local disorders (Goodman & Gilman, 1970). It occurs in products for the treatment of the effects of poison-ivy and poison-oak and for other skin applications. Total sales in the US for such uses are estimated to be about 10 thousand kg annually.

In addition to its natural occurrence in coffee and tea, tannic acid is added as a flavouring agent to beverages, ice cream, sweets, baked goods and liquors. It is also used as a clarifying agent in the brewing and wine industries and as a refining agent for rendered fats. It is estimated that the total US population consumes about 500 thousand kg annually of intentionally added tannic acid in foods and beverages, over half being in wine and beers.

2.2 Occurrence

Practically all wood and vegetation contain some form of tannin in leaves, twigs, bark, wood or fruit. Examples with relatively high tannin contents are the bark of oak, eucalyptus, mangrove, hemlock, pine and willow; the wood of quebracho, chestnut and oak; the fruits of tara, myrobalans and divi-divi; the leaves of sumac and gambier; and the roots of canaigre and palmetto (O'Flaherty & Stubbings, 1967).

2.3 Analysis

A titrimetric method (Kaushik & Prosad, 1973) and colorimetric methods (Haslam, 1966; Willemot & Parry, 1970) have been used to estimate total tannin content.

3. Biological Data Relevant to the Evaluation of Carcinogenic Risk to Man

3.1 Carcinogenicity and related studies in animals

(a) Skin application

Rat: When burn-induced ulcers on the skin of 20 white rats were painted daily with a fresh 5% aqueous solution of tannic acid (USP), no tumours were observed in 11 animals surviving 400 days (Korpássy & Mosonyi, 1950).

(b) Subcutaneous and/or intramuscular administration

Mouse: Tannin extracts prepared from various plant materials (sulphited quebracho, mimosa, Myrtle, chestnut, myrobalans and valonia) and tannic acid (BP) were injected subcutaneously at a dose of 0.25 ml in stock mice weekly for 12 weeks. After one year it was observed that condensed tannins evoked local sarcomas and liver tumours and that hydrolysable tannins produced only liver tumours. With tannic acid and myrobalans, chestnut and valonia tannins, 7, 4, 4 and 1 liver tumours occurred, respectively, but the original number of mice used was not stated. With Myrtle, quebracho and mimosa tannins, the numbers of sarcomas and liver tumours were 5 and 7, 8 and 5, and 2 and 9, respectively. No controls were reported (Kirby, 1960).

A group of 30 male and 30 female young C_3H/A mice was injected i.m. every second week with 0.75 mg/kg bw tannic acid for 12 months. The tannic acid used was nut gall tannic acid, a complex of esters of D-glucose with gallo-tannic acid and galloyl gallo-tannic acid. The experiment was terminated after 18 months, 6 months after the last injection; no local tumours were found (Bichel & Bach, 1968).

Rat: A group of 14 male and 14 female white rats, 2-months old, was injected subcutaneously with an aqueous solution of tannic acid (USP) every 5th day for 290 days (initial dose, 150 mg/kg bw; later, 200 mg/kg bw); 23 rats survived 100 days. The experiment was terminated after 388 days, and 5/28 rats examined had hepatomas and 6/28 had cholangiomas. These tumours occurred rarely in untreated rats of that colony (Korpássy & Mosonyi, 1950). The same authors found that four weekly doses of 200 or 250 mg/kg bw tannic acid, injected subcutaneously, enhanced the hepatocarcinogenic effect of 2-acetylaminofluorene (Mosonyi & Korpássy, 1953).

Tannin extracts prepared from plant materials (sulphited quebracho, mimosa and myrobalans) and tannic acid (BP) were injected subcutaneously in groups of 10 August rats at doses of 1 ml weekly during 12 weeks. One rat injected with quebracho extract and 1 injected with mimosa extract developed local sarcomas after 1 year (Kirby, 1960).

3.2 Other relevant biological data

The oral LD_{50}'s of tannic acid are about 3.50 g/kg bw in mice (Robinson & Graessle, 1943) and 2.26 g/kg bw in rats (Boyd, 1965). Its s.c. LD_{50} in rats is 1.5 g/kg bw (Cameron et al., 1943); that in mice after i.v. injection is 0.04 g/kg bw (Robinson & Graessle, 1943). Armstrong et al. (1957) reported s.c. LD_{50} values in mice ranging from 0.1 g/kg bw for hydrolysable tannins (myrobalans and chestnut) to 1.6 g/kg bw for condensed tannins (quebracho and mimosa).

No liver damage was observed in 7 male Wistar rats fed 60 mg/kg bw/day tannic acid (DAB.6) during 152 days (Blumenberg et al., 1960). A single s.c. dose of 250 mg/kg bw tannic acid to rats resulted in centrilobular necrosis of the liver (Horvath et al., 1960); similar results were obtained in rabbits (Arhelger et al., 1965).

Korpassy et al. (1951) found an increased concentration of tannic acid in the blood of rabbits and dogs given tannic acid by stomach tube, with a maximum level after three hours. Absorption of tannic acid from the colon, as shown by rising blood levels, was demonstrated in rabbits, sheep, goats, rats and dogs (Dollahite et al., 1962; McAlister et al., 1963).

Tannic acid administered by i.p. or s.c. injection to rats appeared in the liver 1 hour after administration and was concentrated in the nuclei as early as 3 hours later. The sequence of events was concentration of tannic acid in the nuclei, inhibition of nuclear RNA synthesis, inhibition of protein synthesis and production of necrosis (Badawy et al., 1969; Horvath et al., 1960; Reddy & Svoboda, 1968; Reddy et al., 1970).

In autopsied human burn cases, Wells et al. (1942) observed liver necrosis attributable to the absorption of tannic acid through burned skin surfaces. Eight deaths due to acute liver failure have been suggested to be associated with the use of barium enemas containing tannic acid (Lucke et al., 1963; McAlister et al., 1963).

3.3 Observations in man

No case reports or epidemiological studies concerning cancer in relation to human exposure to tannic acid or tannins were available.

4. Comments on Data Reported and Evaluation[1]

4.1 Animal data

Tannic acid is carcinogenic in rats following its subcutaneous injection; it produced liver tumours. In mice, subcutaneous injection of hydrolysable tannins produced liver tumours, and that of condensed tannins produced both local sarcomas and liver tumours. No adequate published studies involving oral administration of tannins were available to the Working Group.

4.2 Human data

No case reports or epidemiological studies were available to the Working Group.

---

[1] See also the section "Animal Data in Relation to the Evaluation of Risk to Man" in the introduction to this volume, p. 15.

5. References

Anon. (1971) *Oil, Paint and Drug Reporter*, May 3, pp. 13-14

Arhelger, R.B., Broom, J.S. & Boler, R.K. (1965) Ultrastructural hepatic alterations following tannic acid administration to rabbits. *Amer. J. Path.*, 46, 409-434

Armstrong, D.M.G., Clarke, E.G.C. & Cotchin, E. (1957) A note on the acute toxicity of hydrolysable and condensed tannins. *J. Pharm. Pharmacol.*, 9, 98-101

Badawy, A.A.B., White, A.E. & Lathe, G.H. (1969) The effect of tannic acid on the synthesis of protein and nucleic acid by rat liver. *Biochem. J.*, 113, 307-313

Bichel, J. & Bach, A. (1968) Investigation on the toxicity of small chronic doses of tannic acid with special reference to possible carcinogenicity. *Acta pharmacol. toxicol.*, 26, 41-45

Blumenberg, F.W., Enneker, C. & Kessler, F.J. (1960) Zur Frage der hepatotoxischen Wirkung oral verabreichten Tannins und seiner Galloyl-Bausteine. *Arzneimittel-Forsch.*, 10, 223-226

Boyd, E.M. (1965) The acute toxicity of tannic acid administered intragastrically. *Canad. med. Ass. J.*, 92, 1292-1297

British Pharmacopeia Commission (1973) *British Pharmacopoeia*, London, HMSO, p. 461

Cameron, G.R., Milton, R.F. & Allen, J.W. (1943) Toxicity of tannic acid. An experimental investigation. *Lancet*, ii, 179-186

Council of Europe (1969) *European Pharmacopoeia*, European Treaty Series No. 50, Vol. 1, Paris, Maisonneuve, p. 202

Dollahite, J.W., Pigeon, R.F. & Camp, B.J. (1962) The toxicity of gallic acid, pyrogallol, tannic acid and *Quercus havardi* in the rabbit. *Amer. J. vet. Res.*, 23, 1264-1267

Goodman, L.S. & Gilman, A., eds (1970) *The Pharmacological Basis of Therapeutics*, 4th ed., London, Toronto, MacMillan, p. 992

Haslam, E. (1966) *Chemistry of Vegetable Tannins*, London, New York, Academic Press

Haworth, R.D. (1961) Some problems in the chemistry of the gallotannins. *Proc. chem. Soc.*, 401-412

Horvath, E., Sólyom, A. & Korpássy, B. (1960) Histochemical and biochemical studies in acute poisoning with tannic acid. Brit. J. exp. Path., 41, 298-304

Kaushik, R.L. & Prosad, R. (1973) Periodate as an analytical reagent. VI. Estimation of Hg (II) and its application in the indirect determination of glucose, fructose, maltose, lactose, furfural, gallic acid, tannic acid, formaldehyde, acetaldehyde and benzaldehyde. J. Ind. chem. Soc., 50, 17-18

Kirby, K.S. (1960) Induction of tumours by tannin extracts. Brit. J. Cancer, 14, 147-150

Korpássy, B. & Mosonyi, M. (1950) The carcinogenic activity of tannic acid. Liver tumours induced in rats by prolonged subcutaneous administration of tannic acid solutions. Brit. J. Cancer, 4, 411-420

Korpássy, B., Horvai, R. & Koltay, M. (1951) On the absorption of tannic acid from the gastro-intestinal tract. Arch. int. Pharmacodyn., 88, 368-377

Lucke, H.H., Hodge, K.E. & Patt, N.L. (1963) Fatal liver damage after barium enemas containing tannic acid. Canad. med. Ass. J., 89, 1111-1114

McAlister, W.H., Anderson, M.S., Bloomberg, G.R. & Margulis, A.R. (1963) Lethal effects of tannic acid in the barium enema. Radiology, 80, 765-773

Mosonyi, M. & Korpássy, B. (1953) Rapid production of malignant hepatomas by simultaneous administration of tannic acid and 2-acetylaminofluorene. Nature (Lond.), 171, 791

O'Flaherty, F. & Stubbings, R.L. (1967) Leather. In: Kirk, R.E. & Othmer, D.F., eds, Encyclopedia of Chemical Technology, 2nd ed., Vol. 12, New York, John Wiley and Sons, pp. 314-315

Reddy, J. & Svoboda, D. (1968) The relationship of nucleolar segregation to ribonucleic acid synthesis following the administration of selected hepatocarcinogens. Lab. Invest., 19, 132-145

Reddy, J.K., Chiga, M., Hariss, C.C. & Svoboda, D.J. (1970) Polyribosome disaggregation in rat liver following administration of tannic acid. Cancer Res., 30, 58-65

Roberts, E.A.H. & Myers, M. (1959) The phenolic substances of manufactured tea. IV. Enzymic oxidations of individual substrates. J. Sci. Fd Agric., 10, 167-179

Roberts, E.A.H. & Myers, M. (1960) The phenolic substances of manufactured tea. VII. The preparation of individual flavanols. J. Sci. Fd Agric., 11, 153-163

Robinson, H.J. & Graessle, O.E. (1943) Toxicity of tannic acid. J. Pharmacol. exp. Ther., 77, 63-69

US International Trade Commission (1975) Synthetic Organic Chemicals, US Production and Sales, 1973, ITC Publication 728, Washington DC, US Government Printing Office, p. 212

US Pharmacopeial Convention, Inc. (1970) The US Pharmacopeia, 18th rev., Easton, Pa, Mack, pp. 1013-1014

US Tariff Commission (1971) Summaries of Trade and Tariff Information, TC Publication 408, Washington DC, US Government Printing Office, pp. 105-108

Walker, E.A., Pignatelli, B. & Castegnaro, M. (1975) Effects of gallic acid on nitrosamine formation. Nature (Lond.), 258, 176

Wells, D.B., Humphrey, H.D. & Coll, J.S. (1942) The relation of tannic acid to the liver necrosis occurring in burns. New Engl. J. Med., 226, 629-635

Willemot, J. & Parry, G. (1970) Une nouvelle réaction colorée applicable au dosage photocolorimétrique de l'acide tannique. Ann. pharm. franç., 28, 391-395

PYRROLIZIDINE ALKALOIDS

HYDROXYSENKIRKINE

1. Chemical and Physical Data

1.1 Synonyms and trade names

Chem. Abstr. Reg. Serial No.: 26782-43-4

Chem. Abstr. Name: 8,12,18-Trihydroxy-4-methyl-11,16-dioxo-senecionanium

Stereoisomer of 4-ethylidene-7-hydroxy-7α-(hydroxymethyl)-6,14-dimethyl-2,9-dioxa-1,14-azabicyclo (9.5.1) heptadec-11-ene-3,8,17-trione; *trans*-15-ethylidene-12β-hydroxy-12α-hydroxymethyl-4,13β-dimethyl-8-oxo-4,8-secosenec-1-enine

1.2 Chemical formula and molecular weight

$C_{19}H_{27}NO_7$ Mol. wt: 381.4

1.3 Chemical and physical properties of the pure substance

(a) Description: Colourless plates

(b) Melting-point: 124-125°C (as a 1:1 solvate from acetone)

(c) Optical rotation: $[\alpha]_D^{26}$ +5.3° (in ethanol)

(d) Spectroscopy data: For infra-red and nuclear magnetic resonance spectral data see Crout (1972).

(e) Identity and purity test: Melting-point and mixed melting-point; thin-layer and gas chromatographic comparison with the authentic compound (Crout, 1972)

(f) Solubility: Soluble in water, ethanol, chloroform and hot acetone

(g) *Volatility*: Sublimes at 136°C at 0.01 mm

(h) *Stability*: Stable at room temperature in closed containers; but it is best stored for lengthy periods under nitrogen at -15°C.

(i) *Reactivity*: Readily hydrolysed with alkali (Crout, 1972)

1.4 Technical products and impurities

No data were available to the Working Group.

2. Production, Use, Occurrence and Analysis

2.1 Production and use

Hydroxysenkirkine is not produced commercially.

2.2 Occurrence

Hydroxysenkirkine has been isolated from the plant *Crotalaria laburnifolia* L. *eldomae* (family Leguminosae) (Crout, 1972). This plant is used as a medicinal herb in Tanzania (Schoental & Coady, 1968).

2.3 Analysis

No specific methods for the determination of hydroxysenkirkine are available, however, the analysis of plant material may be carried out by general methods developed for pyrrolizidine alkaloids (see section "General Information and Conclusions on Pyrrolizidine Alkaloids", p. 335).

3. Biological Data Relevant to the Evaluation of Carcinogenic Risk to Man

3.1 Carcinogenicity and related studies in animals

Intraperitoneal administration

Of 5 male weanling Wistar-Porton rats given single i.p. injections of 100-300 mg/kg bw hydroxysenkirkine, 1 that had been given 300 mg/kg bw and killed after 14.5 months, showed 3 apparently separate tumours of the cerebrum, all of an astrocytic form. Tumours of the CNS are reported to be rare in rats of the colony used (Schoental & Cavanagh, 1972).

3.2 _Other relevant biological data_

Weanling rats given 300 mg/kg bw hydroxysenkirkine by stomach tube died within a few days with liver lesions typical of those induced by pyrrolizidine alkaloids; 1-4 day-old rats were more sensitive and died within a few days after receiving a dose of 50 mg/kg bw hydroxysenkirkine by s.c. or i.p. injection (Schoental, 1970).

The metabolism of hydroxysenkirkine is expected to be similar to that of other hepatotoxic pyrrolizidine alkaloids as described in the section "General Information and Conclusions on Pyrrolizidine Alkaloids", p. 336.

3.3 _Observations in man_

No data were available to the Working Group.

4. Comments on Data Reported and Evaluation

4.1 _Animal data_

Hydroxysenkirkine was tested only by the intraperitoneal route in five male rats, producing tumours of the brain in one animal. The available information is insufficient to evaluate the carcinogenicity of this compound (see also section "General Information and Conclusions on Pyrrolizidine Alkaloids", p. 333).

4.2 _Human data_

No case reports or epidemiological studies were available to the Working Group.

5. References

Crout, D.H.G. (1972) Pyrrolizidine and seco-pyrrolizidine alkaloids of *Crotalaria laburnifolia* L. subspecies *eldomae*. J. chem. Soc., 1602-1607

Schoental, R. (1970) Hepatotoxic activity of retrorsine, senkirkine and hydroxysenkirkine in newborn rats, and the role of epoxides in carcinogenesis by pyrrolizidine alkaloids and aflatoxins. Nature (Lond.), 227, 401-402

Schoental, R. & Cavanagh, J.B. (1972) Brain and spinal cord tumours in rats treated with pyrrolizidine alkaloids. J. nat. Cancer Inst., 49, 665-671

Schoental, R. & Coady, A. (1968) The hepatotoxicity of some Ethiopian and East African plants, including some used in traditional medicines. E. Afr. med. J., 45, 577-580

ISATIDINE

1. Chemical and Physical Data

1.1 Synonyms and trade names

Chem. Abstr. Reg. Serial No.: 15503-86-3

Chem. Abstr. Name: 12,18-Dihydroxysenecionan-11,16-dione-4-oxide

trans-15-Ethylidene-12β-hydroxy-12α-hydroxymethyl-13β-methylsenec-1-enine-4-oxide; retrorsine N-oxide

1.2 Chemical formula and molecular weight

$C_{18}H_{25}NO_7$ Mol. wt: 367.4

1.3 Chemical and physical properties of the pure substance

(a) Description: Colourless prisms

(b) Melting-point: 138°C (decomposition)

(c) Optical rotation: $[\alpha]_D^{22}$ -8.2° (in water)

(d) Spectroscopy data: λ_{max} 217 nm; E_1^1 = 172 (in water) (Leisegang, 1950); no infra-red or nuclear magnetic resonance spectral data have been published, but reduction with zinc and sulphuric acid readily converts isatidine to retrorsine, for which characterization data have been recorded separately (Culvenor & Smith, 1955).

(e) Identity and purity test: Melting-point and mixed melting-point; thin-layer and gas chromatographic comparison of the zinc-sulphuric acid reduction product with retrorsine (Chalmers *et al.*, 1965)

(f) _Solubility_: Soluble in water and ethanol; sparingly soluble in non-polar solvents

(g) _Volatility_: Very low

(h) _Stability_: Decomposes slowly at room temperature

(i) _Reactivity_: Reduced by zinc and sulphuric acid to retrorsine; readily hydrolysed with alkali; dehydrated to dehydroretrorsine with acetic anhydride and related reagents (Mattocks, 1969)

1.4 Technical products and impurities

No data were available to the Working Group.

2. Production, Use, Occurrence and Analysis

2.1 Production and use

Isatidine is not produced commercially. Some of the *Senecio* species in which isatidine occurs have been used as medicinal herbs. *S. bupleuroids* DC. is an ingredient of an African herbal remedy (Watt & Breyer-Brandwijk, 1962). *S. isatideus* is a high-yielding source suitable for preparative purposes (Koekemoer & Warren, 1951).

2.2 Occurrence

Isatidine has been isolated from *Senecio bupleuroids* DC., *S. isatideus* DC., *S. paucicalyculatus* Klett, *S. retrorsus* DC. and *S. sceleratus* Schweickerdt (family Compositae) (Bull et al., 1968; de Waal, 1939). Since isatidine is the N-oxide of retrorsine, it is also expected to occur in all plant species from which retrorsine has been isolated; these include *Crotalaria* (family Leguminosae) as well as *Senecio* species.

2.3 Analysis

No specific method of analysis exists for this compound. However, the analysis of plant material for isatidine may be carried out by the general methods developed for pyrrolizidine alkaloids (see section "General Information and Conclusions on Pyrrolizidine Alkaloids, p. 335).

3. Biological Data Relevant to the Evaluation of Carcinogenic Risk to Man

3.1 Carcinogenicity and related studies in animals

(a) Oral administration

Rat: Of 22 albino Wistar rats (8 male and 14 female) treated with isatidine in the drinking-water at concentrations of 0.05 then 0.03 mg/ml on 3 days/week for about 20 months, 5 had nodular hyperplasia of the liver and 5 males and 5 females had multiple hepatomas with atypical hyperplasia of the endothelial cells. In one of these rats, which died 14 months after the start of treatment, multiple metastases were found (Schoental et al., 1954).

Of 7 rats (3 male and 4 female) surviving 14-21 months of treatment with isatidine and a choline-supplemented diet, 6 showed nodular hyperplasia of the liver; trabecular hepatomas were observed in 4 females (Schoental et al., 1954).

(b) Other experimental systems

Of 5 rats (2 male and 3 female) given single i.p. injections of 2 mg isatidine in tricaprylin, followed by skin applications on the neck of a 0.5% solution of isatidine in ethanol 3 times weekly for 15 months, and surviving 11-18 months after the start of the treatment, 1 rat developed liver nodules which appeared to be hepatomas; no lesions occurred on the painted areas (Schoental et al., 1954).

3.2 Other relevant biological data

The acute i.v. LD_{50} of isatidine in mice was found to be 835 mg/kg bw (Harris et al., 1942). The acute LD_{50}'s in rats were 48 mg/kg bw orally and 250 mg/kg bw following i.p. injection (Mattocks, 1971).

Weanling rats given 0.1 or 0.2 mg/ml isatidine in their drinking-water on 3 or 5 days a week for 3 or 6 weeks showed liver lesions, including necrosis, fatty infiltration, fibrosis and nodular hyperplasia. In some animals there was stunting of growth, anaemia, drastic reduction in serum proteins, ascites, congestion of the lungs, immaturity of the sex organs and damage to the spleen, pancreas and kidneys (Schoental, 1955).

Isatidine is not converted into pyrrolic metabolites by isolated rat liver microsomes. It is, however, reduced to retrorsine in the intestinal tract of rats, possibly by the gut flora, thus accounting for the large increase in toxicity when isatidine is administered by mouth rather than parenterally (Mattocks, 1971). Following its reduction to retrorsine, metabolism proceeds as described for other hepatoxic pyrrolizidine alkaloids (see also section "General Information and Conclusions on Pyrrolizidine Alkaloids", p. 336).

3.3 Observations in man

No data were available to the Working Group.

4. Comments on Data Reported and Evaluation[1]

4.1 Animal data

Isatidine is carcinogenic in rats as shown by a limited study in which it produced liver tumours following its oral administration (see also section "General Information and Conclusions on Pyrrolizidine Alkaloids", p. 333).

4.2 Human data

No case reports or epidemiological studies were available to the Working Group.

---

[1] See also the section "Animal Data in Relation to the Evaluation of Risk to Man" in the introduction to this volume, p. 15.

5. References

Bull, L.B., Culvenor, C.C.J. & Dick, A.T. (1968) <u>The Pyrrolizidine Alkaloids</u>, Amsterdam, North Holland, pp. 238-244

Chalmers, A.H., Culvenor, C.C.J. & Smith, L.W. (1965) Characterisation of pyrrolizidine alkaloids by gas, thin-layer and paper chromatography. <u>J. Chromat.</u>, <u>20</u>, 270-277

Culvenor, C.C.J. & Smith, L.W. (1955) The alkaloids of *Erectites quadridentata* DC. <u>Austr. J. Chem.</u>, <u>8</u>, 556-561

Harris, P.N., Anderson, R.C. & Chen, K.K. (1942) The action of isatidine, pterophine and sceleratine. <u>J. Pharmacol. exp. Ther.</u>, <u>75</u>, 83-88

Koekemoer, M.J. & Warren, F.L. (1951) The *Senecio* alkaloids. VIII. The occurrence and preparation of the N-oxides. An improved method of extraction of the *Senecio* alkaloids. <u>J. chem. Soc.</u>, 66-68

Leisegang, E.C. (1950) *Senecio* alkaloids. The ultra-violet extinction curves of the alkaloids and the 'necic' acids. <u>J.S. Afr. chem. Inst.</u>, <u>3</u>, 73-76

Mattocks, A.R. (1969) Dihydropyrrolizine derivatives from unsaturated pyrrolizidine alkaloids. <u>J. chem. Soc., C</u>, 1115-1162

Mattocks, A.R. (1971) Hepatotoxic effects due to pyrrolizidine alkaloid N-oxides. <u>Xenobiotica</u>, <u>1</u>, 563-565

Schoental, R. (1955) Kwashiorkor-like syndrome and other pathological changes in rats as a result of feeding with *Senecio* alkaloids (isatidine). <u>Voeding</u>, <u>16</u>, 268-285

Schoental, R., Head, M.A. & Peacock, P.R. (1954) *Senecio* alkaloids: primary liver tumours in rats as a result of treatment with (i) a mixture of alkaloids from *S. jacobaea* Lin.; (ii) retrorsine; (iii) isatidine. <u>Brit. J. Cancer</u>, <u>8</u>, 458-465

de Waal, H.L. (1939) The *Senecio* alkaloids. I. The isolation of isatidine from *S. retrorsus* and *S. isatideus*. <u>Onderstepoort J. vet. Sci. Animal Industr.</u>, <u>12</u>, 155-163

Watt, J.M. & Breyer-Brandwijk, M.G., eds (1962) <u>The Medicinal and Poisonous Plants of Southern and Eastern Africa</u>, 2nd ed., Edinburgh, London, E. & S. Livingstone, p. 284

JACOBINE

1. Chemical and Physical Data

1.1 Synonyms and trade names

Chem. Abstr. Reg. Serial No.: 471-14-7

Chem. Abstr. Name: (15α,20R)15,20-Epoxy-15,20-dihydro-12-hydroxy-senecionan-11,16-dione

12β-Hydroxy-12α,13β-dimethylsenec-1-enine-15S-spiro-2'-(3'R-methyl-oxiran); NSC 89936*; stereoisomer of 5,6,9,11,13,14,14a,14b-octahydro-6-hydroxy-3,5,6-trimethyl-spiro[(1,6)dioxacyclododecino-[2,3,4-*gh*]pyrrolizine-3-(2*H*)]-2'-oxirane-2,7(4*H*)-dione

1.2 Chemical formula and molecular weight

$C_{18}H_{25}NO_6$ Mol. wt: 351.4

1.3 Chemical and physical properties of the pure substance

(a) <u>Description</u>: Colourless plates

(b) <u>Melting-point</u>: 228°C

(c) <u>Optical rotation</u>: $[\alpha]_D^{20}$ -40° (in chloroform) (Bradbury & Culvenor, 1954)

(d) <u>Spectroscopy data</u>: For infra-red spectral data, see Culvenor & Dal Bon (1964).

---

*Cancer Chemotherapy National Service Centre Number, NCI, NIH, USA

(e) <u>Identity and purity test</u>: Melting-point and mixed melting-point; thin-layer and gas chromatographic comparison with the authentic compound (Chalmers et al., 1965)

(f) <u>Solubility</u>: Soluble in chloroform; sparingly soluble in ethanol, water and ether

(g) <u>Volatility</u>: Low, but sufficient for gas chromatography and mass spectrometry

(h) <u>Stability</u>: Stable at room temperature in closed containers; for long periods, it is best stored under nitrogen at $-15^{\circ}C$.

(i) <u>Reactivity</u>: Readily hydrolysed with alkali; reacts with hydrochloric acid to form the chlorhydrin, jaconine (Bradbury & Willis, 1956)

1.4 <u>Technical products and impurities</u>

No data were available to the Working Group.

2. Production, Use, Occurrence and Analysis

2.1 <u>Production and use</u>

Jacobine is not produced commercially. *Senecio jacobaea*, in which it occurs, is reported to have been used as a medicinal herb in Europe (Blacow, 1972; Burns, 1972; Schoental & Pullinger, 1972).

2.2 <u>Occurrence</u>

Jacobine occurs in the following *Senecio* species (family Compositae): *S. brasiliensis* DC., *S. cineraria* DC., *S. jacobaea* L. and *S. paludosus* L. (Bull et al., 1968). *S. jacobaea* is a common weed in temperate regions.

2.3 <u>Analysis</u>

No specific method of analysis has been reported for this compound. However, the analysis of plant material for jacobine may be carried out by the general methods developed for pyrrolizidine alkaloids (see section "General Information and Conclusions on Pyrrolizidine Alkaloids", p. 335).

3. Biological Data Relevant to the Evaluation of Carcinogenic Risk to Man

3.1 Carcinogenicity and related studies in animals

Oral administration

Rat: No data relating to the pure alkaloid are available; however, studies have been carried out on plant material and plant extracts containing this alkaloid (see section "General Information and Conclusions on Pyrrolizidine Alkaloids", p. 333).

3.2 Other relevant biological data

LD_{50} values for jacobine have been reported to be 77 mg/kg bw following i.v. injection in mice (Harris et al., 1942) and 138 mg/kg bw following i.p. injection in female rats (Bull et al., 1968).

In mice, large doses of jacobine cause clonic convulsions and death within a few minutes. Lower doses, of the order of the acute LD_{50}, produce death mostly within 1-4 days, with extensive haemorrhagic necrosis of the liver and, sometimes, congestion and oedema of the lungs. Smaller doses, given on 5 days per week and producing death in 26-70 days, give rise to liver necrosis, hypertrophy of liver cells with enlarged nuclei and, sometimes, ascites, pulmonary oedema and hydrothorax (Harris et al., 1942). Doses approaching the LD_{50} also produce haemorrhagic centrilobular necrosis in rats (Bull et al., 1968).

The metabolism of jacobine is expected to be similar to that of other hepatotoxic pyrrolizidine alkaloids described in the section "General Information and Conclusions on Pyrrolizidine Alkaloids", p. 336.

Doses of 0.08 µl of a 20 mM solution of jacobine of unspecified purity in 0.7% sodium chloride were injected into the abdomen of 24-hour old Canton S *Drosophila melanogaster* males. Weak mutagenic effects on the induction of sex-linked recessive lethals were scored (Clark, 1960).

3.3 Observations in man

No data were available to the Working Group.

4. Comments on Data Reported and Evaluation

4.1 Animal data

No data were available concerning the carcinogenicity of pure jacobine. However, see also the section "General Information and Conclusions on Pyrrolizidine Alkaloids", p. 333.

4.2 Human data

No case reports or epidemiological studies were available to the Working Group.

5. References

Blacow, N.W., ed. (1972) *Martindale, The Extra Pharmacopoeia*, 26th ed., London, The Pharmaceutical Press, p. 2038

Bradbury, R.B. & Culvenor, C.C.J. (1954) The alkaloids of *Senecio jacobaea* L. I. Isolation of the alkaloids and identification of jacobine as seneciphylline. *Austr. J. Chem.*, 7, 378-383

Bradbury, R.B. & Willis, J.B. (1956) The alkaloids of *Senecio jacobaea* L. II. The structures of the acids, and the relationship between jacobine and jaconine. *Austr. J. Chem.*, 9, 258-276

Bull, L.B., Culvenor, C.C.J. & Dick, A.T. (1968) *The Pyrrolizidine Alkaloids*, Amsterdam, North Holland, pp. 142, 252

Burns, J. (1972) The heart and pulmonary arteries in rats fed on *Senecio jacobaea*. *J. Path.*, 106, 187-194

Chalmers, A.H., Culvenor, C.C.J. & Smith, L.W. (1965) Characterisation of pyrrolizidine alkaloids by gas, thin-layer and paper chromatography. *J. Chromat.*, 20, 270-277

Clark, A.M. (1960) The mutagenic activity of some pyrrolizidine alkaloids in *Drosophila*. *Z. Vererbungsl.*, 91, 74-80

Culvenor, C.C.J. & Dal Bon, R. (1964) Carbonyl stretching frequencies of pyrrolizidine alkaloids. *Austr. J. Chem.*, 17, 1296-1300

Harris, P.N., Anderson, R.C. & Chen, K.K. (1942) The action of senecionine, integerrimine, jacobine, longilobine and spartioidine, especially on the liver. *J. Pharmacol. exp. Ther.*, 75, 69-77

Schoental, R. & Pullinger, B.D. (1972) On the alleged oestrogenic and other medicinal properties of pyrrolizidine (*Senecio*) alkaloids. *E. Afr. med. J.*, 49, 436-439

LASIOCARPINE

1. Chemical and Physical Data

1.1 Synonyms and trade names

Chem. Abstr. Reg. Serial No.: 303-34-4

Chem. Abstr. Name: Lasiocarpine

(7α-Angelyloxy-5,6,7,8α-tetrahydro-3H-pyrrolizin-1-yl)methyl-2,3-dihydroxy-2-(1'-methoxyethyl)-3-methylbutyrate; 2-butenoic acid, 2-methyl-7{[2,3-dihydroxy-2-(1-methoxyethyl)-3-methyl-1-oxobutoxy]methyl}-2,3,5,7a-tetrahydro-1H-pyrrolizin-1-yl ester{1S-[1α(Z),-7(2S,3R)7aα]}; (z)-2-methylcrotonic acid, 2,3-dihydroxy-2-(1-methoxyethyl)-3-methylbutyrate(ester); NSC 30625*; stereoisomer of 7-[2,3-dihydroxy-2-(1-methoxyethyl)-3-methyl-1-oxobutoxy]methyl-2,3,5,7α-tetrahydro-1H-pyrrolizin-1-yl-2-methyl-2-butenoate; 2,3,5,7αβ-tetrahydro-1-hydroxy-1H-pyrrolizine-7-methanol-1-angelate-7-[2,3-dihydroxy-2(1-methoxyethyl)]-3-methyl-butyrate; (z)-2-methylcrotonic acid, 2,3-dihydroxy-2-(1-methoxyethyl)-3-methylbutyrate(ester)

1.2 Chemical formula and molecular weight

$C_{21}H_{33}NO_7$ Mol. wt: 411.5

1.3 Chemical and physical properties of the pure substance

(a) Description: Colourless plates

(b) Melting-point: 96.4-97°C

(c) Optical rotation: $[\alpha]_D^{16}$ -3.0° (in ethanol)

---

*Cancer Chemotherapy National Service Centre Number, NCI, NIH, USA

(d) <u>Spectroscopy data</u>: For infra-red and nuclear magnetic resonance spectral data see Culvenor & Dal Bon (1964) and Bull *et al.* (1968).

(e) <u>Identity and purity test</u>: Melting-point and mixed melting-point; thin-layer and gas chromatographic comparison with authentic substance (Chalmers *et al.*, 1965)

(f) <u>Solubility</u>: Soluble in most non-polar organic solvents and ethanol; sparingly soluble in water (0.68%) and light petroleum; soluble in water as the hydrochloride

(g) <u>Volatility</u>: Low, but sufficient for gas chromatography and mass spectrometry

(h) <u>Stability</u>: Decomposes slowly on standing in air at room temperature; it is best stored under nitrogen at $-15°C$.

(i) <u>Reactivity</u>: Readily hydrolysed with alkali; reacts readily with oxidizing agents (slowly with atmospheric oxygen) to form a dihydropyrrolizine derivative

1.4 Technical products and impurities

No data were available to the Working Group.

2. Production, Use, Occurrence and Analysis

2.1 Production and use

Lasiocarpine is produced for research purposes from *Heliotropium europaeum* by two firms in Australia. *Heliotropium europaeum* L. is reported to have been used medicinally in India as an emetic and in the treatment of snake bites (Chopra, 1933). It has also been used medicinally in Greece and the eastern Mediterranean (Gunther, 1934).

2.2 Occurrence

Lasiocarpine has been isolated only from plant species of the family Boraginaceae. It is known to occur in *Heliotropium europaeum* L., *H. lasiocarpum* Fisch. et C. Mey. (Bull *et al.*, 1968), *Lappula intermedia* (Man'ko & Vasil'kov, 1968), *Symphytum caucasicum* and *S. officinale* (Man'ko *et al.*, 1969).

In the Central Asian republics of the USSR, contamination of cereal grain for human consumption by seeds of *H. lasiocarpum* occurred at least until 1946. At that time the seeds were shown to be the cause of a disease then known as 'toxic hepatitis with ascites' but re-named 'heliotropic dystrophy of the liver' (Khanin, 1956).

2.3 Analysis

The analysis of plant material and animal tissues for lasiocarpine is carried out by general methods developed for pyrrolizidine alkaloids (see section "General Information and Conclusions on Pyrrolizidine Alkaloids", p. 335).

Lasiocarpine in alkaloid mixtures has been estimated by partition chromatography (Culvenor et al., 1954) and by thin-layer chromatography (Chalmers et al., 1965). The partition system previously employed will probably not separate lasiocarpine adequately from acetyllasiocarpine, which was recently found to occur in *Heliotropium europaeum* (Culvenor et al., 1976). Dann (1960) has estimated lasiocarpine in body tissues and fluids by removing protein, chromatographing on Florisil and estimating colorimetrically with methyl orange.

3. Biological Data Relevant to the Evaluation of Carcinogenic Risk to Man

3.1 Carcinogenicity and related studies in animals

Intraperitoneal administration

Rat: Twenty-five inbred male Fischer 344 rats were given i.p. injections of 7.8 mg/kg bw lasiocarpine (10% of the LD_{50}) twice weekly for 4 weeks then once a week for 52 weeks, whereupon injections were discontinued. Eighteen survived the time of the appearance of the first tumour (56 weeks), and 16 developed tumours 60 to 76 weeks after the beginning of the experiment. Ten rats developed hepatocellular carcinomas, 6 developed well-differentiated squamous-cell carcinomas of the skin of the back, 5 developed pulmonary adenomas, 2 developed well-differentiated adenocarcinomas of the small intestine, 1 developed a cholangiocarcinoma, 1 an adenomyoma of the ileum and 1 an interstitial-cell tumour of the testes. The hepatocellular and squamous-cell carcinomas were transplanted successfully through five generations. Two lung adenomas occurred among 25 controls killed after 76 weeks (Svoboda & Reddy, 1972).

When i.p. injections of lasiocarpine were given to rats fed aflatoxin B_1 in the diet and also pre-treated with lasiocarpine to produce an antimitotic effect, liver tumours developed after a similar time (within 18 weeks) and in similar numbers to those in rats given aflatoxin alone. The tumours were, however, associated with post-necrotic cirrhosis or advanced portal scarring not seen in rats receiving aflatoxin alone (Reddy & Svoboda, 1972).

3.2 Other relevant biological data

The acute i.v. LD_{50}'s were 85 mg/kg bw in mice, 88 mg/kg bw in rats and 67 mg/kg bw in hamsters (Rose *et al.*, 1959). Bull *et al.* (1958) reported the i.p. LD_{50}'s in rats to be 72 mg/kg bw for males and 79 mg/kg bw for females.

Lasiocarpine is also toxic to guinea-pigs and monkeys (Chen *et al.*, 1940; Rose *et al.*, 1959). Very high doses cause rapid death within a few hours, often with convulsions and unrelated to liver damage. Lower doses, of the order of the acute LD_{50}, produce severe haemorrhagic necrosis of the liver, gastro-intestinal haemorrhage, sometimes congestion and oedema of the lungs, congestion of the adrenals and sometimes pyloric, duodenal and rectal ulceration (Bull *et al.*, 1958; 1968; Chen *et al.*, 1940; Schoental & Magee, 1957). Leucocytosis (Chen *et al.*, 1940) and severe but temporary hypoprothrombinaemia (Rose *et al.*, 1959) also occur. Chronic toxicity gives rise to small, nodular livers with megalocytic parenchymal cells which have reduced respiratory enzyme activity (Bull *et al.*, 1968). The megalocytosis develops as a result of long-lasting mitotic inhibition induced in the hepatocytes by the alkaloid (Downing & Peterson, 1968; Jago, 1969). There may also be focal hepatic necrosis and bile-duct proliferation, anaemia, bilirubinaemia, persistent hypoprothrombinaemia, gastro-intestinal haemorrhage, pulmonary, pancreatic, subcutaneous or generalized oedema, splenic enlargement and damaged kidneys, thymus and pancreas (Bull & Dick, 1959; Bull *et al.*, 1968; Schoental & Magee, 1957; 1959).

Sensitivity of rats to lasiocarpine is reduced by feeding a diet low in lipotropes or by simultaneous administration of mercaptoethylamine (Rogers & Newberne, 1971); it is increased by feeding a low-protein diet (Schoental & Magee, 1957) and by the inhibitors of the mixed-function oxidases (Tuchweber *et al.*, 1974).

Most of the toxic effects of hepatotoxic pyrrolizidine alkaloids appeared to be mediated *via* the very reactive dehydroalkaloid metabolites that are produced by the liver mixed-function oxidases. Although the toxicity of some alkaloids is related to the level of activity of this enzyme system, the relationship does not hold for lasiocarpine (Mattocks, 1972; Mattocks & White, 1971). Induction with phenobarbitone or pregnenolone-16-α-carbonitrile, while markedly increasing the rate of microsomal pyrrole production, protects against lasiocarpine toxicity in both male and female rats; whereas inhibition of this enzyme system with SKF-525A increases its toxicity (Jago, 1971; Tuchweber *et al.*, 1974).

Suckling rats showed toxic signs and died with severe liver lesions when their mothers were given total doses of about 125 mg/kg bw lasiocarpine (5-10 mg/dose orally or by i.p. injection) twice or more weekly. The mothers showed no outward ill-effects (Schoental, 1959).

When ^{14}C-lasiocarpine (randomly labelled, 44% in the amino-alcohol) was administered intraperitoneally to a rat (total dose, 5 mg), the distribution of label after 4 hours was as follows: carcass, 6.4%; intestines, 8.6%; testes, 0.1%; lung, 0.05%; kidney, 0.26%; heart, 0.05%; spleen, 0.01%; brain, 0.03%; urine, 27.2%; liver, 2.8%; expired carbon dioxide, 9.3%. Fractionation of the liver resulted in 1.73% in a trichloracetic acid extract, 0.6% in protein, 0.48% in lipids and 0.005% in the nucleic acids (Culvenor *et al.*, 1969).

The metabolism of lasiocarpine is similar to that of other hepatotoxic pyrrolizidine alkaloids described in more detail in the section "General Information and Conclusions on Pyrrolizidine Alkaloids", p. 336. Studies with lasiocarpine have confirmed the formation of pyrrolic metabolites by the mixed-function oxidase system of the microsomal fraction of rat liver (Jago *et al.*, 1970; Mattocks & White, 1971). Dehydroheliotridine has been isolated and identified as a product of microsomal oxidation of lasiocarpine (Jago *et al.*, 1970).

In a urine sample obtained 16 hours after injection of lasiocarpine to rats, Dann (1960) observed unchanged lasiocarpine (1-1.5% of dose), heliotridine (1.5-3%), heliotridine N-oxide (6%) and traces of bases with the chromatographic properties of europine and 7-angelylheliotridine (expected products of partial hydrolysis). Mattocks (1968) estimated that the metabolites in a 24-hour urine sample comprised 8.5% of the administered lasiocarpine.

A high dose of lasiocarpine causes a marked, though temporary, drop in the activity of the DNA-dependent RNA polymerase of rat liver nuclei (Frayssinet & Moulé, 1969; Reddy et al., 1968). However, the alkaloid does not inhibit the transcription of rat liver DNA by *Micrococcus lysodeikticus*-RNA polymerase, a system that is completely inhibited by actinomycin D. Synthesis of DNA in 24-hour regenerating liver is also inhibited to 70-92% by administration of lasiocarpine 1-3 hours before assay (Frayssinet & Moulé, 1969).

Doses of 0.08 µl of a 20 mM solution of lasiocarpine of unspecified purity in 0.7% sodium chloride were injected into the abdomen of 24-hour old Canton S *Drosophila melanogaster* males. Strong mutagenic effects on the induction of recessive sex-linked lethals were scored (Clark, 1960). Suppression mutations of several types have been induced in *Aspergillus nidulans* following treatment of conidia with 20 mM aqueous solutions of lasiocarpine of undefined purity (Alderson & Clark, 1966).

No data were available on the toxicity of pure lasiocarpine in humans. However, as lasiocarpine is the main toxic alkaloid of *Heliotropium lasiocarpum*, reports of toxicity in humans due to the consumption of bread made from wheat, barley or millet contaminated with the seeds of this plant are relevant. Epidemics in the USSR affected groups of agricultural workers and their families in specific regions; men, women and children were equally affected (Dubrovinskii, 1952).

Cardinal signs of heliotrope toxicosis were hepatomegaly, ascites and disturbances of hepatic function; hepatomegaly occurred in all cases, ascites in 85% and jaundice in 2-3%. Recovery was complete in 60% of cases; it was good with slight residual hepatomegaly in 35%; in 3% the hepatomegaly persisted; and recurrent ascites were seen in 2% (Munshkin,

1952). Braginsky & Bobokhodzhaev (1965) reported liver dysfunctions in patients 4 years after the onset of illness. Zheltova (1952) found that the majority of chronic cases had splenomegaly and that some developed cirrhosis.

3.3 Observations in man

No case reports of cancer or epidemiological studies were available to the Working Group.

4. Comments on Data Reported and Evaluation[1]

4.1 Animal data

Lasiocarpine is carcinogenic in rats following its intraperitoneal injection; it produced malignant tumours of the liver, skin and intestine. No other routes of administration or species have been adequately tested (see also the section "General Information and Conclusions on Pyrrolizidine Alkaloids", p. 333).

4.2 Human data

No case reports or epidemiological studies were available to the Working Group.

---

[1] See also the section "Animal Data in Relation to the Evaluation of Risk to Man" in the introduction to this volume, p. 15.

5. References

Alderson, T. & Clark, A.M. (1966) Interlocus specificity for chemical mutagens in *Aspergillus nidulans*. Nature (Lond.), 210, 593-595

Braginsky, B.M. & Bobokhodzhaev, I.Y. (1965) The clinical picture of hepatomegalia of heliotropic origin. Klin. Med. (Moscow), 43, 42

Bull, L.B. & Dick, A.T. (1959) The chronic pathological effects on liver of the rat of the pyrrolizidine alkaloids heliotrine, lasiocarpine and their N-oxides. J. Path. Bact., 78, 483-502

Bull, L.B., Dick, A.T. & McKenzie, J.S. (1958) The acute toxic effects of heliotrine and lasiocarpine and their N-oxides on the rat. J. Path. Bact., 75, 17-25

Bull, L.B., Culvenor, C.C.J. & Dick, A.T. (1968) The Pyrrolizidine Alkaloids, Amsterdam, North Holland, pp. 39, 142, 157-161, 253

Chalmers, A.H., Culvenor, C.C.J. & Smith, L.W. (1965) Characterisation of pyrrolizidine alkaloids by gas, thin-layer and paper chromatography. J. Chromat., 20, 270-277

Chen, K.K., Harris, P.N. & Schulze, H.A. (1940) The toxicity of lasiocarpine. J. Pharmacol. exp. Ther., 68, 123-129

Chopra, R.N., ed. (1933) Indigenous Drugs of India, Calcutta, The Art Press

Clark, A.M. (1960) The mutagenic activity of some pyrrolizidine alkaloids in *Drosophila*. Z. Vererbungsl., 91, 74-80

Culvenor, C.C.J. & Dal Bon, R. (1964) Carbonyl stretching frequencies of pyrrolizidine alkaloids. Austr. J. Chem., 17, 1296-1300

Culvenor, C.C.J., Drummond, L.J. & Price, J.R. (1954) The alkaloids of *Heliotropium europaeum* L. I. Heliotrine and lasiocarpine. Austr. J. Chem., 7, 277-286

Culvenor, C.C.J., Downing, D.T., Edgar, J.A. & Jago, M.V. (1969) Pyrrolizidine alkaloids as alkylating and antimitotic agents. Ann. N.Y. Acad. Sci., 163, 837-847

Culvenor, C.C.J., Johns, S.R. & Smith, L.W. (1976) Acetyllasiocarpine, an alkaloid from *Heliotropium europaeum*. Austr. J. Chem., 28, 2319-2322

Dann, A.T. (1960) Detection of N-oxides of the pyrrolizidine alkaloids. Nature (Lond.), 186, 1051

Downing, D.T. & Peterson, J.E. (1968) Quantitative assessment of the persistent antimitotic effect of certain hepatotoxic pyrrolizidine alkaloids on rat liver. Austr. J. exp. Biol. med. Sci., 46, 493-502

Dubrovinskii, J.B. (1952) The etiology of toxic hepatitis with ascites. In: Milenkov, S.M. & Kizhaikin, Y., eds, Symposium on Toxic Hepatitis with Ascites, Tashkent, V.M. Molotov Medical Institute, p. 74

Frayssinet, C. & Moulé, Y. (1969) Effect of lasiocarpine on transcription in liver cells. Nature (Lond.), 217, 659-661

Gunther, R.T. (1934) Greek Herbal of Dioscorides, Oxford, Oxford University Press

Jago, M.V. (1969) The development of the hepatic megalocytosis of chronic pyrrolizidine alkaloid poisoning. Amer. J. Path., 56, 405-421

Jago, M.V. (1971) Factors affecting the chronic hepatotoxicity of pyrrolizidine alkaloids. J. Path. Bact., 105, 1-11

Jago, M.V., Edgar, J.A., Smith, L.W. & Culvenor, C.C.J. (1970) Metabolic conversion of heliotridine-based pyrrolizidine alkaloids to dehydroheliotridine. Molec. Pharmacol., 6, 402-406

Khanin, M.N. (1956) The aetiology and pathogenesis of toxic hepatitis with ascites. Arkhiv Pathologii, 18, 35

Man'ko, I.V. & Vasil'kov, P.N. (1968) The alkaloids of *Lappula intermedia* I. Tr. Leningrad Khim-Farm.Inst., 26, 166-173

Man'ko, I.V., Korotkova, M.P. & Shevtsova, N.M. (1969) Alkaloids of some *Symphytum* species. Rast. Resur., 5, 508-512

Mattocks, A.R. (1968) Toxicity of pyrrolizidine alkaloids. Nature (Lond.), 217, 723-728

Mattocks, A.R. (1972) Acute hepatotoxicity and pyrrolic metabolites in rats dosed with pyrrolizidine alkaloids. Chem.-biol. Interact., 5, 227-242

Mattocks, A.R. & White, I.N.H. (1971) The conversion of pyrrolizidine alkaloids to N-oxides and to dihydropyrrolizidine derivatives by rat liver microsomes *in vitro*. Chem.-biol. Interact., 3, 383-396

Munshkin, A.S. (1952) The clinical aspects, pathogenesis and treatment of toxic hepatitis with ascites. In: Milenkov, S.M. & Kizhaikin, Y., eds, Symposium on Toxic Hepatitis with Ascites, Tashkent, V.M. Molotov Medical Institute, p. 83

Reddy, J.K. & Svoboda, D. (1972) Effect of lasiocarpine on aflatoxin B_1 carcinogenicity in rat liver. Arch. Path., 93, 55-60

Reddy, J., Harris, C. & Svoboda, D. (1968) Inhibition by lasiocarpine of RNA synthesis, RNA polymerase and induction of tryptophan pyrrolase activity. Nature (Lond.), 217, 659-661

Rogers, A.E. & Newberne, P.M. (1971) Lasiocarpine: factors influencing its toxicity and effects on liver cell division. Toxicol. appl. Pharmacol., 18, 356-366

Rose, C.L., Harris, P.N. & Chen, K.K. (1959) Some pharmacological actions of supinine and lasiocarpine. J. Pharmacol. exp. Ther., 126, 179-184

Schoental, R. (1959) Liver lesions in young rats suckled by mothers treated with the pyrrolizidine (Senecio) alkaloids, lasiocarpine and retrorsine. J. Path. Bact., 77, 485-495

Schoental, R. & Magee, P.N. (1957) Chronic liver changes in rats after a single dose of lasiocarpine, a pyrrolizidine (Senecio) alkaloid. J. Path. Bact., 74, 305-319

Schoental, R. & Magee, P.N. (1959) Further observations on the sub-acute and chronic liver changes in rats after a single dose of various pyrrolizidine (Senecio) alkaloids. J. Path. Bact., 78, 471-482

Svoboda, D.J. & Reddy, J.K. (1972) Malignant tumours in rats given lasiocarpine. Cancer Res., 32, 908-912

Tuchweber, B., Kovacs, K., Jago, M.V. & Beaulieu, T. (1974) Effect of steroidal and nonsteroidal microsomal enzyme inducers on the hepatotoxicity of pyrrolizidine alkaloids in rats. Res. Comm. chem. Path. Pharmacol., 7, 459-480

Zheltova, L.I. (1952) The clinical course of toxic hepatitis. In: Milenkov, S.M. & Kizhaikin, Y., eds, Symposium on Toxic Hepatitis with Ascites, Tashkent, V.M. Molotov Medical Institute, p. 79

MONOCROTALINE

1. Chemical and Physical Data

1.1 Synonyms and trade names

Chem. Abstr. Reg. Serial No.: 315-22-0

Chem. Abstr. Name: Monocrotaline

14,19-Dihydro-12,13-dihydroxy-(13α,14α)-20-norcrotalanan-11,15-dione; 12β,13β-dihydroxy-12α,13α,14α-trimethylcrotal-1-enine; NSC 28693*; stereoisomer of 4,5,8,10,12,13,13a,13b-octahydro-4,5-dihydroxy-3,4,5-trimethyl-2H-(1,6)dioxacycloundecino[2,3,4-gh]pyrrolizine-2,6(3H)-dione

1.2 Chemical formula and molecular weight

$C_{16}H_{23}NO_6$ Mol. wt: 325.3

1.3 Chemical and physical properties of the pure substance

(a) Description: Colourless prisms; bitter taste

(b) Melting-point: 202-203°C

(c) Optical rotation: $[\alpha]_D^{20}$ -15° (in ethanol)

(d) Spectroscopy data: Infra-red and nuclear magnetic resonance spectral data are given by Culvenor & Dal Bon (1964) and Bull et al. (1968).

(e) Identity and purity test: Melting-point and mixed melting-point; thin-layer and gas chromatographic comparison with authentic substance (Chalmers et al., 1965)

---

*Cancer Chemotherapy National Service Centre Number, NCI, NIH, USA

(f) *Solubility*: Slightly soluble in water (1.2%); sparingly soluble in non-polar organic solvents (0.09% in oleyl alcohol, 0.012% in dodecane); soluble in ethanol and chloroform; readily soluble in water as the hydrochloride (Bull *et al.*, 1968)

(g) *Volatility*: Very slight, but sufficient for gas chromatography and mass spectrometry

(h) *Stability*: Stable for long periods at room temperature in closed containers, but best stored under nitrogen at $-15^\circ C$

(i) *Reactivity*: Readily hydrolysed with alkali; reacts readily with oxidizing agents (slowly with atmospheric oxygen) to form dihydropyrrolizine and other derivatives

1.4 Technical products and impurities

No data were available to the Working Group.

2. Production, Use, Occurrence and Analysis

2.1 Production and use

Monocrotaline is produced for research purposes by one company in the US by extraction from the seeds of *Crotalaria spectabilis*. It has been used mostly in investigations of its toxicity and tumour-inhibiting properties.

The seeds of *C. retusa*, *C. sericea* and *C. spectabilis* contain high levels of monocrotaline and are good sources for isolation purposes.

C. retusa has been widely used as a dye plant and possibly as a vegetable in some parts of East Africa. In West Africa the root is crushed and mixed with spices as a colic remedy, and a decoction of the leaf, or sometimes the fresh juice of the plant, is taken for the relief of fever. In India, the root has been used as a remedy for haemoptysis, the leaf as a vegetable and a preparation of the plant as a local application in skin diseases (Dalziel, 1948; Watt & Breyer-Brandwijk, 1962).

C. recta is used against childhood malaria in Tanzania (Schoental & Coady, 1968).

2.2 Occurrence

Monocrotaline occurs in *Crotalaria* species (family Leguminosae) and has been isolated from *C. crispata* F. Muell. ex Benth., *C. grahamiana* R. Wight et Walk.-Arn., *C. mitchellii* Benth., *C. mysorensis* Roth, *C. novae-hollandiae* DC., *C. quinquefolia* L., *C. retusa* L., *C. sericea* Retz., *C. spectabilis* Roth (Atal *et al.*, 1969; Bull *et al.*, 1968; Sawhney & Atal, 1968), *C. lechnaultii* (Suri & Atal, 1967), *C. leioloba* Bartl. (*C. ferruginea* Wall.), *C. stipularia* Desv. (Puri *et al.*, 1974), *C. recta* Steud. ex A. Rich. (Crout, 1968) and *C. sagittalis* L. (Willette & Cammarato, 1972).

A major exposure of humans to monocrotaline and related alkaloids has occurred in the West Indies through the consumption of extracts of *Crotalaria* species as 'bush teas' (see also section 3.2). An educational campaign to stop consumption of *Crotalaria* 'teas', which began in 1959, has apparently been successful in reducing the incidence of veno-occlusive disease (Kay & Heath, 1969).

2.3 Analysis

No specific method of analysis has been reported for this compound. However, the analysis of plant material and animal tissues for monocrotaline may be carried out by the general methods developed for pyrrolizidine alkaloids (see section "General Information and Conclusions on Pyrrolizidine Alkaloids", p. 335).

3. Biological Data Relevant to the Evaluation of Carcinogenic Risk to Man

3.1 Carcinogenicity and related studies in animals

(a) <u>Oral administration</u>

<u>Rat</u>: A group of 50 male weanling Sprague-Dawley (CD) rats was given weekly doses of monocrotaline by gastric intubations, 25 mg/kg bw for 4 weeks then 8 mg/kg bw for 38 weeks. Of 42 rats surviving at the time of appearance of the first tumour (55 weeks) 10 developed liver-cell carcinomas; all survivors were killed after 72 weeks. Of a group of 50 rats fed a diet marginally deficient in lipotropes and given monocrotaline on the

same dosing schedule as above, 14/35 survivors at the time of the appearance of the first tumour (46 weeks) developed liver-cell carcinomas. Lung metastases occurred in both groups, but the numbers were not given. No liver tumours occurred in 45 controls surviving 40-72 weeks (Newberne & Rogers, 1973).

3.2 <u>Other relevant biological data</u>

The oral LD_{50} values for Swiss Webster mice are 166 mg/kg bw for males and 170 mg/kg bw for females (Goldenthal et al., 1964), while the i.v. LD_{50} for albino mice is 261 mg/kg bw (Harris et al., 1942). For rats, Rose et al. (1945) reported an i.v. LD_{50} value of 92 mg/kg bw, and Bull et al. (1968) gave i.p. values of 175 mg/kg bw for males and 189 mg/kg bw for females.

Monocrotaline has been shown to be toxic to rabbits (Gardiner et al., 1965) and monkeys (Allen & Carstens, 1971; Allen & Chesney, 1972). Guinea-pigs show no clinical or pathological effects when given a dose of monocrotaline about four times the LD_{50} for rats (240 mg/kg bw) (Chesney & Allen, 1973a).

It causes severe pulmonary, vascular, hepatic and renal lesions. Pulmonary oedema, hydrothorax and congestion and occlusion of the pulmonary blood vessels occur (Harris et al., 1942; Schoental & Head, 1955), resulting in pulmonary hypertension and cardiac hypertrophy (Allen & Chesney, 1972; Chesney & Allen, 1973b; Hayashi & Lalich, 1967). This is followed by intimal hyalinization and medial muscular hypertrophy of the pulmonary arteries and arterioles (Hayashi et al., 1967). Fractures of the endothelial linings of the larger pulmonary arteries predispose to the accumulation of blood components throughout the wall and to the development of fibrin thrombi within the lumen of the affected vessels. Enlarged alveolar epithelial cells also appear. The liver necrosis of the acute lesion, with congested and thrombosed vessels (Harris et al., 1942; Schoental & Head, 1955), progresses to a veno-occlusive lesion (Allen & Carstens, 1971) with increased portal pressure. There is a decrease in total serum proteins, a shift in the albumin:globulin ratio, an increase in prothrombin time and sometimes a rise in serum bilirubin. Megalocytic parenchymal cells may also develop (Allen & Chesney, 1972).

With monocrotaline poisoning, however, lung damage is sometimes more prominent than liver damage. Of 25 male Sprague-Dawley rats given s.c. injections of 60 mg/kg bw monocrotaline, all developed lung lesions, while only 1 showed haemorrhagic necrosis of the liver and 4, hepatic megalocytosis (Hayashi et al., 1967). S.c. administration of 30 mg/kg bw monocrotaline followed by 60 mg/kg bw during the 2nd, 4th and 6th month of the experiment to infant *Macaca arctoides* (stumptail) monkeys produced severe lung lesions and cardiac hypertrophy but little liver damage (Allen & Chesney, 1972). On the other hand, the same dosages of monocrotaline given to adolescent monkeys caused severe hepatic veno-occlusive lesions. Seven adult *Macaca speciosa* monkeys given 1 g monocrotaline (about 250 mg/kg bw) by gastric intubation on days 1 and 14 of the experiment also developed severe hepatic veno-occlusive lesions (Allen et al., 1967).

Some reports have recorded damage to kidneys and thymus. A single s.c. injection of 120 mg/kg bw monocrotaline to 22 Sprague-Dawley rats, 14 days of age, produced a renal haemosiderosis and glomerular necrosis with hyaline thrombosis in glomerular capillaries and afferent arterioles (Hayashi & Lalich, 1967). Of 13 albino mice given a single high dose (over 200 mg/kg bw) intravenously, 8 had necrosis of the thymic cortex (Harris et al., 1942). Protection against monocrotaline poisoning is given by co-administration of mercaptoethylamine or L-cysteine (Hayashi & Lalich, 1968).

A study of the distribution and excretion of monocrotaline and its metabolites in rats, using normal and tritiated alkaloid, has been reported briefly (Hayashi, 1966). After s.c. administration of monocrotaline, 50-70% of the dose was found in urine as unchanged monocrotaline (estimated by the methyl orange method). After administration of the tritiated alkaloid, about 30% of the radioactivity was detected in the bile as an unknown metabolite. Monocrotaline (or metabolite) concentrations were highest in the liver, kidney and stomach.

Studies with monocrotaline have confirmed the formation of pyrrolic metabolites by the mixed-function oxidase system of the microsomal fraction of rat liver (Mattocks & White, 1971). Dehydromonocrotaline (monocrotaline pyrrole) is highly cytotoxic, producing pulmonary, cardiac, vascular and hepatic lesions similar to those produced by the parent alkaloid (Butler *et al.*, 1970; Chesney *et al.*, 1974). It is a highly reactive alkylating agent which, on formation within the cell, reacts immediately with cell constituents to give soluble or bound secondary metabolites or hydrolyses to the dehydroaminoalcohol, dehydroretronecine (Culvenor *et al.*, 1970; Mattocks, 1973). It also combines with and cross-links DNA *in vitro* (White & Mattocks, 1972). On current evidence, the toxic reactions of the hepatotoxic pyrrolizidine alkaloids are mediated by the pyrrolic metabolites; this is discussed in more detail in the section "General Information and Conclusions on Pyrrolizidine Alkaloids", p. 333.

Dehydroretronecine has been isolated as a metabolite of monocrotaline in rat urine (Hsu *et al.*, 1973).

The toxicity of monocrotaline appears to be directly related to the level of activity of the hepatic mixed-function oxidases that convert it to dehydromonocrotaline. Thus, induction of these enzymes with phenobarbitone or pregnenolone-16α-carbonitrile increases toxicity, whereas inhibition by SKF-525A reduces it (Mattocks, 1972; Tuchweber *et al.*, 1974). Toxicity is also reduced by feeding a diet very low in protein (Ratnoff & Mirick, 1949) or one low in lipotropes (Newberne *et al.*, 1971) and by co-administration of chloramphenicol (Allen *et al.*, 1972), all of which may be related to decreased levels of activity of the hepatic mixed-function oxidases.

Following the administration of monocrotaline to rats, liver, lung and kidney tissues gave positive reactions with Ehrlich's reagent, suggesting binding of the pyrrolic metabolites to cellular constituents, in particular to proteins (Mattocks, 1972).

Monocrotaline of unspecified purity was dissolved in 0.7% sodium chloride at a concentration of 20 mM, and 0.08 µl were injected into the abdomen of 24-hour-old Canton S *Drosophila melanogaster* males. Strong effects on the induction of sex-linked recessive lethals were scored (Clark, 1960). The same results were obtained in Oregon K and Oregon R males (Cook & Holt, 1966).

There is no information available concerning the toxicity of pure monocrotaline in man. However, it is reasonably clear that the hepatic veno-occlusive disease of humans in the West Indies was due to consumption of extracts of *Crotalaria* species containing monocrotaline and related alkaloids

(Bras *et al.*, 1957; Fishman, 1974; Hill *et al.*, 1951; Kay & Heath, 1969; Stuart & Bras, 1957). Two of the species reported were *C. retusa* and *C. spectabilis*, which contain monocrotaline as the only alkaloid.

Although persons of all age groups were affected, the disease occurred mainly in children. The acute phase was characterized by abdominal discomfort, ascites and hepatomegaly, often accompanied by massive pleural effusion; the small hepatic veins became occluded, and there was severe centrilobular congestion and necrosis. In the subacute stage there was often symptomless hepatomegaly and centrilobular fibrosis; the chronic phase showed post-necrotic cirrhosis. Death often occurred after an oesophageal haemorrhage. Pancreatic changes similar to those in kwashiorkor were common (Bras & Hill, 1956; Stuart & Bras, 1957).

A recent report (Lyford & Moeller, 1974) documents the diagnosis of a case of human veno-occlusive disease in the United States in a 35-year old woman from Ecuador with a 6-month history of ingestion of *Crotalaria* extracts taken as medicinal remedies. Pertinent findings included hypoalbuminaemia, transudative ascitic fluid and an elevated portal vein pressure. Liver biopsy showed marked centrizonal congestion.

3.3 Observations in man

No case reports of cancer or epidemiological studies were available to the Working Group.

4. Comments on Data Reported and Evaluation[1]

4.1 Animal data

Monocrotaline is carcinogenic in rats following its oral administration, the only species and route of administration tested; it produced carcinomas of the liver (see also the section "General Information and Conclusions on Pyrrolizidine Alkaloids", p. 333).

---

[1]See also the section "Animal Data in Relation to the Evaluation of Risk to Man" in the introduction to this volume, p. 15.

4.2 Human data

No case reports or epidemiological studies were available to the Working Group.

5. References

Allen, J.R. & Carstens, L.A. (1971) Monocrotaline-induced Budd-Chiari syndrome in monkeys. Amer. J. dig. Dis., 16, 111-121

Allen, J.R. & Chesney, C.F. (1972) Effect of age on development of cor pulmonale in non-human primates following pyrrolizidine alkaloid intoxication. Exp. molec. Path, 17, 220-232

Allen, J.R., Carstens, L.A. & Olsen, B.E. (1967) Veno-occlusive disease in *Macaca speciosa* monkeys. Amer. J. Path., 50, 653-659

Allen, J.R., Chesney, C.F. & Frazee, W.J. (1972) Modifications of pyrrolizidine alkaloid intoxication resulting from altered hepatic microsomal enzymes. Toxicol. appl. Pharmacol., 23, 470-479

Atal, C.K., Culvenor, C.C.J., Sawhney, R.S. & Smith, C.W. (1969) The alkaloids of *Crotalaria grahamiana*. Grahamine, the 3'-[(-)-2-methylbutyryl] ester of monocrotaline. Austr. J. Chem., 72, 1773-1777

Bras, G. & Hill, K.R. (1956) Veno-occlusive disease of the liver. Essential pathology. Lancet, ii, 161-163

Bras, G., Berry, D.M. & György, P. (1957) Plants as aetiological factor in veno-occlusive disease of the liver. Lancet, i, 960-962

Bull, L.B., Culvenor, C.C.J. & Dick, A.T. (1968) The Pyrrolizidine Alkaloids, Amsterdam, North Holland, pp. 38, 46, 142, 254, 279

Butler, W.H., Mattocks, A.R. & Barnes, J.M. (1970) Lesions in the liver and lungs of rats given pyrrole derivatives of pyrrolizidine alkaloids. J. Path. Bact., 100, 169-175

Chalmers, A.H., Culvenor, C.C.J. & Smith, L.W. (1965) Characterisation of pyrrolizidine alkaloids by gas, thin-layer and paper chromatography. J. Chromat., 20, 270-277

Chesney, C.F. & Allen, J.R. (1973a) Resistance of the guinea pig to pyrrolizidine alkaloid intoxication. Toxicol. appl. Pharmacol., 26, 385-392

Chesney, C.F. & Allen, J.R. (1973b) Monocrotaline-induced pulmonary vascular lesions in non-human primates. Cardiovasc. Res., 7, 508-518

Chesney, C.F., Allen, J.R. & Hsu, I.C. (1974) Right ventricular hypertrophy in monocrotaline pyrrole treated rats. Exp. molec. Pharmacol., 20, 257-268

Clark, A.M. (1960) The mutagenic activity of some pyrrolizidine alkaloids in *Drosophila*. Z. Vererbungsl., 91, 74-80

Cook, L.M. & Holt, A.C.E. (1966) Mutagenic activity of two pyrrolizidine alkaloids. J. Genet., 59, 273-274

Crout, D.H.G. (1968) Pyrrolizidine alkaloids. The co-occurrence of monocrotaline and trichodesmine in *Crotalaria recta* Steud. A. Rich. Phytochem., 7, 1425-1427

Culvenor, C.C.J. & Dal Bon, R. (1964) Carbonyl stretching frequencies of pyrrolizidine alkaloids. Austr. J. Chem., 17, 1296-1300

Culvenor, C.C.J., Edgar, J.A., Smith, L.W. & Tweeddale, H.J. (1970) Dihydropyrrolizines. III. Preparation and reactions of derivatives related to pyrrolizidine alkaloids. Austr. J. Chem., 23, 1853-1867

Dalziel, J.M. (1948) Useful plants of West Tropical Africa. Appendix to: Hutchinson, J. & Dalziel, J.M., Flora of West Tropical Africa, London, Crown Agents for the Colonies, pp. 235-237

Fishman, A.P. (1974) Dietary pulmonary hypertension. Circulation Res., 36, 657-660

Gardiner, M.R., Royce, R. & Bokor, A. (1965) Studies on *Crotalaria crispata*, a newly recognized cause of Kimberley horse disease. J. Path. Bact., 89, 43-55

Goldenthal, E.I., D'Aguanno, W. & Lynch, J.F. (1964) Hormonal modification of the sex differences following monocrotaline administration. Toxicol. appl. Pharmacol., 6, 434-441

Harris, P.N., Anderson, R.C. & Chen, K.K. (1942) The action of monocrotaline and retronecine. J. Pharmacol. exp. Ther., 75, 78-82

Hayashi, Y. (1966) Excretion and alteration of monocrotaline in rats after a subcutaneous injection. Fed. Proc., 25, 688

Hayashi, Y. & Lalich, J.J. (1967) Renal and pulmonary alterations induced in rats by a single injection of monocrotaline. Proc. Soc. exp. Biol. (N.Y.), 124, 392-396

Hayashi, Y. & Lalich, J.J. (1968) Protective effect of mercaptoethylamine and cysteine against monocrotaline intoxication in rats. Toxicol. appl. Pharmacol., 12, 36-43

Hayashi, Y., Hussa, J.F. & Lalich, J.J. (1967) Cor pulmonale in rats. Lab. Invest., 16, 875-881

Hill, K.R., Rhodes, K., Stafford, J.L. & Aub, R. (1951) Liver disease in Jamaican children. W. Ind. med. J., 1, 49-63

Hsu, I.C., Allen, J.R. & Chesney, C.F. (1973) Identification and toxicological effects of dehydroretronecine, a metabolite of monocrotaline. Proc. Soc. exp. Biol. (N.Y.), 144, 834-838

Kay, J.M. & Heath, D. (1969) *Crotalaria spectabilis*, Springfield, Thomas

Lyford, C.L. & Moeller, D.D. (1974) *Crotalaria*-induced hepatic veno-occlusive disease (VOD) diagnosed in the United States. Gastroenterology, 66, 734

Mattocks, A.R. (1972) Acute hepatotoxicity and pyrrolic metabolites in rats dosed with pyrrolizidine alkaloids. Chem.-biol. Interact., 5, 227-242

Mattocks, A.R. (1973) Mechanisms of pyrrolizidine alkaloid toxicity. In: Loomis, T.A., ed., Pharmacology and the Future of Man, Proceedings of 5th International Congress on Pharmacology, San Francisco, 1972, Vol. 2, Toxicological Problems, White Plains, NY, Phiebig, p. 114

Mattocks, A.R. & White, I.N.H. (1971) The conversion of pyrrolizidine alkaloids to N-oxides and to dihydropyrrolizine derivatives by rat liver microsomes *in vitro*. Chem.-biol. Interact., 3, 383-396

Newberne, P.N. & Rogers, A.E. (1973) Nutrition, monocrotaline and aflatoxin B_1 in liver carcinogenesis. In: Newman, P.N., ed., Plant Foods for Man, pp. 23-31

Newberne, P.N., Wilson, R. & Rogers, A.E. (1971) Effects of a low-lipotrope diet on the response of young male rats to the pyrrolizidine alkaloid monocrotaline. Toxicol. appl. Pharmacol., 18, 387-397

Puri, S.C., Sawhney, R.S. & Atal, C.K. (1974) Genus *Crotalaria*. XVI. Pyrrolizidine alkaloids of *C. leioloba* Bartl., *C. stipularia* Desv. and *C. tetragona* Roxb. J. Ind. chem. Soc., 51, 628-629

Ratnoff, O.D. & Mirick, G.S. (1949) Influence of sex upon the lethal effects of an hepatotoxic alkaloid, monocrotaline. Bull. Johns Hopkins Hospital, 84, 507-525

Rose, C.L., Fink, R.D., Harris, P.N. & Chen, K.K. (1945) The effect of hepatotoxic alkaloids on the prothrombin time of rats. J. Pharmacol. exp. Ther., 83, 265-269

Sawhney, R.S. & Atal, C.K. (1968) Phytochemical studies on the genus *Crotalaria*. VIII. Chemical constituents of *Crotalaria mysorensis*. J. Ind. chem. Soc., 45, 1052-1053

Schoental, R. & Coady, A. (1968) The hepatotoxicity of some Ethiopian and East African plants, including some used in traditional medicines. E. Afr. med. J., 45, 577-580

Schoental, R. & Head, M.A. (1955) Pathological changes in rats as a result of treatment with monocrotaline. Brit. J. Cancer, 9, 229-237

Stuart, K.L. & Bras, G. (1957) Veno-occlusive disease of the liver. Q. J. Med., 26, 291-315

Suri, O.P. & Atal, C.K. (1967) Isolation of monocrotaline and crispatine from *Crotalaria lechnaultii*. Current Sci. (India), 36, 614-615

Tuchweber, B., Kovacs, K., Jago, M.V. & Beaulieu, T. (1974) Effect of steroidal and nonsteroidal microsomal enzyme inducers on the hepatotoxicity of pyrrolizidine alkaloids in rats. Res. Comm. chem. Path. Pharmacol., 7, 459-480

Watt, J.M. & Breyer-Brandwijk, M.G., eds (1962) The Medicinal and Poisonous Plants of Southern and Eastern Africa, 2nd ed., Edinburgh, London, E. & S. Livingstone, p. 284

White, I.N.H. & Mattocks, A.R. (1972) Reaction of dihydropyrrolizines with deoxyribonucleic acids *in vitro*. Biochem. J., 128, 291-297

Willette, R.E. & Cammarato, L.V. (1972) Phytochemical survey of Connecticut. I. Isolation of monocrotaline from *Crotalaria sagittalis* L. fruit. J. pharm. Sci., 61, 122

RETRORSINE

1. Chemical and Physical Data

1.1 Synonyms and trade names

Chem. Abstr. Reg. Serial No.: 480-54-6

Chem. Abstr. Name: 12,18-Dihydroxysenecionan-11,16-dione

3-Ethylidene-3,4,5,6,9,11,13,14,14α,14β-decahydro-6-hydroxy-6-hydroxymethyl-5-methyl(1,6)dioxacyclododeca[2,3,4-gh]pyrrolizidine-2,7-dione; $trans$-15-ethylidene-12β-hydroxy-12α-hydroxymethyl-13β-methylsenec-1-enine; β-longilobine

1.2 Chemical formula and molecular weight

$C_{18}H_{25}NO_6$ Mol. wt: 351.4

1.3 Chemical and physical properties of the pure substance

(a) Description: Colourless prisms

(b) Melting-point: 219-220°C ($in\ vacuo$); 216°C (at 760 mm Hg)

(c) Optical rotation: $[\alpha]_D^{20}$ -61.4° (in chloroform)

(d) Spectroscopy data: λ_{max} 217 nm; E_1^1 = 201 (in water) (Bull et al., 1968); infra-red and nuclear magnetic resonance spectral data are given by Culvenor & Smith (1955)

(e) Identity and purity test: Melting-point and mixed melting-point; thin-layer and gas chromatographic comparison with authentic substance (Chalmers et al., 1965)

(f) <u>Soluble</u>: Soluble in chloroform; slightly soluble in acetone, ethanol and water

(g) <u>Volatility</u>: Low, but sufficient for gas chromatography and mass spectrometry

(h) <u>Stability</u>: Stable at room temperature in closed containers; for long periods the substance is best stored under nitrogen at $-15^\circ C$

(i) <u>Reactivity</u>: Readily hydrolysed with alkali; reacts with oxidizing agents (slowly with atmospheric oxygen) to form dihydropyrrolizine and other derivatives

1.4 Technical products and impurities

No data were available to the Working Group.

2. Production, Use, Occurrence and Analysis

2.1 Production and use

Retrorsine is not produced commercially. Some of the *Senecio* species in which it occurs have been used as medicinal herbs; e.g., *S. discolor* (S.W.)DC. was used against coughs, colds, fevers and indigestion in Jamaica (Asprey & Thornton, 1955); *S. bupleuroids* DC. was reported to be an ingredient in an African remedy for chest troubles; and *S. vulgaris* was used in Europe for dysmenorrhea and amenorrhea and in the US as a diaphoretic, diuretic, tonic and emmenagogue (Watt & Breyer-Brandwijk, 1962). *S. isatideus* is a high-yielding source suitable for preparative purposes (Koekemoer & Warren, 1951).

2.2 Occurrence

Retrorsine is a common constituent of *Senecio* species (family Compositae) and has been isolated from *S. ambrosioides*, *S. ampullaceus* Hook., *S. bupleuroides* DC., *S. discolor* DC., *S. douglasii* DC., *S. eremophilus* Richards, *S. glaberrimus* DC., *S. graminifolius* N.J. Jacq., *S. ilicifolius* Thunb., *S. isatideus* DC., *S. longilobus* Benth., *S. paucicalyculatus* Klatt, *S. pterophorus* DC., *S. quadridentatus* Labill., *S. retrorsus* DC., *S. riddellii* Torr. et A. Gray var. *parksii* (Cory), *S. ruderalis* Harvey, *S. sceleratus* Schweickerd

S. venosus Harvey, *S. vulgaris* L. (Bull *et al.*, 1968), *S. bipinnatisectus* Belcher (White, 1969), *S. brasiliensis* Less. (Montedome & Ferreira, 1966a), *S. grisebachii* (Montedome & Ferreira, 1966b) and *S. swaziensis* Compton (Gordon-Gray & Wells, 1972). Retrorsine has also been isolated from *Crotalaria usaramoensis* E.G. Baker and *C. spartioides* DC. (family Leguminosae) (Bull *et al.*, 1968).

Senecio ilicifolius and other *Senecio* species grow in cornfields in the S.W. Cape District of South Africa, and seed and plant fragments sometimes contaminate the corn and cause 'bread poisoning' in humans (de Waal, 1940). Retrorsine is one of the main alkaloids in *S. ilicifolius* (de Waal, 1941), but other alkaloids are also partly responsible for 'bread poisoning'.

2.3 Analysis

The analysis of plant material and animal tissues for retrorsine may be carried out by general methods developed for pyrrolizidine alkaloids (see the section "General Information and Conclusions on Pyrrolizidine Alkaloids, p. 335).

3. Biological Data Relevant to the Evaluation of Carcinogenic Risk to Man

3.1 Carcinogenicity and related studies in animals

Oral administration

Rat: Ten male and 4 female albino Wistar rats weighing 55-150 g were given retrorsine in drinking-water at a concentration of 0.03 mg/ml on 3 days per week until death at 10-24 months. Six male rats showed nodular hyperplasia, and in 4 of these the nodules were confirmed as hepatomas. The liver of one male rat showed a haemorrhagic tumour. One female rat killed at 23 months showed regenerative liver changes and a papillary adenoma in the lung (Schoental *et al.*, 1954).

In an attempt to ascertain whether the chronic liver lesions produced in rats by retrorsine could develop into liver tumours with a suitable stimulus, weanling Porton Wistar rats were given single doses of 30 mg/kg bw retrorsine by stomach tube (a) with no other treatment, in 95 rats;

(b) with whole body irradiation of 400 rads 100 days after dosing, in 31 rats; and (c) 9 days after partial hepatectomy, in 10 rats. Animals surviving 12 months or more developed the following tumours: Group (a): in the 29 survivors there were 5 hepatomas and 1 case each of mammary tumour, carcinoma of the lung, haemangioendothelioma of the spleen, carcinoma of the uterus, retroperitoneal sarcoma and squamous-cell carcinoma of the jaw; Group (b): in 25 survivors there were 5 hepatomas, 5 mammary tumours, 2 renal carcinomas and 1 case each of carcinoma of the liver with pulmonary metastases, carcinoma of the lung, carcinoma of the colon, haemangioendothelioma of the spleen, osteosarcoma of the humerus, leukaemia and spindle-cell tumour of the neck; Group (c): in the 9 survivors there were 2 hepatomas and a squamous-cell carcinoma of the jaw. There was no clear evidence for synergistic effects of the two treatments, since 2 cases of leukaemia, 1 osteosarcoma and 1 renal adenoma occurred in 6 rats given X-irradiation alone (Schoental & Bensted, 1963).

3.2 Other relevant biological data

Four or 7-day LD_{50} values for retrorsine in various species have been determined as follows (mg/kg bw): mice, 58.8 i.v. (Anon., 1949), 65 for males i.p. and 69 for females i.p. (White *et al.*, 1973); rats, 34 for males i.p. and 153 for females i.p. (Mattocks, 1972); hamsters, 81 for males i.p.; guinea-pigs, >800 for males i.p.; fowl, 85 for males i.p.; quail, 279 for males i.p. (White *et al.*, 1973); monkeys, 46 by gastric intubation (10-day LD_{50}) (van der Watt & Purchase, 1970).

The primary toxic effect of retrorsine was reported to be on liver parenchyma and on the central and hepatic veins, with the production of centrilobular haemorrhagic necrosis. This was followed by an apparent proliferation of the endothelium of the central and sublobular veins, leading to partial or complete occlusion of the lumen (Selzer *et al.*, 1951). Enlargement of surviving hepatocytes sometimes occurred. There was also loss of weight, ascites, congestion of the spleen and haemorrhage of the gastrointestinal tract. In some instances there was pleural effusion and pulmonary veno-occlusion (Davidson, 1935; Schoental *et al.*, 1954; White *et al.*, 1973).

Suckling rats died with severe liver and other typical pyrrolizidine-induced lesions when their mothers were given 20-84 mg/animal retrorsine in doses of 5-10 mg orally or i.p. twice weekly or more often. The mothers survived, although liver lesions developed (Schoental, 1959).

The liver lesions produced in vervet monkeys by gastric intubation of retrorsine were comparable to those observed in rats: mainly central and hepatocellular midzonal necrosis and haemorrhage from the central vein. One monkey surviving the dose of 46 mg/kg bw developed isolated giant cells (van der Watt & Purchase, 1970). Monkeys dosed intragastrically with 20 mg/kg bw retrorsine once weekly for 30 weeks and once every two weeks thereafter, survived 20-72 weeks; death was preceded by dullness, incoordination and hepatic coma. The livers became atrophic and megalocytic, necrosis being observed occasionally and in single cells. Focal regeneration appeared after one year. Megalocytosis in the renal tubules and veno-occlusion in the liver were observed, but lung lesions were minimal (van der Watt et al., 1972).

The metabolism of retrorsine is similar to that of other hepatotoxic pyrrolizidine alkaloids and is described in more detail in the section "General Information and Conclusions on Pyrrolizidine Alkaloids", p. 336.

Studies with retrorsine have confirmed the formation of the N-oxide and pyrrolic metabolites by the mixed-function oxidase system of the microsomal fraction of rat liver (Mattocks & White, 1971).

Butler et al. (1970) demonstrated that injection of dehydroretrorsine (retrorsine pyrrole) into the tail vein of rats produced lung lesions typical of pyrrolizidine alkaloid poisoning, while administration via the mesenteric vein produced the characteristic liver lesion. Dehydroretrorsine, like other dehydroalkaloids, is a highly reactive alkylating agent, reacting immediately after formation with cell constituents to give soluble or bound secondary metabolites or hydrolysing to the dehydroaminoalcohol (Culvenor et al., 1970; Mattocks, 1969).

Administration of 40 mg/kg bw retrorsine by stomach tube to rats caused a severe and rapid inhibition of the synthesis of liver and serum proteins (Villa-Trevino & Leaver, 1968).

Although most of the toxic effects of retrorsine appear to be mediated via the very reactive metabolite dehydroretrorsine (retrorsine pyrrole), which is produced in the liver by the mixed-function oxidases, the toxicity of this alkaloid does not always relate directly to the activity of the enzymes. Pre-treatment with phenobarbitone (PB), which increases the rate of *in vitro* microsomal production of pyrroles from retrorsine three-fold and that of N-oxides two-fold, protected male rats against retrorsine poisoning (i.p. LD_{50}'s, 34 mg/kg bw alone, 67 mg/kg bw with PB) but increased its toxicity in female rats (i.p. LD_{50}'s, 153 mg/kg bw alone, 87 mg/kg bw with PB). However, there were delayed toxic effects, including congestion and oedema of the lungs, which are rarely seen after retrorsine (Mattocks, 1972; Mattocks & White, 1971). Similar increases in the rate of pyrrole production and N-oxidation were observed with retrorsine for the liver microsomal enzymes of mice and guinea-pigs after pre-treatment with PB. This resulted in a decrease in toxicity in both male and female mice but in an increase in toxicity in guinea-pigs (White *et al.*, 1973).

In male rats, protection against acute deaths was given when mixed-function oxidases were inhibited by SKF-525A (i.p. LD_{50}, 53 mg/kg bw) and by a 4-day sucrose diet (i.p. LD_{50}, 120 mg/kg bw), but chronic hepatic and pulmonary lesions developed subsequently (Mattocks, 1972; Mattocks & White, 1971).

Retrorsine is one of the main alkaloids present in the *Senecio* species which have contaminated grain and so caused the often fatal 'bread poisoning' of humans in South Africa (Selzer & Parker, 1951; de Waal, 1940; 1941). The most common symptoms were severe abdominal pain, rapidly developing ascites and hepatomegaly. In some outbreaks there were extreme emaciation, nausea and diarrhoea. At necropsy, the liver was found to be congested, with an occlusive lesion in the central and sub-lobular hepatic veins and with blood pools replacing large areas of centrilobular parenchymal tissue; there was often marked oedema of the large intestine. Males and females were affected with equal frequency. Over 80 cases of *Senecio* poisoning, mainly in the young and mostly fatal, occurred in the George and Mossel Bay districts around 1910-1920 (Willmott & Robertson, 1920); 12 cases were hospitalized in one area in 1931-1941 (Sapeika, 1952; Selzer & Parker, 1951).

3.3 Observations in man

No case reports of cancer or epidemiological studies were available to the Working Group.

4. Comments on Data Reported and Evaluation[1]

4.1 Animal data

Retrorsine is carcinogenic in rats following its oral administration; it produced a variety of tumours. No other species or routes of administration were adequately tested (see also the section "General Information and Conclusions on Pyrrolizidine Alkaloids", p. 333).

4.2 Human data

No case reports or epidemiological studies were available to the Working Group.

---

[1] See also the section "Animal Data in Relation to the Evaluation of Risk to Man" in the introduction to this volume, p. 15.

5. References

Anon. (1949) *Senecio* and related alkaloids. Research Today, 5, 55

Asprey, G.F. & Thornton, P. (1955) Medicinal plants of Jamaica. IV. W. Ind. med. J., 4, 145-168

Bull, L.B., Culvenor, C.C.J. & Dick, A.T. (1968) The Pyrrolizidine Alkaloids, Amsterdam, North Holland, pp. 37, 255-256, 280

Butler, W.H., Mattocks, A.R. & Barnes, J.M. (1970) Lesions in the liver and lungs of rats given pyrrole derivatives of pyrrolizidine alkaloids. J. Path., 100, 169-175

Chalmers, A.H., Culvenor, C.C.J. & Smith, L.W. (1965) Characterisation of pyrrolizidine alkaloids by gas, thin-layer and paper chromatography. J. Chromat., 20, 270-277

Culvenor, C.C.J. & Smith, L.W. (1955) The alkaloids of *Erectites quadridentata* DC. Austr. J. Chem., 8, 556-561

Culvenor, C.C.J., Edgar, J.A., Smith, L.W. & Tweeddale, H.J. (1970) Dihydropyrrolizines. III. Preparation and reactions of derivatives related to pyrrolizidine alkaloids. Austr. J. Chem., 23, 1853-1867

Davidson, J. (1935) The action of retrorsine on rat's liver. J. Path., 40, 285-295

Gordon-Gray, C.G. & Wells, R.B. (1972) Swazine, a new alkaloid from *S. swaziensis*. Chemical and X-ray crystal study of a novel spiro dilactone. Tetrahedron Lett., 707-710

Koekemoer, M.J. & Warren, F.L. (1951) The *Senecio* alkaloids. VIII. The occurrence and preparation of the *N*-oxides. An improved method of extraction of the *Senecio* alkaloids. J. chem. Soc., 66-68

Mattocks, A.R. (1969) Dihydropyrrolizine derivatives from unsaturated pyrrolizidine alkaloids. J. chem. Soc., C, 1155-1162

Mattocks, A.R. (1972) Acute hepatotoxicity and pyrrolic metabolites in rats dosed with pyrrolizidine alkaloids. Chem.-biol. Interact., 5, 227-242

Mattocks, A.R. & White, I.N.H. (1971) The conversion of pyrrolizidine alkaloids to *N*-oxides and to dihydropyrrolizine derivatives by rat liver microsomes *in vitro*. Chem.-biol. Interact., 3, 383-396

Montedome, M. & Ferreira, P.C. (1966a) Alkaloids from *Senecio brasiliensis* Less. Rev. Fac. Farm. Bioquím. Univ. Sao Paulo, 4, 13-44

Montedome, M. & Ferreira, P.C. (1966b) Alkaloids from the genus *Senecio*. Rev. Fac. Farm. Bioquím. Univ. Sao Paulo, 4, 175-179

Sapieka, N. (1952) The *Senecio* alkaloids. S. Afr. med. J., 26, 485-488

Schoental, R. (1959) Liver lesions in young rats suckled by mothers treated with the pyrrolizidine (*Senecio*) alkaloids, lasiocarpine and retrorsine. J. Path. Bact., 77, 485-495

Schoental, R. & Bensted, J.P.M. (1963) Effects of whole body irradiation and of partial hepatectomy on the liver lesions induced in rats by a single dose of retrorsine, a pyrrolizidine (*Senecio*) alkaloid. Brit. J. Cancer, 17, 242-251

Schoental, R., Head, M.A. & Peacock, P.R. (1954) *Senecio* alkaloids: primary liver tumours in rats as a result of treatment with (i) a mixture of alkaloids from *S. jacobaea* Linn., (ii) retrorsine, (iii) isatidine. Brit. J. Cancer, 8, 458-465

Selzer, G. & Parker, R.G.F. (1951) *Senecio* poisoning exhibiting as Chiari's syndrome. Amer. J. Path., 27, 885-907

Selzer, G., Parker, R.G.F. & Sapeika, N. (1951) An experimental study of *Senecio* poisoning in rats. Brit. J. exp. Path., 32, 14-20

Villa-Trevino, S. & Leaver, D.D. (1968) Effects of the hepatotoxic agents retrorsine and aflatoxin B_1 on hepatic protein synthesis in the rat. Biochem. J., 109, 87-91

de Waal, H.L. (1940) *Senecio* alkaloids. III. Chemical investigations upon the *Senecio* species responsible for 'bread-poisoning'. The isolation of senecionine from *Senecio ilicifolius* Thunb. and a new alkaloid, 'rosmarinine', from *Senecio rosmarinifolius* Linn. Onderstepoort J. vet. Sci. animal Ind., 15, 241

de Waal, H.L. (1941) South African *Senecio* alkaloids. V. Notes on isatidine, rosmarinine and pterophine, and on the structure of their necines and necic acids. Onderstepoort J. vet. Sci. animal Ind., 16, 149

van der Watt, J.J. & Purchase, I.F.H. (1970) The acute toxicity of retrorsine, aflatoxin and sterigmatocystin in vervet monkeys. Brit. J. exp. Path., 51, 183-190

van der Watt, J.J., Purchase, I.F.H. & Tustin, R.C. (1972) The chronic toxicity of retrorsine, a pyrrolizidine alkaloid, in vervet monkeys. J. Path., 107, 279-287

Watt, J.M. & Breyer-Brandwijk, M.G., eds (1962) The Medicinal and Poisonous Plants of Southern and Eastern Africa, 2nd ed., Edinburgh, London, E. & S. Livingstone, p. 284

White, E.P. (1969) Alkaloids of some herbaceous *Senecio* species in New Zealand. N.Z. J. Sci., 12, 165-170

White, I.N.H., Mattocks, A.R. & Butler, W.H. (1973) The conversion of the pyrrolizidine alkaloid retrorsine to pyrrolic derivatives *in vivo* and *in vitro* and its acute toxicity to various animal species. Chem.-biol. Interact., 6, 207-218

Willmott, F.C. & Robertson, G.W. (1920) *Senecio* disease or cirrhosis of the liver due to *Senecio* poisoning. Lancet, ii, 848-849

RIDDELLIINE

1. Chemical and Physical Data

1.1 Synonyms and trade names

Chem. Abstr. Reg. Serial No.: 23246-96-0

Chem. Abstr. Name: 13,19-Didehydro-12,18-dihydroxysenecionan-11,16-dione

trans-15-Ethylidene-12β-hydroxy-12α-hydroxymethyl-13-methylenesenec-1-enine; stereoisomer of 3-ethylidene-3,4,5,6,9,11,13,14,14α,14β-decahydro-6-hydroxy-6-(hydroxymethyl)-5-methylene(1,6)dioxacyclodo-decino[2,3,4-*gh*]-pyrrolizidine-2,7-dione; riddelline

1.2 Chemical formula and molecular weight

$C_{18}H_{23}NO_6$ Mol. wt: 349.4

1.3 Chemical and physical properties of the pure substance

(a) Description: Colourless prisms

(b) Melting-point: 198°C

(c) Optical rotation: $[\alpha]_D^{25}$ -109.5° (in chloroform) (Bull *et al.*, 1968)

(d) Spectroscopy data: For infra-red spectral data see Culvenor & Dal Bon (1964)

(e) Identity and purity test: Melting-point and mixed melting-point; thin-layer and gas chromatographic comparison with authentic material (Chalmers *et al.*, 1965)

(f) <u>Solubility</u>: Soluble in chloroform; slightly soluble in acetone, ethanol and water; soluble in water as the hydrochloride

(g) <u>Volatility</u>: Low, but sufficient for gas chromatography and mass spectrometry

(h) <u>Stability</u>: Stable at room temperature in closed containers; for long periods it is best stored under nitrogen at $-15°C$.

(i) <u>Reactivity</u>: Readily hydrolysed in aqueous alkali; reacts readily with oxidizing agents (slowly with atmospheric oxygen) to form dihydropyrrolizine and other derivatives

1.4 Technical products and impurities

No data were available to the Working Group.

2. Production, Use, Occurrence and Analysis

2.1 Production and use

Riddelliine is not produced commercially. *Crotalaria juncea*, in which it occurs, is cultivated in India and East Africa for its fibre. In East India the root of *C. juncea* is taken as a haemoptysis remedy; the leaf and seeds have been used as food (Watt & Breyer-Brandwijk, 1962). In India, *C. juncea* has been used against impetigo, psoriasis and as an emmenagogue (Chopra, 1933).

2.2 Occurrence

Riddelliine has been isolated from *Crotalaria juncea* L. (family Leguminosae) and from several *Senecio* species (family Compositae), including *S. douglassii* DC., *S. eremophilus* Richards, *S. longilobus* Benth., *S. riddellii* Torr. et A. Gray and *S. riddellii* Torr. et A. Gray var. *parksii* (Cory) (Bull *et al.*, 1968).

2.3 Analysis

The analysis of plant material and animal tissues for riddelliine may be carried out by general methods developed for pyrrolizidine alkaloids (see the section "General Information and Conclusions on Pyrrolizidine Alkaloids", p. 335).

3. Biological Data Relevant to the Evaluation of Carcinogenic Risk to Man

3.1 Carcinogenicity and related studies in animals

Oral and intraperitoneal administration

Rat: Fourteen female and 6 male Wistar rats were given drinking-water containing 0.02 mg/ml riddelliine twice weekly for 6 months. Five of the females and the 5 surviving males were given 3 i.p. injections of 25 mg/kg bw riddelliine during the 7th month. The remaining 9 females continued to receive solutions of the alkaloid, presumably in the drinking-water. One year after the beginning of treatment all surviving rats, 12 females and 4 males, received an i.p. injection of 30 mg/kg bw riddelliine and were left without further treatment until death. The 4 males that survived the full course of treatment died or were killed 6-16 months after the last injection. Liver nodules were observed in all 4; one of these showed a trabecular arrangement; one liver had bile-duct proliferation. Nodules were seen in the livers of 5 of the females, and in 1 there was a sarcoma of the liver arising from the wall of a tapeworm cyst. No nodules or tumours were observed in the livers of 8 male and 7 female controls which survived 18-33 months (Schoental & Head, 1957).

3.2 Other relevant biological data

The i.v. LD_{50} of riddelliine in mice is 105 mg/kg bw (Anon., 1949). The course of development of chronic liver lesions in rats given single doses of riddelliine was essentially the same as that in rats given lasiocarpine, retrorsine or seneciphylline; the characteristic feature is megalocytosis (Schoental & Magee, 1959). Nodular hyperplasia, fibrosis and bile-duct proliferation were also observed.

The metabolism of riddelliine is expected to be similar to that of other hepatotoxic pyrrolizidine alkaloids as described in the section "General Information and Conclusions on Pyrrolizidine Alkaloids", p. 336.

3.3 Observations in man

No data were available to the Working Group.

4. Comments on Data Reported and Evaluation

4.1 Animal data

The available information is insufficient to evalute the carcinogenicity of riddelliine. However, see also the section "General Information and Conclusions on Pyrrolizidine Alkaloids", p. 333.

4.2 Human data

No case reports or epidemiological studies were available to the Working Group.

5. References

Anon. (1949) *Senecio* and related alkaloids. Research Today, 5, 55

Bull, L.B., Culvenor, C.C.J. & Dick, A.T. (1968) The Pyrrolizidine Alkaloids, Amsterdam, North Holland, pp. 256, 280

Chalmers, A.H., Culvenor, C.C.J. & Smith, L.W. (1965) Characterisation of pyrrolizidine alkaloids by gas, thin-layer and paper chromatography. J. Chromat., 20, 270-277

Chopra, R.N., ed. (1933) Indigenous Drugs of India, Calcutta, The Art Press

Culvenor, C.C.J. & Dal Bon, R. (1964) Carbonyl stretching frequencies of pyrrolizidine alkaloids. Austr. J. Chem., 17, 1296-1300

Schoental, R. & Head, M.A. (1957) Progression of liver lesions produced in rats by temporary treatment with pyrrolizidine (*Senecio*) alkaloids and the effects of betaine and high casein diet. Brit. J. Cancer, 11, 535-544

Schoental, R. & Magee, P.N. (1959) Evolution of liver lesions in the rat after a single dose of pyrrolizidine alkaloids. Acta un. int. cancr., 15, 212-215

Watt, J.M. & Breyer-Brandwijk, M.G., eds (1962) The Medicinal and Poisonous Plants of Southern and Eastern Africa, 2nd ed., Edinburgh, London, E. & S. Livingstone, p. 284

SENECIPHYLLINE

1. Chemical and Physical Data

1.1 Synonyms and trade names

Chem. Abstr. Reg. Serial No.: 480-81-9

Chem. Abstr. Name: 13,19-Didehydro-12-hydroxysenecionan-11,16-dione

trans-15-Ethylidene-12β-hydroxy-12α-methyl-13-methylenesenec-1-enine; jacodine; NSC 30622*

1.2 Chemical formula and molecular weight

$C_{18}H_{23}NO_5$ Mol. wt: 333.4

1.3 Chemical and physical properties of the pure substance

(a) Description: Colourless prisms

(b) Melting-point: 217°C

(c) Optical rotation: $[\alpha]_D^{26}$ -139° (in chloroform) (Bull et al., 1968)

(d) Spectroscopy data: λ_{max} 281 nm; E_1^1 = 238 (in methanol) (Bull et al., 1968); for infra-red and nuclear magnetic resonance spectral data see Culvenor & Dal Bon (1964) and Bull et al. (1968)

---

*Cancer Chemotherapy National Service Centre Number, NCI, NIH, USA

(e) <u>Identity and purity test</u>: Melting-point and mixed melting-point; thin-layer and gas chromatographic comparison with the authentic substance (Chalmers *et al.*, 1965)

(f) <u>Solubility</u>: Soluble in chloroform; sparingly soluble in ethanol and acetone; slightly soluble in water. The hydrochloride is soluble in water.

(g) <u>Volatility</u>: Low, but sufficient for gas chromatography and mass spectrometry

(h) <u>Stability</u>: Stable at room temperature in closed containers; for long periods it is best stored under nitrogen at -15°C.

(i) <u>Reactivity</u>: Readily hydrolysed with alkali; reacts readily with oxidizing agents (slowly with atmospheric oxygen) to form dihydropyrrolizine and other derivatives

1.4 Technical products and impurities

No data were available to the Working Group.

2. Production, Use, Occurrence and Analysis

2.1 Production and use

Seneciphylline is not produced commercially. *Crotalaria juncea*, from which it has been isolated, is cultivated in India and East Africa for its fibre. In East Africa the root of *C. juncea* has been reported to be used as a haemoptysis remedy, and the leaf and seeds may be used as food (Watt & Breyer-Brandwijk, 1962). In India *C. juncea* was used against impetigo, psoriasis and as an emmenogogue (Chopra, 1933).

Seneciphylline is a minor constituent of *S. jacobaea*, which has been used as a medicinal herb in Europe (Blacow, 1972; Burns, 1972; Schoental & Pullinger, 1972).

2.2 Occurrence

Seneciphylline has been isolated from *Crotalaria juncea* L. (L.) Rafin. (family Leguminosae) and from a large number of species in the tribe Senecioneae (family Compositae), including: *Erechtites hieracifolia* (L.)

Raf. ex DC., *Senecio ambrosioides*, *S. ampullaceus* Hook., *S. aquaticus* Hill, *S. borysthenicus*, *S. brasiliensis* DC., *S. cannabifolius*, *S. carthamoides* Greene, *S. chrysanthemoides*, *S. cineraria* DC., *S. douglasii* DC., *S. eremophilus* Richards, *S. erraticus* Bertol. subsp. *barbaraeifolius* Krock., *S. erucifolius* L., *S. fremontii* Torr. et A. Gray, *S. grandifolius*, *S. ilicifolius* Thunb., *S. jacobaea* L., *S. latifolius*, *S. longilobus* Benth., *S. othonnae* Bieb., *S. palmatus* Pall., *S. paludosus* L., *S. paucifolius* S.G. Gmel, *S. platyphylloides* Somm. et Lev., *S. pterophorus* DC., *S. quadridentatus* Labill., *S. racemosus*, *S. renardii* Winkl., *S. rhombifolius* (Willd.) Sch. Bip., *S. spartioides* Torr. et A. Gray, *S. stenocephalus* Maxim., *S. subalpinus* C. Koch., *S. vulgaris* L. (Bull *et al.*, 1968); *S. alpinus* L. (Scop.) (Klasek *et al.*, 1968); *S. desfontainei* Druce (Gharbo & Habib, 1969); *S. fluviatilis* Wallr. (Klasek *et al.*, 1973); *S. incanus* L. subsp. *carniolicus* Willd. Br. (Klasek *et al.*, 1968); *S. krylovii* (Sapunova & Ban'kovskii, 1968); *S. minimus* Poir. (White, 1969); *S. propinquus* (Khalilov *et al.*, 1972).

Plant fragments and seeds of *S. ilicifolius* and possibly *S. latifolius*, which are among the *Senecio* species growing in cornfields in the S.W. Cape district of South Africa, sometimes contaminate corn and cause 'bread poisoning' in humans (de Waal, 1940; 1941).

2.3 Analysis

The analysis of plant material and animal tissues for seneciphylline may be carried out by general methods developed for pyrrolizidine alkaloids (see the section "General Information and Conclusions on Pyrrolizidine Alkaloids", p. 335).

3. Biological Data Relevant to the Evaluation of Carcinogenic Risk to Man

3.1 Carcinogenicity and related studies in animals

No data relating to the pure alkaloid are available; however, studies have been carried out on mixtures of alkaloids containing seneciphylline (see the section "General Information and Conclusions on Pyrrolizidine Alkaloids", p. 333).

3.2 *Other relevant biological data*

One to 7-day i.v. LD_{50}'s in mice and rats are about 90 and 80 mg/kg bw, respectively (Anon., 1949). In rats, 3-day i.p. LD_{50} doses for males and females are 77 and 83 mg/kg bw, respectively (Bull *et al.*, 1968).

High i.v. doses cause rapid death with tonic convulsions. Lower doses lead to delayed deaths and produce haemorrhagic necrosis of the liver in mice, rats and, to a lesser extent, in guinea-pigs. Some guinea-pigs show reticuloendothelial hyperplasia in the spleen (Chen *et al.*, 1940). A chronic liver lesion, which is characterized by megalocytosis, is produced in rats that survive for a long period (Schoental & Magee, 1959). In 14-day old rats, an i.p. dose of 8 mg/kg bw seneciphylline induces megalo-cytosis of the liver at 30 days, and an i.p. dose of 33 mg/kg bw causes acute deaths with liver necrosis (Culvenor *et al.*, 1976).

The metabolism of seneciphylline is expected to be similar to that of other hepatotoxic pyrrolizidine alkaloids as described in the section "General Information and Conclusions on Pyrrolizidine Alkaloids", p. 336.

Seneciphylline is one of the main alkaloids present in the *Senecio* species which have contaminated grain and so caused 'bread poisoning' of humans in South Africa (de Waal, 1940; 1941). The most common symptoms were severe abdominal pain, rapidly developing ascites and hepato-megaly. In some outbreaks there were extreme emaciation, nausea and diarr-hoea. At necropsy, the liver was found to be congested, with an occlusive lesion in the central and sublobular hepatic veins and with blood pools replacing large areas of centrilobular parenchymal tissue; there was often marked oedema of the large intestine. Males and females were affected with equal frequency. Over 80 cases of *Senecio* poisoning, mainly in the young and mostly fatal, occurred in the George and Mossel Bay districts around 1910-1920 (Willmott & Robertson, 1920); 12 cases were hospitalized in one area in 1931-1941 (Sapeika, 1952; Selzer & Parker, 1951).

3.3 *Observations in man*

No case reports of cancer or epidemiological studies were available to the Working Group.

4. Comments on Data Reported and Evaluation

4.1 Animal data

No data on the carcinogenicity of pure seneciphylline were available. However, see also the section "General Information and Conclusions on Pyrrolizidine Alkaloids", p. 333.

4.2 Human data

No case reports or epidemiological studies were available to the Working Group.

5. References

Anon. (1949) *Senecio* and related alkaloids. Research Today, 5, 55

Blacow, N.W., ed. (1972) Martindale, The Extra Pharmacopoeia, 26th ed., London, The Pharmaceutical Press, pp. 2038-2039

Bull, L.B., Culvenor, C.C.J. & Dick, A.T. (1968) The Pyrrolizidine Alkaloids, Amsterdam, North Holland, pp. 37, 142, 258-260

Burns, J. (1972) The heart and pulmonary arteries in rats fed on *Senecio jacobaea*. J. Path., 106, 187-194

Chalmers, A.H., Culvenor, C.C.J. & Smith, L.W. (1965) Characterisation of pyrrolizidine alkaloids by gas, thin-layer and paper chromatography. J. Chromat., 20, 270-277

Chen, K.K., Harris, P.N. & Rose, C.L. (1940) The action and toxicity of platyphylline and seneciphylline. J. Pharmacol. exp. Ther., 68, 130-140

Chopra, R.N., ed. (1933) Indigenous Drugs of India, Calcutta, The Art Press,

Culvenor, C.C.J. & Dal Bon, R. (1964) Carbonyl stretching frequencies of pyrrolizidine alkaloids. Austr. J. Chem., 17, 1296-1300

Culvenor, C.C.J., Edgar, J.A., Jago, M.V., Outteridge, A., Peterson, J.E. & Smith, L.W. (1976) Hepato- and pneumotoxicity of pyrrolizidine alkaloids and derivatives in relation to molecular structure. Chem.-biol. Interact., 12, 299-324

Gharbo, S.A. & Habib, A.A.M. (1969) Phytochemical investigation of Egyptian *Senecio*. II. Alkaloids of *Senecio aegyptius*, *Senecio desfontainei*, *Senecio vulgaris*, *Senecio petasitis* and *Senecio mikanioides*. Lloydia, 32, 503-508

Khalilov, D.S., Damirov, I.A. & Telezhenetskaya, M.V. (1972) Seneciphylline from *Senecio propinquus*. Khim. prir. soedin., 5, 656

Klasek, A., Reichstein, T. & Santavy, F. (1968) Pyrrolizidine alkaloids. XIII. Pyrrolizidine alkaloids from *Senecio alpinus*, *Senecio subalpinus* and *Senecio incarnus*. Helv. chim. acta, 51, 1089-1096

Klasek, A., Sula, B. & Santavy, F. (1973) Pyrrolizidine alkaloids. XXI. Alkaloids from *Senecio fluviatilis*. Coll. Czech. Chem. Commun., 38, 2658-2660

Sapeika, N. (1952) The *Senecio* alkaloids. S. Afr. med. J., 26, 485-488

Sapunova, L.A. & Ban'kovskii, A.I. (1968) Alkaloids of *Senecio krylovii*. Khim. prir. soedin., 4, 389

Schoental, R. & Magee, P.N. (1959) Evolution of liver lesions in the rat after a single dose of pyrrolizidine alkaloids. Acta un. int. cancr., 15, 212-215

Schoental, R. & Pullinger, B.D. (1972) On the alleged oestrogenic and other medicinal properties of pyrrolizidine (*Senecio*) alkaloids. E. Afr. med. J., 49, 436-439

Selzer, G. & Parker, R.G.F. (1951) *Senecio* poisoning exhibiting as Chiari's syndrome. Amer. J. Path., 27, 884-907

de Waal, H.L. (1940) *Senecio* alkaloids. III. Chemical investigations upon the *Senecio* species responsible for 'bread poisoning'. The isolation of senecionine from *Senecio ilicifolius* Thunb. and a new alkaloid 'rosmarinine' from *Senecio rosmarinifolius* Linn. Onderstepoort J. vet. Sci. animal Ind., 15, 241

de Waal, H.L. (1941) South African *Senecio* alkaloids. V. Notes on isatidine, rosmarinine and pterophine, and on the structure of their necines and necic acids. Onderstepoort J. vet. Sci. animal Ind., 16, 149

Watt, J.M. & Breyer-Brandwijk, M.G., eds (1962) The Medicinal and Poisonous Plants of Southern and Eastern Africa, 2nd ed., Edinburgh, London, E. & S. Livingstone, p. 284

White, E.P. (1969) Alkaloids of some herbaceous *Senecio* species in New Zealand. N.Z. J. Sci., 17, 165-170

Willmott, F.C. & Robertson, G.W. (1920) *Senecio* disease or cirrhosis of the liver due to *Senecio* poisoning. Lancet, ii, 848-849

SENKIRKINE

1. Chemical and Physical Data

1.1 Synonyms and trade names

Chem. Abstr. Reg. Serial No.: 6882-01-5

Chem. Abstr. Name: 8,12-Dihydroxy-4-methyl-11,16-dioxosenecionanium

trans-15-Ethylidene-12β-hydroxy-4,12α,13β-trimethyl-8-oxo-4,8-secosenec-1-enine; NSC-89945*; renardine; stereoisomer of 3-ethylidene-2,3,4,5,6,7,9,11,13,14,14a,14b-dodecahydro-16,14b-dihydroxy-5,6,12-trimethyl-2,7-dioxo(1,6)dioxacyclododecino[2,3,4-*gh*]pyrrolizinium

1.2 Chemical formula and molecular weight

$C_{19}H_{27}NO_6$ Mol. wt: 365.4

1.3 Chemical and physical properties of the pure substance

(a) Description: Colourless plates

(b) Melting-point: 198°C

(c) Optical rotation: $[\alpha]_D^{15}$ -6.2° (in chloroform)

(d) Spectroscopy data: λ_{max} 215 nm; E_1^1 = 286; for infra-red and nuclear magnetic resonance spectral data see Briggs *et al.* (1965)

---

*Cancer Chemotherapy National Service Centre Number, NCI, NIH, USA

(e) <u>Identity and purity test</u>: Melting-point and mixed melting-point; thin-layer and gas chromatographic comparison with authentic substance (Chalmers *et al.*, 1965)

(f) <u>Solubility</u>: Readily soluble in ethyl acetate and chloroform; less soluble in water, ethanol, acetone and benzene

(g) <u>Volatility</u>: Low, but sufficient for gas chromatography and mass spectrometry

(h) <u>Stability</u>: Stable at room temperature in closed containers; for lengthy periods it is best stored under nitrogen at $-15^{\circ}C$

(i) <u>Reactivity</u>: Readily hydrolysed with alkali

1.4 Technical products and impurities

No data were available to the Working Group.

2. Production, Use, Occurrence and Analysis

2.1 Production and use

Senkirkine is not produced commercially. *Farfugium japonicum*, in which senkirkine occurs, is used in Japanese folk medicine for treatment of suppuration and eczema (Furuya *et al.*, 1971).

The dried flowering shoots of *Tussilago farfara* have been used in Europe in anti-irritants for the relief of coughs and chest complaints (Blacow, 1972), and the young flowers, which have been shown to contain senkirkine, are used medicinally in the Peoples' Republic of China and Japan (Culvenor *et al.*, 1976). *Tussilago farfara* is also used in cleansing gels and shampoos.

2.2 Occurrence

Senkirkine occurs in several species of the tribe Senecioneae (family Compositae) including *Brachyglottis repanda* Forst. et Forst. F.; *Petasites laevigatus* (Willd.) Reichenb. [*Nardosmia laevigata* (Willd.) DC.]; *Senecio kirkii* Hook. f. ex Kirk; *S. kleinia* Sch. Bip.; *S. renardii* Winkl. (Bull *et al.*, 1968); *S. antieuphorbium* (L.) Sch. bip. (Rodriguez & Gonzales, 1971); *Farfugium japonicum* Kitam. (Furuya *et al.*, 1971); and *Tussilago farfara* (Culvenor *et al.*, 1976). It also occurs in *Crotalaria laburnifolia* subsp. *eldomae* (family Leguminosae) (Crout, 1972).

2.3 Analysis

The analysis of plant material for senkirkine may be carried out by general methods developed for pyrrolizidine alkaloids (see the section "General Information and Conclusions on Pyrrolizidine Alkaloids", p. 335).

3. Biological Data Relevant to the Evaluation of Carcinogenic Risk to Man

3.1 Carcinogenicity and related studies in animals

No data relating to the pure alkaloid were available to the Working Group. However, studies have been carried out on plant material containing this alkaloid (see the section "General Information and Conclusions on Pyrrolizidine Alkaloids", p. 333).

3.2 Other relevant biological data

Weanling rats given 300 mg/kg bw senkirkine by stomach tube died within a few days with liver lesions typical of those induced by pyrrolizidine alkaloids; 1-4 day-old rats were more sensitive and died within a few days of receiving 50 mg/kg bw senkirkine by s.c. or i.p. injection (Schoental, 1970).

The metabolism of senkirkine is expected to be similar to that of other hepatotoxic pyrrolizidine alkaloids as described in the section "General Information and Conclusions on Pyrrolizidine Alkaloids", p. 336.

3.3 Observations in man

No data were available to the Working Group.

4. Comments on Data Reported and Evaluation

4.1 Animal data

No carcinogenicity studies on pure senkirkine were available. However, see the section "General Information and Conclusions on Pyrrolizidine Alkaloids", p. 333.

4.2 **Human data**

No case reports or epidemiological studies were available to the Working Group.

5. References

Blacow, N.W., ed. (1972) *Martindale, The Extra Pharmacopoeia*, 26th ed. London, The Pharmaceutical Press, p. 1494

Briggs, L.H., Cambie, R.C., Candy, B.J., O'Donovan, G.M., Russell, R.H. & Seelye, R.N. (1965) Alkaloids of New Zealand *Senecio* species. II. Senkirkine. *J. chem. Soc.*, 2492-2498

Bull, L.B., Culvenor, C.C.J. & Dick, A.T. (1968) *The Pyrrolizidine Alkaloids*, Amsterdam, North Holland, p. 260

Chalmers, A.H., Culvenor, C.C.J. & Smith, L.W. (1965) Characterisation of pyrrolizidine alkaloids by gas, thin-layer and paper chromatography. *J. Chromat.*, 20, 270-277

Crout, D.H.G. (1972) Pyrrolizidine and seco-pyrrolizidine alkaloids of *Crotalaria laburnifolia* L. subspecies *eldomae*. *J. chem. Soc.*, 1602-1607

Culvenor, C.C.J., Edgar, J.A., Smith, L.W. & Hirono, I. (1976) The occurrence of senkirkine in *Tussilago farfara*. *Austr. J. Chem.*, 29, 229-233

Furuya, T., Murakami, K. & Hikichi, M. (1971) Constituents of crude drugs. III. Senkirkine, a pyrrolizidine alkaloid from *Farfugium japonicum*. *Phytochemistry*, 10, 3306-3307

Rodriguez, D.F. & Gonzalez, G.A. (1971) Alcaloides de plantes canarias. XII. Alcaloides del *Senecio antieuphorbium* (L.) Sch. Bip. *Farm. nueva*, 36, 810-811

Schoental, R. (1970) Hepatotoxic activity of retrorsine, senkirkine and hydroxysenkirkine in newborn rats and the role of epoxides in carcinogenesis by pyrrolizidine alkaloids and aflatoxins. *Nature (Lond.)*, 227, 401-402

GENERAL INFORMATION AND CONCLUSIONS ON PYRROLIZIDINE ALKALOIDS

Two relevant reviews are available (Bull *et al.*, 1968; McLean, 1970).

(a) <u>Toxicity and carcinogenicity studies on plants and plant extracts containing pyrrolizidine alkaloids and alkaloid mixtures</u>

Senecio jacobaea alkaloids

Eleven albino rats were each given a solution of 0.1 or 0.05 mg/ml mixed *Senecio jacobaea* L. alkaloids as drinking-water intermittently during 1,2,3,4,5,6,7,8,9,10, or 11 months, respectively. The 3 rats treated for longer than 8 months developed tumour-like masses which were regarded as hepatomas (Cook *et al.*, 1950).

Of 13 male and 12 female Wistar rats given a solution of 0.05 mg/ml mixed *S. jacobaea* L. alkaloids as drinking-water for 1 or 2 weeks and water only for 7 weeks, 9 males and 1 female survived. These were then given a solution containing 0.03 mg/ml alkaloids thrice weekly until death. All rats survived for 11.5-17 months from the start of treatment, and all developed nodular hyperplasia of the liver, some nodules being described as early trabecular hepatomas. Such changes were not reported in 7 male and 7 female controls surviving 18.5-25.5 months (Schoental *et al.*, 1954).

Twenty-four chickens were given an alkaloid mixture from *S. jacobaea* hydrochlorides (stated to be substantially seneciphylline) in weekly i.v. doses of 35 then 20 mg/kg bw for periods of up to 8 weeks or until death. Liver tumours developed in 6/18 birds which had died by the time of reporting (234 days); 3 of the tumours were considered to be malignant (Campbell, 1956).

Petasites japonicus

Petasites japonicus, a form of coltsfoot, which is reported to be used as a herbal remedy and as food in Japan, induced haemangioendothelial sarcomas of the liver in 3/25 and 8/19 ACI rats fed diets containing 4% then 8% for 430 days or 4% for 220 days of dried flower stalks of the plant. Six and 4 liver-cell adenomas and 2 and 1 hepatocellular carcinomas were also observed in the 2 groups, respectively (Hirono *et al.*, 1973).

Senecio longilobus

Two large-scale experiments were carried out in Harlan rats by Harris & Chen (1970) on the carcinogenicity of diets containing dried, ground *Senecio longilobus*, of which seneciphylline is a major alkaloidal constituent (Adams & Govindachari, 1949). In the first series, 295 rats received diets containing 0.25-5% *S. longilobus*; 4 male and 2 female rats treated for 133-446 days developed hepatomas adjacent to and invading veins. An additional male rat treated for 479 days had a rounded tumour composed of well-differentiated cells.

In the second series, 4 treatment groups consisting of 50 males and 50 females were used. The first group was given a diet containing 0.75% *S. longilobus*, but all animals died within 131 days. The second group received 0.5% *S. longilobus*, but only 4 rats survived longer than 200 days. The third group was given 0.5% *S. longilobus* in the diet for 1 month, alternating with 2 weeks on a *S. longilobus*-free diet, for 1 year. A total of 23 rats survived longer than 200 days, and 3 males and 1 female developed hepatocarcinomas between 428 and 657 days; 1 had metastases in the lungs. The fourth group was given 0.5% *S. longilobus* for 1 week, alternating with 1 week on a *S. longilobus*-free diet, for 1 year. Forty-seven rats survived longer than 200 days, and 14 males and 3 females developed malignant liver tumours within 217-470 days; 16 of these had hepatocarcinomas and 1 had 3 angiosarcomas in the liver; 2 rats had pulmonary and 4 had hepatic metastases. Liver tumours were reported to be rare in 20 contemporary and many other non-contemporary controls.

Tussilago farfara L.

Dried and milled pre-blooming flowers of coltsfoot, *Tussilago farfara* L., were administered in the diet to 3 groups of 1.5-month-old ACI rats in the following proportions: 6 females and 6 males received 32% then 16% in the diet; 5 females and 5 males, 8% in the diet; and 5 females and 6 males, 4% in the diet. A group of 8 females and 9 males served as controls. The experiment was terminated after 600 days. In the first group 8/12 rats developed haemangioendothelial sarcomas of the liver; 3 of these 8 rats developed additional tumours (1 hepatocellular carcinoma, 1 hepatocellular adenoma and 1 urinary bladder papilloma). In the second group, only 1 rat developed a haemangioendothelial sarcoma in the liver; and in the third group all rats survived longer than 455 days, and none had tumours. No tumours of the type observed in the first group were observed in contemporary controls nor in 150 rats used as controls in previous long-term experiments (Hirono et al., 1976).

Senecio jacobaea

Mice fed *Senecio jacobaea* for 193 days developed diffuse megalocytosis in the liver, pulmonary lesions characterized by enlarged cells in the alveoli and bronchi (1 mouse had alveolar epithelialization) and moderate cellular enlargement of the renal tubular epithelium (Hooper, 1974). Chronic effects in rats fed a ration containing 8% *S. jacobaea* included general megalocytosis in the liver and moderate haemorrhagic extravasation (Bull et al., 1968). Pulmonary arterial hypertension has also been observed in rats fed a diet containing *S. jacobaea* (Burns, 1972). Dietary protein, S-amino acid or glutamic acid supplements increased the survival time of rats fed *S. jacobaea* (Cheeke & Garman, 1974). Hypertrophy of the epithelial cells of the proximal convoluted tubules of the kidney was observed in pigs fed *S. jacobaea* (Harding et al., 1964).

Mixed seneciphylline and senecionine

The effects in mice of pterophine, a mixture of seneciphylline and a smaller amount of senecionine (Culvenor & Smith, 1954), and of longilobine, a mixture of seneciphylline and retrorsine (Adams & Govindachari, 1949), have been described. Total doses of the order of the LD_{50} cause haemorrhagic necrosis of the liver and sometimes ascites, pulmonary oedema and hydrothorax (Harris et al., 1942a, b).

(b) General methods of analysis

The analysis of plant material for pyrrolizidine alkaloids is based on a general procedure for extraction of the tertiary base alkaloids before and after reduction of the alkaloid *N*-oxides which are also usually present (Culvenor & Smith, 1955). The difference in the two results is an approximate measure of the N-oxide content of the plant material. The levels of both tertiary base and N-oxide forms of the alkaloid are relevant to an evaluation of the toxicity of the plant material. The individual bases are separated and estimated by partition chromatography (Culvenor et al., 1954) or thin-layer, paper or gas chromatography (Chalmers et al., 1965). Comparative R_F values and retention times are given by the latter-mentioned authors. The electrophoretic mobilities of many of the alkaloids have also been recorded and are useful in resolving alkaloid mixtures (Frahn, 1969). Some of the precautions required are discussed by Bull et al. (1968).

Pyrrolizidine alkaloids may be estimated in animal tissues and fluids by removing protein, chromatographing on Florisil and estimating colorimetrically with methyl orange (Dann, 1960). A more sensitive procedure for estimating 1,2-dehydropyrrolizidine alkaloids in metabolic studies utilizes oxidation to pyrrolic derivatives and colour development with a modified Ehrlich reagent (Mattocks, 1967; 1968a). The method may be used to give an approximate figure for total alkaloid in mixtures and in plant material and has been modified for use as a field test for hepatotoxic pyrrolizidine N-oxides in plants (Mattocks, 1971a) and for estimating pyrrolic metabolites bound to animal tissue (Mattocks & White, 1970).

(c) General metabolism and hepatotoxicity of pyrrolizidine alkaloids

In general, the hepatotoxic pyrrolizidine alkaloids are metabolized in rat liver to give hydrolysis products, N-oxides (Bull et al., 1968; Jago et al., 1969) and dehydropyrrolizidine (pyrrolic) derivatives (Jago et al., 1970; Mattocks, 1973). The latter group appears on current evidence to mediate most of the toxic reactions of the alkaloids. These pyrrolic derivatives are produced by the mixed-function oxidases of liver cells (Mattocks & White, 1971). The initial product formed from alkaloids that are esters of heliotridine (e.g., lasiocarpine) or retronecine (e.g., jacobine, monocrotaline, retrorsine, riddelliine and seneciphylline) is very probably the dehydroalkaloid (Jago et al., 1970; Mattocks, 1973) (see also diagram). The dehydroalkaloids are highly reactive alkylating agents which react immediately with cell constituents to give soluble or bound secondary metabolites or which hydrolyse to the dehydroaminoalcohol (Culvenor et al., 1970; Mattocks, 1969).

Alkaloids that are esters of otonecine (e.g., hydroxysenkirkine and senkirkine) are also converted into dehydroretronecine and probably undergo demethylation to an intermediate which changes spontaneously into a metabolite of the dehydroalkaloid type (Culvenor et al., 1971). Alkaloid N-oxides (e.g., isatidine) are not readily converted into pyrrolic metabolites by liver enzymes (Jago et al., 1970; Mattocks, 1968b), but when administered orally they are reduced to the parent alkaloid in the gut or rumen (Bull et al., 1968; Mattocks, 1971b). Alkaloids that are esters of supinidine (similar to retronecine esters, but with no substitution at C7) are readily converted to the corresponding pyrrolic metabolites (Bull et al., 1968).

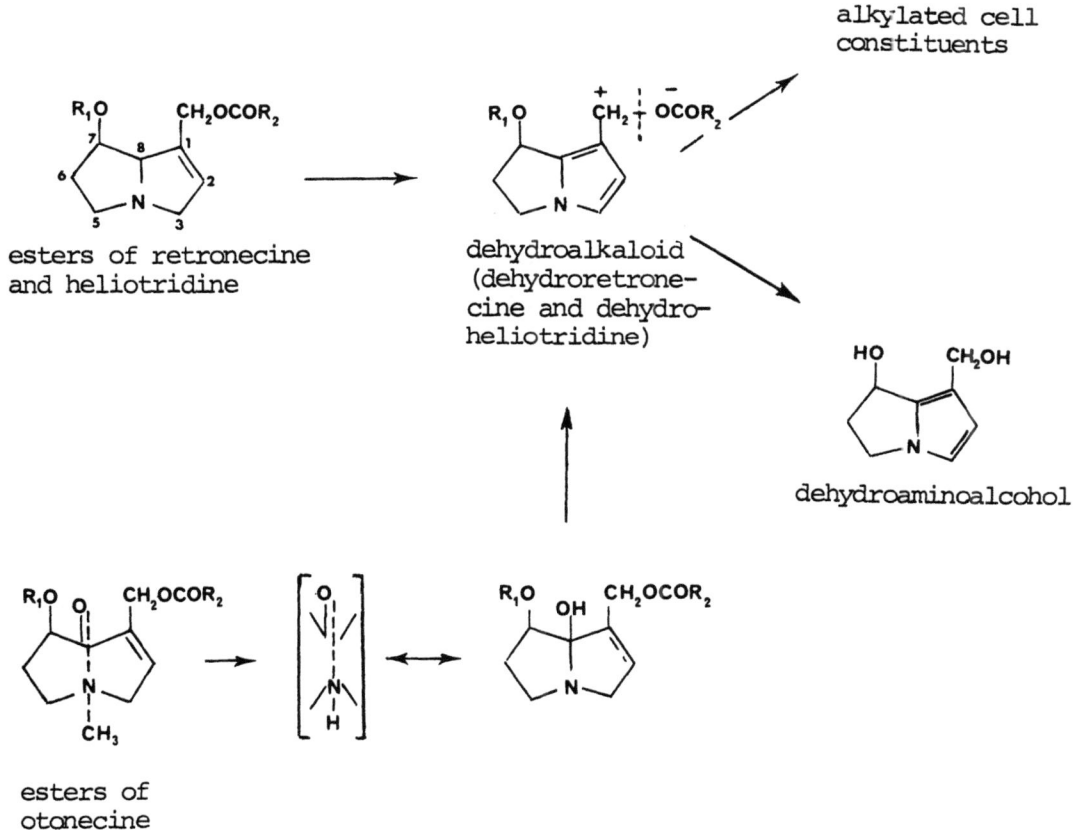

All alkaloids in these structural groups appear to be capable of conversion into toxic pyrrolic metabolites, and a large majority of those tested (33/36) were demonstrably hepatotoxic (Bull et al., 1968; Culvenor et al., 1976). Dehydroheliotridine has been isolated and identified as a product of microsomal oxidation of lasiocarpine (Jago et al., 1970). The enantiomeric compound, dehydroretronecine, has been isolated as a metabolite of monocrotaline in rat urine (Hsu et al., 1973). Dehydroheliotridine and dehydroretronecine show only small differences in toxic effects, and these differences are probably due to age of animals used and other experimental conditions (Allen & Hsu, 1974; Hsu et al., 1973; Peterson et al., 1972). They do not cause liver necrosis but exert an antimitotic effect on rat liver and on tissues in which there is active cell division, e.g., bone marrow, gastrointestinal mucosa, thymus, spleen, testis and hair follicles. The antimitotic effect in rat liver is long-lasting, persisting for at least 6 weeks after administration of dehydroretronecine. Dehydroheliotridine and dehydroretronecine have been shown to be capable of inducing, under appropriate circumstances, the chronic megalocytic liver lesion produced by administration of the parent alkaloids (Hsu et al., 1973; Peterson et al., 1972).

The liver tissue of animals administered pyrrolizidine alkaloids gives positive reactions to colour reagents which indicate binding of the pyrrolic metabolites to cellular constituents, in particular to proteins. In rats, the level of such metabolites in the liver after 2 hours is roughly proportional to acute toxicity (Mattocks, 1972), but toxicity is not always related to the activity of the mixed-function oxidases. In some instances (e.g., monocrotaline), toxicity is enhanced by enzyme induction and decreased by enzyme inhibition; whereas in other cases (e.g., lasiocarpine), the reverse applies. Retrorsine and monocrotaline are considerably more toxic to male than to female rats (Jago, 1971; Mattocks, 1972; Mattocks & White, 1971; Tuchweber et al., 1974). The effect of diet on toxicity probably depends, therefore, on the specific alkaloid concerned. Both dehydroalkaloids and dehydroaminoalcohols combine with and cross link DNA in vitro (Black & Jago, 1970; Mattocks, 1972).

(d) Carcinogenicity of metabolites

Dehydroretronecine, the main water-soluble pyrrolic metabolite of jacobine, monocrotaline, retrorsine, riddelliine and seneciphylline, and the putative metabolite of hydroxysenkirkine and senkirkine, has been shown to be carcinogenic. In young, male Sprague-Dawley rats, given biweekly s.c. injections of 20 mg/kg bw dehydroretronecine for 4 months then 10 mg/kg bw for 8 months and killed when moribund over the next 10 months, local rhabdomyosarcomas developed in 31/60 animals. Metastases were observed in 5 animals (Allen et al., 1975).

Dehydroheliotridine, the corresponding metabolite from lasiocarpine and the enantiomer of dehydroretronecine, has not been tested for carcinogenicity.

(e) General conclusions

Up to now, about 30 pyrrolizidine alkaloids have been found to be hepatotoxic, mostly in rodents. There is also circumstantial evidence for the hepatotoxicity of some of these alkaloids in man. The available evidence in animals suggests that hepatotoxicity is due to, and is indicative of, the formation of toxic pyrrolic metabolites, one of which has been shown to be carcinogenic in rats.

Four pure alkaloids have been found to be carcinogenic in rats[1], but adequate tests are not available for the others. Some plant materials known to contain pyrrolizidine alkaloids, the identity of which is not or is only partly established, have also been shown to be carcinogenic in experimental animals. On the present evidence, it seems justified that carcinogenicity tests should be undertaken on the untested hepatotoxic pyrrolizidine alkaloids to which humans may possibly be exposed.

---

[1]See also the section "Animal Data in Relation to the Evaluation of Risk to Man" in the introduction to this volume, p. 15.

References

Adams, R. & Govindachari, T.R. (1949) *Senecio* alkaloids: α- and β-longilobine from *Senecio longilobus*. J. Amer. chem. Soc., 71, 1180-1186

Allen, J.R. & Hsu, I.C. (1974) Antimitotic effects of dehydroretronecine pyrrole. Proc. Soc. exp. Biol. (N.Y.), 147, 546-550

Allen, J.R., Hsu, I.C. & Carstens, L.A. (1975) Dehydroretronecine-induced rhabdomyosarcomas in rats. Cancer Res., 35, 997-1002

Black, D.N. & Jago, M.V. (1970) Interaction of dehydroheliotridine, a metabolite of heliotridine-based pyrrolizidine alkaloids, with native and heat-denatured deoxyribonucleic acid *in vitro*. Biochem. J., 118, 347-353

Bull, L.B., Culvenor, C.C.J. & Dick, A.T. (1968) The Pyrrolizidine Alkaloids, Amsterdam, North Holland

Burns, J. (1972) The heart and pulmonary arteries in rats fed on *Senecio jacobaea*. J. Path., 106, 187-194

Campbell, J.G. (1956) An investigation of the hepatotoxic effects in the fowl of ragwort (*Senecio jacobaea* Linn.) with special reference to the induction of liver tumours with seneciphylline. Proc. roy. Soc. Edinb., 66B, 111-130

Chalmers, A.H., Culvenor, C.C.J. & Smith, L.W. (1965) Characterisation of pyrrolizidine alkaloids by gas, thin-layer and paper chromatography. J. Chromat., 20, 270-277

Cheeke, P.R. & Garman, G.R. (1974) Influence of dietary protein and sulfur amino acid levels on the toxicity of *Senecio jacobaea* (tansy ragwort) to rats. Nutr. Rep. Int., 9, 197-207

Cook, J.W., Duffy, E. & Schoental, R. (1950) Primary liver tumours in rats following feeding with alkaloids of *Senecio jacobaea*. Brit. J. Cancer, 4, 405-410

Culvenor, C.C.J. & Smith, L.W. (1954) The separation of *Senecio* alkaloids and the nature of hieracifoline and pterophine. Chemistry & Industry, November 6, p. 1386

Culvenor, C.C.J. & Smith, L.W. (1955) The alkaloids of *Erectites quadridentata* DC. Austr. J. Chem., 8, 556-561

Culvenor, C.C.J., Drummond, L.J. & Price, J.R. (1954) The alkaloids of *Heliotropium europaeum* L. Austr. J. Chem., 7, 277-297

Culvenor, C.C.J., Edgar, J.A., Smith, L.W. & Tweeddale, H.J. (1970) Dihydropyrrolizines. III. Preparation and reactions of derivatives related to pyrrolizidine alkaloids. Austr. J. Chem., 23, 1853-1867

Culvenor, C.C.J., Edgar, J.A., Smith, L.W., Jago, M.V. & Peterson, J.E. (1971) Active metabolites in the chronic hepatotoxicity of pyrrolizidine alkaloids, including otonecine esters. Nature (Lond.), 229, 255-256

Culvenor, C.C.J., Edgar, J.A., Jago, M.V., Outteridge, A., Peterson, J.E. & Smith, L.W. (1976) Hepato- and pneumotoxicity of pyrrolizidine alkaloids and derivatives in relation to molecular structure. Chem.-biol. Interact., 12, 299-324

Dann, A.T. (1960) Detection of N-oxides of the pyrrolizidine alkaloids. Nature (Lond.), 186, 1051

Frahn, J.L. (1969) Paper electrophoresis of pyrrolizidine alkaloids. Austr. J. Chem., 22, 1655-1667

Harding, J.D.J., Lewis, G., Done, J.T. & Allcroft, R. (1964) Experimental poisoning by *Senecio jacobaea* in pigs. Path. Vet., 1, 204-220

Harris, P.N. & Chen, K.K. (1970) Development of hepatic tumors in rats following ingestion of *Senecio longilobus*. Cancer Res., 30, 2881-2886

Harris, P.N., Anderson, R.C. & Chen, K.K. (1942a) The action of senecionine, integerrimine, jacobine, longilobine and spartioidine, especially on the liver. J. Pharmacol. exp. Ther., 75, 69-77

Harris, P.N., Anderson, R.C. & Chen, K.K. (1942b) The action of isatidine, pterophine and sceleratine. J. Pharmacol. exp. Ther., 75, 83-88

Hirono, I., Shimizu, M., Fushimi, K., Mori, H. & Kato, K. (1973) Carcinogenic activity of *Petasites japonicus* Maxim., a kind of coltsfoot. Gann, 64, 527-528

Hirono, I., Mori, H. & Culvenor, C.C.J. (1976) Carcinogenic activity of coltsfoot, *Tussilago farfara* L. in rat liver. Gann (in press)

Hooper, P.T. (1974) The pathology of *Senecio jacobaea* poisoning of mice. J. Path., 113, 227-230

Hsu, I.C., Allen, J.R. & Chesney, C.F. (1973) Identification and toxicological effects of dehydroretronecine, a metabolite of monocrotaline. Proc. Soc. exp. Biol. (N.Y.), 144, 834-838

Jago, M.V. (1971) Factors affecting the chronic hepatotoxicity of pyrrolizidine alkaloids. J. Path., 105, 1-11

Jago, M.V., Lanigan, G.W., Bingley, J.B., Piercy, D.W.T., Whittem, J.H. & Titchen, D.A. (1969) Excretion of the pyrrolizidine alkaloid heliotrine in the urine and bile of sheep. J. Path., 98, 115-128

Jago, M.V., Edgar, J.A., Smith, L.W. & Culvenor, C.C.J. (1970) Metabolic conversion of heliotridine-based pyrrolizidine alkaloids to dehydroheliotridine. Molec. Pharmacol., 6, 402-406

Mattocks, A.R. (1967) Detection of pyrrolizidine alkaloids on thin-layer chromatograms. J. Chromat., 27, 505-508

Mattocks, A.R. (1968a) Spectrophotometric determination of pyrrolizidine alkaloids. Some improvements. Analyt. Chem., 40, 1749-1750

Mattocks, A.R. (1968b) Toxicity of pyrrolizidine alkaloids. Nature (Lond.), 217, 723-728

Mattocks, A.R. (1969) Dihydropyrrolizine derivatives from unsaturated pyrrolizidine alkaloids. J. chem. Soc., C, 1155-1162

Mattocks, A.R. (1971a) A field test for N-oxides of unsaturated pyrrolizidine alkaloids. Trop. Sci., 13, 65-70

Mattocks, A.R. (1971b) Hepatotoxic effects due to pyrrolizidine alkaloid N-oxides. Xenobiotica, 1, 563-565

Mattocks, A.R. (1972) Acute hepatotoxicity and pyrrolic metabolites in rats dosed with pyrrolizidine alkaloids. Chem.-biol. Interact., 5, 227-242

Mattocks, A.R. (1973) Mechanism of pyrrolizidine alkaloid toxicity. In: Loomis, T.A., ed., Pharmacology and the Future of Man, Proceedings of the 5th International Congress on Pharmacology, San Francisco, 1972, Vol. 2, Toxicological Problems, White Plains, NY, Phiebig, p. 114

Mattocks, A.R. & White, I.N.H. (1970) Estimation of metabolites of pyrrolizidine alkaloids in animal tissues. Analyt. Biochem., 38, 529-535

Mattocks, A.R. & White, I.N.H. (1971) The conversion of pyrrolizidine alkaloids to N-oxides and to dihydropyrrolizidine derivatives by rat-liver microsomes *in vitro*. Chem.-biol. Interact., 3, 383-396

Peterson, J.E., Samuel, A. & Jago, M.V. (1972) Pathological effects of dehydroheliotridine, a metabolite of heliotridine-based pyrrolizidine alkaloids, in the young rat. J. Path., 107, 175-189

Schoental, R., Head, M.A. & Peacock, P.R. (1954) *Senecio* alkaloids: primary liver tumours in rats as a result of treatment with (i) a mixture of alkaloids from *S. jacobaea* Linn., (ii) retrorsine, (iii) isatidine. Brit. J. Cancer, 8, 458-465

Tuchweber, B., Kovacs, K., Jago, M.V. & Beaulieu, T. (1974) Effect of steroidal and non-steroidal microsomal enzyme inducers in the hepatotoxicity of pyrrolizidine alkaloids in rats. Res. Comm. chem. Path. Pharmacol., 7, 459-480

SUPPLEMENTARY CORRIGENDA TO VOLUMES 1 - 9

A corrigenda covering Volumes 1 - 7 appeared in Volume 8. The present one covers a further error which has since been brought to our attention.

Volume 1

p. 75   3.1(a)
      para 3   line 8   *replace* for life *by* for 2 years, 10 months or 3 years, 1 month, *and replace* 2 bladder papillomatoses *by* 3 bladder papillomas

CUMULATIVE INDEX TO IARC MONOGRAPHS ON THE EVALUATION OF CARCINOGENIC RISK OF CHEMICALS TO MAN

Numbers underlined indicate volume, and numbers in italics indicate page. References to corrigenda are given in parentheses.

Acetamide	_7_,*197*
Actinomycins	_10_,*29*
Adriamycin	_10_,*43*
Aflatoxins	_1_,*145* (corr. _7_,*319*)
	(corr. _8_,*349*)
	_10_,*51*
Aldrin	_5_,*25*
Amaranth	_8_,*41*
para-Aminoazobenzene	_8_,*53*
ortho-Aminoazotoluene	_8_,*61*
4-Aminobiphenyl	_1_,*74*
2-Amino-5-(5-nitro-2-furyl)-1,3,4-thiadiazole	_7_,*143*
Amitrole	_7_,*31*
Amosite	_2_,*17*
Aniline	_4_,*27* (corr. _7_,*320*)
Anthophyllite	_2_,*17*
Apholate	_9_,*31*
Aramite^R	_5_,*39*
Arsenic (inorganic)	_2_,*48*
Arsenic pentoxide	_2_,*48*
Arsenic trioxide	_2_,*48*
Asbestos (mixed)	_2_,*17* (corr. _7_,*319*)
Auramine	_1_,*69* (corr. _7_,*319*)
Azaserine	_10_,*73*
Aziridine	_9_,*37*
2-(1-Aziridinyl)ethanol	_9_,*47*
Aziridyl benzoquinone	_9_,*51*
Azobenzene	_8_,*75*
Barium chromate	_2_,*102*

345

Benz[c]acridine	3,241
Benz[a]anthracene	3,45
Benzene	7,203
Benzidine	1,80
Benzo[b]fluoranthene	3,69
Benzo[j]fluoranthene	3,82
Benzo[a]pyrene	3,91
Benzo[e]pyrene	3,137
Beryl ore	1,18
Beryllium	1,17
Beryllium oxide	1,17
Beryllium phosphate	1,25
Beryllium sulphate	1,18
BHC (technical grades)	5,47
Bis(1-aziridinyl)morpholinophosphine sulphide	9,55
Bis(2-chloroethyl)ether	9,117
N,N'-Bis(2-chloroethyl)-2-naphthylamine	4,119
Bis(chloromethyl)ether	4,231
1,4-Butanediol dimethanesulphonate	4,247
Cadmium acetate	2,92
Cadmium carbonate	2,74
Cadmium chloride	2,74
Cadmium oxide	2,74
Cadmium powder	2,74
Cadmium sulphate	2,74
Cadmium sulphide	2,74
Calcium arsenate	2,48
Calcium arsenite	2,48
Calcium chromate	2,100
Cantharidin	10,79
Carbon tetrachloride	1,53
Carmoisine	8,83
Chlorambucil	9,125
Chloramphenicol	10,85

Chlormadinone acetate	6,149
Chlorobenzilate	5,75
Chloroform	1,61
Chloromethyl methyl ether	4,239
Cholesterol	10,99
Chromic chromate	2,113
Chromic oxide	2,100
Chromium	2,100
Chromium acetate	2,102
Chromium carbonate	2,102
Chromium dioxide	2,101
Chromium phosphate	2,102
Chromium trioxide	2,101
Chrysene	3,159
Chrysoidine	8,91
Chrysotile	2,17
C.I. Disperse Yellow 3	8,97
Citrus Red No. 2	8,101
Coumarin	10,113
Crocidolite	2,17
Cycasin	1,157 (corr. 7,319)
	10,121
Cyclochlorotine	10,139
Cyclophosphamide	9,135
Daunomycin	10,145
D & C Red No. 9	8,107
DDD (TDE)	5,83 (corr. 7,320)
DDE	5,83
DDT	5,83
Diacetylaminoazotoluene	8,113
2,6-Diamino-3-(phenylazo)pyridine (hydrochloride)	8,117
Diazomethane	7,223
Dibenz[a,h]acridine	3,247
Dibenz[a,j]acridine	3,254

Dibenz[*a,h*]anthracene	3,178
7H-Dibenzo[*c,g*]carbazole	3,260
Dibenzo[*h,rst*]pentaphene	3,197
Dibenzo[*a,e*]pyrene	3,201
Dibenzo[*a,h*]pyrene	3,207
Dibenzo[*a,i*]pyrene	3,215
Dibenzo[*a,l*]pyrene	3,224
ortho-Dichlorobenzene	7,231
para-Dichlorobenzene	7,231
3,3'-Dichlorobenzidine	4,49
Dieldrin	5,125
1,2-Diethylhydrazine	4,153
Diethylstilboestrol	6,55
Diethyl sulphate	4,277
Dihydrosafrole	1,170
	10,233
Dimethisterone	6,167
3,3'-Dimethoxybenzidine (*o*-Dianisidine)	4,41
para-Dimethylaminoazobenzene	8,125
para-Dimethylaminobenzenediazo sodium sulphonate	8,147
trans-2[(Dimethylamino)methylimino]-5-[2-(5-nitro-2-furyl)vinyl]-1,3,4-oxadiazole	7,147
3,3'-Dimethylbenzidine (*o*-Tolidine)	1,87
1,1-Dimethylhydrazine	4,137
1,2-Dimethylhydrazine	4,145 (corr. 7,320)
Dimethyl sulphate	4,271
Endrin	5,157
Ethinyloestradiol	6,77
Ethylenethiourea	7,45
Ethyl methanesulphonate	7,245
Ethynodiol diacetate	6,173
Evans blue	8,151
2-(2-Formylhydrazino)-4-(5-nitro-2-furyl)thiazole	7,151
Griseofulvin	10,153
Haematite	1,29

Heptachlor and its epoxide	5,173
Hydrazine	4,127
4-Hydroxyazobenzene	8,157
Hydroxysenkirkine	10,265
Indeno[1,2,3-cd]pyrene	3,229
Iron-dextran complex	2,161
Iron-dextrin complex	2,161 (corr. 7,319)
Iron oxide	1,29
Iron-sorbitol-citric acid complex	2,161
Isatidine	10,269
Isonicotinic acid hydrazide	4,159
Isosafrole	1,169
	10,232
Jacobine	10,275
Lasiocarpine	10,281
Lead acetate	1,40
Lead arsenate	1,41
Lead carbonate	1,41
Lead chromate	2,101
Lead phosphate	1,48
Lead salts	1,40 (corr. 7,319)
	(corr. 8,349)
Lead subacetate	1,40
Lindane	5,47
Luteoskyrin	10,163
Magenta	4,57 (corr. 7,320)
Maleic hydrazide	4,173
Mannomustine (dihydrochloride)	9,157
Medphalan	9,167
Medroxyprogesterone acetate	6,157
Melphalan	9,167
Merphalan	9,167
Mestranol	6,87
Methoxychlor	5,193

2-Methylaziridine	<u>9</u>,61
Methylazoxymethanol acetate	<u>1</u>,164
N-Methyl-N,4-dinitrosoaniline	<u>1</u>,141
4,4'-Methylene bis(2-chloroaniline)	<u>4</u>,65
4,4'-Methylene bis(2-methylaniline)	<u>4</u>,73
4,4'-Methylenedianiline	<u>4</u>,79 (corr. <u>7</u>,320)
Methyl methanesulphonate	<u>7</u>,253
N-Methyl-N'-nitro-N-nitrosoguanidine	<u>4</u>,183
Methyl red	<u>8</u>,161
Methylthiouracil	<u>7</u>,53
Mirex	<u>5</u>,203
Mitomycin C	<u>10</u>,171
Monocrotaline	<u>10</u>,291
5-(Morpholinomethyl)-3-[(5-nitrofurfurylidene)amino]-2-oxazolidinone	<u>7</u>,161
Mustard gas	<u>9</u>,181
1-Naphthylamine	<u>4</u>,87 (corr. <u>8</u>,349)
2-Naphthylamine	<u>4</u>,97
Native carrageenans	<u>10</u>,181
Nickel	<u>2</u>,126
Nickel acetate	<u>2</u>,126
Nickel carbonate	<u>2</u>,126
Nickel carbonyl	<u>2</u>,126 (corr. <u>7</u>,319)
Nickelocene	<u>2</u>,126
Nickel oxide	<u>2</u>,126
Nickel powder	<u>2</u>,145
Nickel subsulphide	<u>2</u>,126
Nickel sulphate	<u>2</u>,127
4-Nitrobiphenyl	<u>4</u>,113
5-Nitro-2-furaldehyde semicarbazone	<u>7</u>,171
1[(5-Nitrofurfurylidene)amino]-2-imidazolidinone	<u>7</u>,181
N-[4-(5-Nitro-2-furyl)-2-thiazolyl]acetamide	<u>1</u>,181
	<u>7</u>,185
Nitrogen mustard (hydrochloride)	<u>9</u>,193
Nitrogen mustard N-oxide (hydrochloride)	<u>9</u>,209

N-Nitroso-di-*n*-butylamine	<u>4</u>,197
N-Nitrosodiethylamine	<u>1</u>,107
N-Nitrosodimethylamine	<u>1</u>,95
Nitrosoethylurea	<u>1</u>,135
Nitrosomethylurea	<u>1</u>,125
N-Nitroso-*N*-methylurethane	<u>4</u>,211
Norethisterone	<u>6</u>,179
Norethisterone acetate	<u>6</u>,179
Norethynodrel	<u>6</u>,191
Norgestrel	<u>6</u>,201
Ochratoxin A	<u>10</u>,191
Oestradiol-17β	<u>6</u>,99
Oestradiol mustard	<u>9</u>,217
Oestriol	<u>6</u>,117
Oestrone	<u>6</u>,123
Oil orange SS	<u>8</u>,165
Orange I	<u>8</u>,173
Orange G	<u>8</u>,181
Parasorbic acid	<u>10</u>,199
Patulin	<u>10</u>,205
Penicillic acid	<u>10</u>,211
Phenoxybenzamine (hydrochloride)	<u>9</u>,223
Polychlorinated biphenyls	<u>7</u>,261
Ponceau MX	<u>8</u>,189
Ponceau 3R	<u>8</u>,199
Ponceau SX	<u>8</u>,207
Potassium arsenate	<u>2</u>,48
Potassium arsenite	<u>2</u>,49
Potassium chromate	<u>2</u>,102
Potassium dichromate	<u>2</u>,101
Progesterone	<u>6</u>,135
1,3-Propane sultone	<u>4</u>,253
β-Propiolactone	<u>4</u>,259
Propylthiouracil	<u>7</u>,67

Quintozene (Pentachloronitrobenzene)	5,*211*
Reserpine	10,*217*
Retrorsine	10,*303*
Riddelliine	10,*313*
Saccharated iron oxide	2,*161*
Safrole	1,*169*
	10,*231*
Scarlet red	8,*217*
Selenium and selenium compounds	9,*245*
Seneciphylline	10,*319*
Senkirkine	10,*327*
Sodium arsenate	2,*49*
Sodium arsenite	2,*49*
Sodium chromate	2,*102*
Sodium dichromate	2,*102*
Soot, tars and shale oils	3,*22*
Sterigmatocystin	1,*175*
	10,*245*
Streptozotocin	4,*221*
Strontium chromate	2,*102*
Sudan I	8,*225*
Sudan II	8,*233*
Sudan III	8,*241*
Sudan brown RR	8,*249*
Sudan red 7B	8,*253*
Sunset yellow FCF	8,*257*
Tannic acid	10,*253*
Tannins	10,*254*
Terpene polychlorinates (Strobane^R)	5,*219*
Testosterone	6,*209*
Tetraethyllead	2,*150*
Tetramethyllead	2,*150*
Thioacetamide	7,*77*
Thiouracil	7,*85*

Thiourea	7,95
Trichlorotriethylamine hydrochloride	9,229
Tris(aziridinyl)-*para*-benzoquinone	9,67
Tris(1-aziridinyl)phosphine oxide	9,75
Tris(1-aziridinyl)phosphine sulphide	9,85
2,4,6-Tris(1-aziridinyl)-*s*-triazine	9,95
Tris(2-methyl-1-aziridinyl)phosphine oxide	9,107
Trypan blue	8,267
Uracil mustard	9,235
Urethane	7,111
Vinyl chloride	7,291
Yellow AB	8,279
Yellow OB	8,287
Zinc chromate hydroxide	2,102

www.ingramcontent.com/pod-product-compliance
Ingram Content Group UK Ltd.
Pitfield, Milton Keynes, MK11 3LW, UK
UKHW051258180426
11947UKWH00020B/1782

9 789283 212102